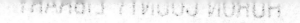

Determinants of Health

ADULTS AND SENIORS

CANADA HEALTH ACTION: BUILDING ON THE LEGACY
PAPERS COMMISSIONED BY THE NATIONAL FORUM ON HEALTH

Determinants of Health

ADULTS AND SENIORS

ÉDITIONS
MULTIMONDES

FORUM NATIONAL
SUR LA SANTÉ

NATIONAL FORUM
ON HEALTH

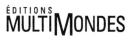

Canadian Cataloguing in Publication Data

Main entry under title:

Canada Health Action: Building on the Legacy

Issued also in French under title: La santé au Canada: un héritage à faire fructifier
To be complete in 5 v.
Includes bibliographical references.
Contents: v. 1. Children and Youth – v. 2. Adults and Seniors.

ISBN 2-921146-62-2 (set)
ISBN 2-921146-47-9 (v. 2)

1. Public health – Canada. 2. Medicine, Preventive – Canada. 3. Children – Health
and hygiene – Canada. 4. Adulthood – Health and hygiene – Canada. 5. Aged –
Health and hygiene – Canada. I. National Forum on Health (Canada).

RA449.C28 1998   362.1'0971   C97-941659-0

Linguistic Revision: Traduction Tandem
Proofreading: Traduction Tandem and Robert Paré
Cover Design: Gérard Beaudry
Graphics: Emmanuel Gagnon

Volume 2: Adults and Seniors
ISBN 2-921146-47-9   Cat. No.: H21-126/6-2-1997E
Legal Deposit– Bibliothèque nationale du Québec, 1998
Legal Deposit – National Library of Canada, 1998
© Her Majesty the Queen in Right of Canada, 1998

The series The National Forum on Health can be ordered at this address:
Éditions MultiMondes
930, rue Pouliot
Sainte-Foy (Québec)
G1V 3N9 CANADA
Telephone: (418) 651-3885; toll free in North America: 1 800 840-3029
Fax: (418) 651 6822; toll free in North America: 1 888 303-5931
E-mail: multimondes@multim.com
Internet: http://www.multim.com

Published by Éditions MultiMondes in co-operation with the National Forum on Health, Health
Canada, and Canadian Government Publishing, Public Works and Government Services Canada.

In this publication the masculine form is used solely for ease of readability.

FOREWORD

In October 1994, the Prime Minister of Canada, The Right Honourable Jean Chrétien, launched the National Forum on Health to involve and inform Canadians and to advise the federal government on innovative ways to improve the health system and the health of Canada's people. The Forum was set up as an advisory body with the Prime Minister as Chair, the federal Minister of Health as Vice Chair, and 24 volunteer members who contributed a wide range of knowledge founded on involvement in the health system as professionals, consumers and volunteers.

To fulfil their mandate, the Forum focused on long-term and systemic issues. They saw their task as formulating advice appropriate to the development of national policies, and divided the work into four key areas – Values, Striking a Balance, Determinants of Health, and Evidence-Based Decision Making.

The complete report of the National Forum on Health consists of two volumes:

> *Canada Health Action: Building on the Legacy*
> The Final Report of the National Forum on Health

and

> *Canada Health Action: Building on the Legacy*
> Synthesis Reports and Issues Papers

Copies available from: Publications Distribution Centre, Health Canada Communications, PL. 090124C, Brooke Claxton Building, Tunney's Pasture, Ottawa, Ontario K1A 0K9. Telephone: (613) 954-5995. Fax: (613) 941-5366. *(Aussi disponible en français.)*

The Forum based its recommendations on 42 research papers written by the most eminent specialists in the field. The papers are brought together in a five-volume series:

VOLUME 1 – CHILDREN AND YOUTH
VOLUME 2 – ADULTS AND SENIORS
VOLUME 3 – SETTINGS AND ISSUES
VOLUME 4 – HEALTH CARE SYSTEMS IN CANADA AND ELSEWHERE
VOLUME 5 – EVIDENCE AND INFORMATION

Individual volumes or the complete series can be ordered from: Editions MultiMondes, 930, rue Pouliot, Sainte-Foy (Québec) G1V 3N9. Telephone: 1 800 840-3029. Fax: 1 888 303-5931. *(Aussi disponible en français.)*

Values

The Values working group sought to understand the values and principles that Canadians hold about health and health care, so that the system continues to reflect and respond to these values. To explore Canadian core values that are connected to the health care system and to understand the implications for decision making, the group conducted some original public opinion research, using scenarios or short stories which addressed many of the issues being investigated by the other working groups of the Forum. The scenarios were tested in focus groups. Quantitative research supplemented the focus groups making the findings more generalizable. The group also contributed to a review of public opinion research on health and social policy. Finally, a review of Canadian and international experience with ethics bodies was commissioned to identify the contribution that such groups can make to continuing the discusssion of values in decision making.

Striking a Balance

The Striking a Balance working group considered how to allocate society's limited resources to best protect, restore and promote the health of Canadians. Attention was given to the balance of resources within the health sector and other sectors of the economy. The group commissioned a series of papers to assist in their deliberations. They conducted a thorough review of international trends in health expenditures, use of resources, and outcomes. They paid considerable attention to public and private financing issues, health system oganization and federal-provicial transfers. The group produced a separate discussion paper on public and private financing, and a position paper on the Canada Health and Social Transfer.

Determinants of Health

The Determinants of Health working group sought to answer the question: In these times of economic and social hardship, what actions must be taken to allow Canadians to continue to enjoy a long life and, if possible, to increase their health status? The group consulted specialists to assist in identifying appropriate actions on the non-medical determinants of health. Specialists were asked to prepare papers on issues of concern to the health of the population related to the macro-economic environment, the contexts in which people live (i.e. families, schools, work and communities), as well as on issues of concern to people's health at different life stages. Each paper presents a review of the literature, examples of success stories or failures, and relevant policy implications.

Evidence-Based Decision Making

The working group on Evidence-Based Decision Making considered how individually practioners and policy makers can have access to, and utilize the best available evidence in making decisions. The group held two workshops with leading authorities to discuss how health information can be used to support and encourage a culture of evicence-based decision making, and to consider what information Canadians need to be better health care consumers and how to get that information to them. The group commissioned papers to: examine the meaning and concepts of evidence and evidence-based decision making as well as cases that illustrate opportunities for improvement; identify the health information infrastructure needed to support evidence-based decision making; examine tools which support more effective health care decision making; and identify strategies for assisting and increasing the role of Canadians in decision making in health and health care.

Members

William R.C. Blundell, B.A.Sc. (Ont.)
Richard Cashin, LL.B. (Nfld.)
André-Pierre Contandriopoulos, Ph.D. (Que.)
Randy Dickinson (N.B.)
Madeleine Dion Stout, M.A. (Ont.)
Robert G. Evans, Ph.D. (B.C.)
Karen Gainer, LL.B. (Alta.)
Debbie L. Good, C.A. (PEI)
Nuala Kenny, M.D. (N.S.)
Richard Lessard, M.D. (Que.)
Steven Lewis (Sask.)
Gerry M. Lougheed Jr. (Ont.)

Margaret McDonald, R.N. (NWT)
Eric M. Maldoff, LL.B. (Que.)
Louise Nadeau, Ph.D. (Que.)
Tom W. Noseworthy, M.D. (Alta.)
Shanthi Radcliffe, M.A. (Ont.)
Marc Renaud, Ph.D. (Que.)
Judith A. Ritchie, Ph.D. (N.S.)
Noralou P. Roos, Ph.D. (Man.)
Duncan Sinclair, Ph.D. (Ont.)
Lynn Smith, LL.B., Q.C. (B.C.)
Mamoru Watanabe, M.D. (Alta.)
Roberta Way-Clark, M.A. (N.S.)

Secretary and Deputy Minister, Health Canada

Michèle S. Jean

Secretariat Staff

Executive Director
Marie E. Fortier

Joyce Adubofuor
Lori Alma
Rachel Bénard
Kathy Bunka
Barbara Campbell
Marlene Campeau
Carmen Connolly
Lise Corbett
John Dossetor
Kayla Estrin
Rhonda Ferderber
Annie Gauvin
Patricia Giesler
Sylvie Guilbault
Janice Hopkins

Lucie Lacombe
Johanne LeBel
Elizabeth Lynam
Krista Locke
John Marriott
Maryse Pesant
Marcel Saulnier
Liliane Sauvé
Linda St-Amour
Judith St-Pierre
Nancy Swainson
Catherine Swift
Josée Villeneuve
Tim Weir
Lynn Westaff

We extend our sincere thanks to all those who participated in the various production stages of this series of publications.

TABLE OF CONTENTS – VOLUME 2

Adults

The Health Consequences of Unemployment

WILLIAM R. AVISON, PH.D.

*Professor of Sociology, Psychiatry, and Epidemiology and Biostatistic
Director, Centre for Health and Well-Being
Ontario Mental Health Foundation Senior Research Fellow
The University of Western Ontario*

SUMMARY

It is widely known that job loss and subsequent periods of unemployment exert severe economic strains on families. Increasingly, it has become clear that these strains have an impact on both the physical and mental health of individuals. This position paper summarizes the research that is available on the health consequences of unemployment. It then reviews selected initiatives that have met with some success in addressing the needs of unemployed individuals. In the final section of this position paper, a number of policies are suggested to address the health problems of unemployed Canadians.

Key Conclusions from the Literature

The review of the literature clearly demonstrates that unemployment has a pernicious effect on individuals' health. Across an array of studies in different countries, it is clear that job loss is a significant risk factor for physical and mental health problems. There is overwhelming evidence that unemployment is a significant risk factor for mortality. Similarly, there is no doubt that involuntary job loss results in elevated levels of mental health problems. Unemployed individuals experience higher levels of psychological distress than do their stably employed counterparts. They also suffer from higher rates of diagnosable disorders such as depression, panic and substance abuse. It also appears that the health costs of job loss are not immediately reversed by reemployment. Physical and mental health problems that are the consequences of unemployment persist for some years after reemployment.

While the evidence is somewhat fragmentary, recent research suggests that job loss has detrimental effects on the health of other family members. Spouses of unemployed workers experience increased emotional problems. As well, there is some indication that children, especially teens, whose parents are unemployed are at higher risk of emotional and behavioural problems than are children whose parents are stably employed.

Finally, this review highlights some of the pathways that link unemployment to health problems. It appears that job loss simultaneously results in increases in stressors (principally, experiences of financial strain and family conflict) and the erosion of self-esteem, self-efficacy, and feelings of social support. These experiences contribute directly to emotional and physical health problems.

Success Stories

The next section of this position paper describes four programs that have been successful in addressing barriers to employment among various groups. Over the last decade, the Michigan Prevention Research Center has developed a preventive intervention, the Michigan JOBS Program, to assist unemployed individuals in gaining new employment and in reducing the psychological distress associated with job loss and reemployment.

Three local initiatives that assist individuals in finding employment are also reviewed. Women Immigrants of London was established in London, Ontario to provide counselling and support services to immigrant and visible minority women in response to the unique barriers that confront these women. The Learning Enrichment Foundation is located in the City of York in the Metropolitan Toronto area. These programs include the operation of 13 daycare centres and an industrial kitchen to provide meals to the staff and clients of these centres. In addition, programs are provided for training in microcomputer skills, English as a second language, and job training in a variety of skilled trades. The Foundation also supports clients in venture programs to start small businesses. Niigwin Skills Development and Placement Centre is a community-based training program that was established in London, Ontario, in 1989. Niigwin provides job skills and life skills training to long-term recipients of social assistance who have been classified by the London Department of Social Services as "employment challenged." This program has had considerable success in placing its participants in jobs in the Greater London area.

Policy Implications

The final section of this paper reviews some policy alternatives that might successfully deal with the health consequences of unemployment. While it seems self-evident, education still remains the most effective weapon against *unemployment. There are at least three principles that ought to guide policymaking and program development in this area:*

1. *Youth must be provided greater incentives to further their education and training;*
2. *We need to encourage adult education and training as a strategy for reemployment;*
3. *Educational institutions must be provided with resources to facilitate students' transitions from the classroom to the workplace.*

There are also policies that corporations could adopt which might well reduce unemployment in this country. First, wider acceptance of job sharing might increase the numbers of employed individuals. Second, movement to a shorter work week with a larger workforce might also create more employment at relatively little increase in cost. A more controversial suggestion is that corporations might encourage early retirement and reduced responsibility as a means of creating opportunities for younger workers.

Ultimately, the problem of widespread unemployment is a problem for communities and their governments. High rates of unemployment threaten the well-being of our neighbourhoods and strain the fabric of society. These considerations suggest that a useful response to widespread unemployment in communities may be the development of ecological or community-based programs.

There are also several economic policies that directly influence the unemployment rate in this country. In recent years, virtually every federal and provincial strategy in Canada has focused on balancing budgets and deficit reduction. An alternative policy that deserves consideration and debate is lowering interest rates nationally.

Clearly, if individuals are to be assisted in coping with the stressors arising out of unemployment, treatment and counselling programs are likely to be too inefficient to deal with the volume of need that is being generated by unemployment in Canada. Health promotion and primary prevention hold promise for reducing the health burden resulting from unemployment.

TABLE OF CONTENTS

FIGURE

TABLE

INTRODUCTION

Significant economic change has taken place in the structure of national economies in North America during the 1990s. Patterns of cyclical unemployment, a decline in the vitality of various economic sectors, and resulting plant closings and downsizing in both the private and public sector have contributed to high unemployment rates in Canada for almost a decade. In March of 1993, the unemployment rate was 12.3 percent, the highest rate in post–World War II history. Since then, unemployment in Canada has declined and now hovers just below 9.5 percent. Regional variations in unemployment rates range substantially from as low as 6 percent in Alberta to as high as 20 percent in Newfoundland.

Across Canada government fiscal policies and corporate strategic plans have resulted in unprecedented levels of restructuring of both the private and public sector. Terms such as "downsizing," "vertical cuts" and "outplacement" have become part of the everyday language of the workplace. It is not surprising, therefore, that policymakers, program providers, and social scientists have redoubled their efforts to examine the effect of unemployment on the lives of individuals and to consider what can be done to address the health consequences of this source of economic disadvantage.

It is widely known, of course, that job loss and subsequent periods of unemployment exert severe economic strains on Canadian families. Increasingly, it has become clear that these strains have an impact on both the physical and mental health of individuals. Indeed, given the magnitude of the economic contraction of the Canadian economy and the accompanying shrinkage of the labour force, it seems clear that the relatively long-term levels of high unemployment in Canada have exacted a significant cost from Canadians, both in terms of their own health and in terms of the costs of health services that are required to deal with these problems.

Of course, Canada is not the only country to have experienced these economic challenges. Indeed, there is a large body of research from the United States and from European countries that documents the health costs of unemployment. This position paper summarizes the research that is available on this issue and identifies the key conclusions that can be drawn from this literature. It then reviews selected initiatives that have met with some success in addressing the needs of unemployed individuals. In the final section of this position paper, a number of policies are suggested to address the health problems of unemployed Canadians.

KEY CONCLUSIONS FROM THE RESEARCH LITERATURE

The study of the impact of unemployment on the health of individuals is by no means a new field of research. During the Great Depression of the 1930s, social scientists conducted several research studies that were designed to assess the impact of unemployment on health (Jahoda, Lazarsfeld, and Zeisel 1933; Bakke 1940). These studies clearly demonstrated that job loss and subsequent periods of unemployment were associated with higher rates of physical health problems. Since that time, the effects of unemployment on health have been investigated throughout the industrialized world. Some of the most intensive research on this topic has been conducted in Scandinavian countries and in the United Kingdom. Considerably fewer studies of unemployment and health have been completed in Canada or the United States.

Before summarizing the results of these studies, it is useful to review briefly the research designs that have been used to estimate the impact of job loss on individuals' health status. *Aggregate time series* studies estimate the correlation between rates of unemployment and rates of mortality, morbidity, or health care utilization. Typically, these designs determine whether rates of unemployment at one point in time are associated with changes in health indicators in a subsequent time period. While these aggregate analyses provide evidence that macro-level economic characteristics are correlated with rates of health problems, they leave open the possibility of the ecological fallacy—aggregate data provide no confirmation that those individuals who are unemployed are the same individuals who are experiencing health problems or who are accessing health care. Moreover, aggregate time series data provide no opportunity to study how individuals cope with unemployment or assess other personal dynamics that comprise individuals' reactions to job loss.

In response to this limitation, various micro-level research designs have been used to study the connection between unemployment and health among individuals. Most of these designs are referred to as *case-control* studies in which a sample of unemployed individuals (the "cases") is compared with a sample of employed individuals (the "controls"). Differences between cases and controls in health outcomes can then be attributed to the impact of job loss or unemployment. There are several variations on this design that have been used in research in this area. One approach has been to compare workers who have lost their jobs in a plant closing with workers from a comparable plant that continues to operate. Another strategy involves the selection of a random sample of individuals from a particular community or region; unemployed and employed individuals are then compared with one another on a range of health, social, and psychosocial measures. This approach can be further elaborated by adding a longitudinal component in which these individuals are surveyed over time.

The Physical and Mental Health Consequences of Unemployment

Mortality

Perhaps the best-known work on the link between unemployment and mortality has been conducted by Harvey Brenner (Brenner 1973, 1979, 1984, 1987 a, b, c; Brenner and Mooney 1983). In his now famous aggregate studies of U.S. unemployment and mortality rates, Brenner estimated that a 1 percent increase in unemployment was associated five years later with an increase in mortality of 1.9 percent, an increase of approximately 6,000 deaths. Brenner has also replicated his finding of a link between unemployment and mortality rates in studies of Sweden, Scotland, and England and Wales.

In contrast to these findings, Adams (1981) conducted aggregate time series analyses of Canadian economic and health indicators for the period from 1950 to 1977. Surprisingly, Adams reports that unemployment rates in Canada appear to be inversely associated with mortality rates. Adams speculates that these counterintuitive findings may be the result of a number of factors including fewer work-related deaths in times of declining business activity, and the moderation of the impact of unemployment on mortality by unemployment insurance benefits.

Studies at the individual level of analyses leave little doubt of the detrimental impact of unemployment on mortality. These investigations have involved long-term prospective studies of large samples of unemployed individuals originally identified in population censuses. In their 10-year follow-up of a large cohort of unemployed Danish men and women, Iversen, Andersen, Andersen, Christoffersen, and Keiding (1987) report that both women and men had elevated mortality rates when contrasted with a comparison sample of employed individuals. Moser, Fox, and Jones (1984) and Moser, Goldblatt, Fox, and Jones (1987) have reported similar findings in two studies of British men. As well, Moser et al. report that the spouses of these unemployed men also had elevated mortality rates. Studies in both Italy (Costa and Segman 1987) and Finland (Martikainen 1990) reveal another interesting pattern: the longer the period of unemployment experienced by individuals, the higher their rate of mortality.

Research on the impact of unemployment on cause-specific mortality has focused primarily on *suicide* and *cardiovascular disease*. Platt (1984) reviewed over 90 studies that have estimated the impact of unemployment on suicide. This research clearly reveals that individuals who died from suicide were more likely to be jobless at the time than were those who died from other causes. Of course, this does not necessarily mean that job loss precipitated suicide. Nevertheless, other studies have provided additional evidence to support this inference. For example, Brenner estimates that a

1 percent increase in the unemployment rate in the United States increases mortality due to suicide by 4.1 percent. Moser et al. (1987) report suicide rates in the United Kingdom to be over 50 percent higher among unemployed men compared to those who were employed. In Denmark, Iversen et al. (1987) find suicide to be almost 2.5 times more frequent among unemployed individuals. Morrell, Taylor, and Quine (1993) and Pritchard (1992) have observed that this association appears to be stronger when data are limited to unemployment among young men.

Several studies document the correlation of unemployment and mortality due to cardiovascular disease. Brenner (1987a) has shown that rates of unemployment are associated with rates of death due to heart disease even after the confounding effects of alcohol and tobacco consumption are controlled. Longitudinal studies of unemployed individuals reveal similar patterns (Moser et al. 1984, 1987; Martikainen 1990; Iversen et al. 1987).

Symptoms of Physical Health Problems

The association between unemployment and physical health symptoms is somewhat more difficult to interpret. Cross-sectional studies reveal that the unemployed experience more physical health problems than do the employed (D'Arcy 1986; D'Arcy and Siddique 1984; Kessler, House, and Turner 1987; Kessler, Turner, and House 1988; Verbrugge 1983). However, longitudinal studies find few effects of unemployment on physical health (Kasl and Cobb 1980; Kasl, Gore, and Cobb 1975) although there is evidence that unemployment results in higher levels of health care utilization (Linn, Sandifer, and Stein 1985; Beale and Nethercott 1985). It should be emphasized, however, that those studies which have found no correlation between unemployment and symptoms of physical illness were investigations of plant closings during good economic times. It may be that job loss during economic downturns may have more substantial effects on physical health problems.

Indeed, two studies by Grayson (1985, 1989) of plant closings in Canada during economic recessions suggest that job loss contributes to an increase in physical health problems. In his study of men who had experienced the closure of a manufacturing plant in 1982, Grayson reports that laid-off workers who remained unemployed after two years reported more symptoms than before their layoffs. The absence of any control group, however, makes it difficult to draw any strong conclusions from this study. In a second study of 400 men laid off in 1984 from another plant, both the laid-off employees and their spouses reported more symptoms of physical health problems than did a comparison sample drawn from the Canada Health Survey.

Mental Health Problems

While the evidence that unemployment exacts a physical health cost may be somewhat ambiguous, there is ample evidence that job loss has a substantial impact on symptoms of depression and anxiety, and measures of psychological distress (Kessler et al. 1987; Krause and Stryker 1980; Linn et al. 1985; McLanahan and Glass 1985; Pearlin, Menaghan, Lieberman, and Mullan 1981; Warr 1987; Warr et al. 1988). Of course, a major point of contention in interpreting these findings concerns whether they reflect the health consequences of job loss and unemployment or whether they represent selection effects where people with mental health problems lose their jobs. Studies employing longitudinal research designs have been able to address this interpretational problem. The weight of evidence from these studies appears to support the conclusion that job loss results in higher levels of mental health symptoms (Banks and Jackson 1982; Dew, Bromet, and Schulberg 1987; Dooley, Catalano, and Rook 1988; Jackson, Stafford, Banks, and Warr 1983; Liem and Liem 1988, 1990; Menaghan 1989; Pearlin et al. 1981).

While it seems apparent that unemployment has a significant impact on symptoms of psychological distress, it is also important to know whether job loss also has consequences for diagnosable psychiatric disorders. Few studies have addressed this issue, although evidence from the Epidemiologic Catchment Area Study in the U.S. indicates that unemployment is associated with major depressive disorder (Weissman, Bruce, Leaf, Florio, and Holzer 1991). As well, Catalano and his colleagues (Catalano 1991, 1995; Catalano, Rook, and Dooley 1986) argue that the impact of unemployment on economic insecurity and on help seeking is consistent with the expectation that unemployment is a risk factor for mental disorder.

Alcohol and Other Substance Abuse

The relationship between job loss and alcohol abuse is an extremely controversial topic. There is little doubt that levels of alcohol consumption and rates of alcohol abuse are higher among the unemployed than among the employed. In the Canada Health Survey, D'Arcy (1986) finds that unemployed individuals consume more alcohol than do employed individuals; however, it is impossible to know whether job loss precipitates heavier drinking, or whether heavier drinking results in the loss of the drinker's job.

Catalano and his associates have argued that job loss provokes heavier drinking in response to the stress engendered by unemployment (Catalano 1991; Catalano, Dooley, Novaco, Wilson, and Hough 1993). Several studies have examined the provocation hypothesis and have found clear evidence that job loss leads to increased alcohol consumption and problem drinking

(Catalano, Dooley, Wilson, and Hough 1993; Dooley, Catalano, and Hough 1992; Kasl and Cobb 1982; Buss and Redburn 1983). Indeed, Dooley et al. report that workers experiencing job loss had rates of alcohol-related disorder that were six times higher than stably employed individuals.

Two studies have reported contrary findings. Giesbrecht, Markele, and MacDonald (1982) report no increases in alcohol consumption among Ontario miners who lost their jobs in a layoff. Similarly, Iversen and Klausen (1986) report that laid-off Danish ship workers' levels of consumption were similar before and after job loss. As Catalano (1995) points out, these two studies are distinctive insofar as these workers in Canada and in Denmark received considerable financial support and other resources during their unemployment.

Health Services Utilization

Given the evidence of increased rates of physical and mental health problems among individuals who have experienced job loss, one would also expect to find a higher level of use of health services by the unemployed in Canada. D'Arcy (D'Arcy 1986; D'Arcy and Siddique 1984) reports that individuals who are unemployed are approximately twice as likely as the employed to have a hospital admission in the previous year. In addition, they visit their physicians more frequently. As well, Adams (1981) finds a significant positive correlation between rates of unemployment and admissions to psychiatric hospitals for diagnoses of psychoses.

In the U.S., studies of unemployment and health services utilization provide mixed results, depending on the populations of unemployed that are studied. There are several reasons why studies of unemployment and health services utilization may yield inconsistent results. First, while one might expect positive correlations between unemployment and service utilization in those countries where universal health care services are provided, much of the research in this area has been conducted in locations in the U.S. where fees for service may limit unemployed persons' abilities to access health care. Second, help-seeking behaviours such as accessing medical services may be limited by other factors such as access to transportation and linguistic barriers, even in health systems that provide universal coverage. Third, the use of health services is an indirect effect of unemployment. Not all unemployed individuals will develop symptoms of ill health and not all individuals with symptoms will seek health care. Indeed, it is well established that younger people and those who are less well educated—the very people who are more likely to experience unemployment—tend to be less likely to use health services. Accordingly, these patterns attenuate the association between unemployment and health services utilization.

The Effects of Unemployment on Family Members

While the majority of these studies have focused on job loss among men, there is some evidence that unemployment among women also results in increased symptoms of mental health difficulties (Banks and Jackson 1982; Breakwell, Harrison, and Propper 1984; Warr and Jackson 1983) although some researchers report that the magnitude of these effects may be less among women (Cohn 1978; Perrucci et al. 1985). To date, however, few studies have systematically made these comparisons across different mental health or physical health outcomes. Given recent arguments that men and women differentially express the effects of stress or strain (i.e., drinking, substance abuse, and hostility among men; depression and anxiety among women) (Aneshensel, Rutter, and Lachenbruch 1991), this is an issue that deserves attention.

What of the effects of job loss and unemployment on other family members? Elder and associates (Elder and Caspi 1988; Liker and Elder 1983) report that women whose husbands lost their jobs during the Great Depression experienced greater distress. Cochrane and Stopes-Roe (1981) report elevated symptomatology among women whose husbands had recently lost their jobs. In their study of job losses due to a plant closing, Dew et al. (1987) document the detrimental psychological effects of husbands' unemployment on their sample of women. Recently, Liem and Liem (1988, 1990) have clearly documented elevated levels of anxiety and depression among the wives of unemployed blue-collar and white-collar workers. These symptoms appear to emerge somewhat later among wives than among their husbands. The Liems have also made an important contribution to our understanding of the connections between men's job loss and subsequent distress among their spouses by proposing a dynamic model that specifies the mediating effects of the family's socioeconomic characteristics, the unemployed individual's functioning, and patterns of family interaction.

Studies of the effects of parental job loss on children's health are even more rare. In their study of children of the Great Depression, Elder (1974) and Elder, Nguyen, and Caspi (1985) find that family economic hardships (including job loss) contributed to poor psychosocial functioning among adolescent girls but not boys. Perhaps the most comprehensive investigations of the association between social disadvantage and children's mental health has been conducted by Offord and his colleagues (Offord et al. 1987) in the Ontario Child Health Study (OCHS), a survey of almost 2,700 four- to 16-year-old children in Ontario. Offord et al. (1987) found that the presence of any psychiatric disorder was significantly higher among children whose families are on welfare. This association between welfare status and disorder persisted even when age, sex, income levels, and the presence of family dysfunction were held constant. Furthermore, the importance of this risk factor was most pronounced for conduct disorders (Offord and Boyle 1988) and attention deficit disorder with hyperactivity (Szatmari, Offord, and Boyle 1989). While parental employment was not a focus of this study, it seems likely that substantial numbers of children living in poverty do so as a result of their parents' job losses. Offord et al. (1987) speculate that being on welfare may signify the accumulation of a number of other risk factors that create a family environment that is not conducive to the positive mental health of children. This formulation is consistent with what Rutter and Madge (1976) have described as "inter-generational cycles of disadvantage," in which mothers on welfare or social assistance tend to be very young, poorly educated, and from more economically disadvantaged backgrounds. In turn, their children experience similar circumstances, which significantly increases their risk of emotional and behavioral disorders. In this sense, then, when troubles cluster together, the prognosis for children's emotional well-being is not encouraging.

While these considerations do not directly implicate job loss or unemployment as risk factors for children's health problems, it seems reasonable to expect that the experiences of poverty and economic hardship are consequences of job loss that, in turn, have important influences on children's health. Recent position papers by the Canadian Institute of Child Health and the Vanier Institute of the Family make it clear that whatever its causes, child poverty has a devastating impact on the health of young Canadians.

More recently, social scientists have begun to study the entire family unit to determine the impact of stressors on various family members. For example, in two recent papers, Conger and his associates (Conger, Ge, Elder, Lorenz, and Simons 1994; Ge, Conger, Lorenz, and Simons 1994) report on the ways in which stressors experienced by individuals also have effects on their spouses and children. This work provides a useful analytical framework for understanding the pervasive effects of unemployment on families.

In summary, while there is evidence documenting the negative effects of job loss and subsequent unemployment on the health of individuals themselves, research on the effects on their spouses and children is still somewhat sparse. Moreover, given the tendency of most studies to focus on men's job loss, there remains a substantial gap in our understanding of the effects of unemployment on women and their families.

Preliminary Results from a Canadian Community Survey

In an attempt to estimate the impact of unemployment on the mental health of families, the Centre for Health and Well-Being at the University of Western Ontario is currently conducting a longitudinal investigation of families in London, Ontario, who have experienced job loss over the previous four years. Funding for this project has been provided by the National Health Research and Development Program (NHRDP) of Health Canada.

Our approach involves a multistage sampling design and the recruitment of 897 two-parent families with at least one child under 18 living at home. Each family participated in a home visit during which both spouses and the oldest child took part in a face-to-face structured interview and completed a self-report questionnaire. In each family, we determined if either spouse was currently unemployed (CU), previously unemployed (PU), or stably employed (SE). CU refers to involuntary loss of a steady job where the worker was employed more than 25 hours per week; unemployment must have been for a minimum of four weeks prior to the screening survey interview. PU refers to involuntary unemployment of at least four weeks at some time in the four years prior to the screening survey (roughly the duration of the economic recession at the time) where the individual had returned to a steady 25+ hours per week job. SE refers to steady employment in a 25+ hours per week job with no unemployment exceeding four weeks over the last four years. Thus, when we speak of unemployment in this study, we are focusing specifically on unemployment due to involuntary job loss. Individuals who left jobs or who were unemployed of their own volition were not included. We also excluded first-time job seekers who were unable to secure employment.

In terms of individual employment status, 532 of the women in our study were SE, 97 were CU, 90 were PU, and 178 were categorized as "other." This group consists largely of women who describe themselves as housewives. A very small number of these women are students, physically disabled, or retired. Among men, 560 were SE, 136 were CU, and 177 were PU. Only 24 were categorized as "other."

When we took both spouses' employment status into account to determine each family's status, 456 families (50.8 percent) qualified as SE where there had been no unemployment over the last four years. A total of 209 (23.3 percent) families were CU and another 228 (25.4 percent) were PU. Only four families (0.4 percent) could not be classified in this manner.

Table 1 presents the results of analyses that were conducted to estimate one-year rates of mental health problems for employed and unemployed men and women in this sample. For the men (husbands) in this study, we contrast those who have been stably employed over the last four years with those who have experienced any period of unemployment over the last four years (this group includes currently and previously unemployed individuals). For the women (wives) whom we interviewed, we also contrast those who fall into the "other" category—primarily housewives.

In the left-hand panel of this table, it is clear that husbands who have experienced any period of unemployment over the last four years are significantly more likely than stably employed men to have had a serious mental health problem in the last year. These men are more likely than their stably employed counterparts to have had an episode of major depression (16.1 percent versus 9.3 percent), to have suffered from dysthymia (ongoing depressive feelings) (4.0 percent versus 0.6 percent), to have experienced panic attacks (6.5 percent versus 2.7 percent), and to have abused alcohol or other drugs (10.5 percent versus 2.9 percent). In total, over one-quarter (27.8 percent) of all husbands in our study who had experienced a period of unemployment had also suffered a significant mental health problem.

Table 1

Differences in rates of DSM-III-R disorders by employment status for husbands and wives

Diagnosis	Husbands				Wives		
	SE		UE	SE		UE	Other
Major depression	9.3%	**	16.1%	14.6%	***	26.6%	** 15.8%
Dysthymia	0.6%	**	4.0%	1.7%	***	8.2%	5.8%
				↑_____		**	_____↑
Generalized anxiety	5.2%		8.1%	7.4%	*	12.5%	8.2%
Panic	2.7%	*	6.5%	9.2%	*	14.7%	12.3%
Substance abuse	2.9%	***	10.5%	1.2%	*	3.8%	2.9%
Any disorder	15.9%	***	27.8%	23.0%	***	35.9%	27.6%
N	442		248	513		184	170

*   p≤ .05
**   p≤ .01
***   p≤ .001

Among the women in our study, those who had experienced job loss within the last four years also had significantly higher rates of all diagnosed disorders. This is displayed in the right-hand panel of table 1. What is particularly significant for the wives in our study is their elevated rates of depression and dysthymia associated with their unemployment. Over one-quarter of women who had experienced job loss were also depressed in the last year; almost 1 in 10 had experienced dysthymia. Taking all diagnoses together, more than one in every three women (35.9 percent) who had been unemployed in the last four years had suffered a mental health problem in the last 12 months. By contrast, 23 percent of stably employed women had experienced a mental health problem during that time period. Women in the "other" category (who described themselves mainly as housewives) fall between the stably employed and unemployed groups.

These comparisons contrast stably employed women and men with those who have experienced job loss within the last four years; they do not take into account whether or not these individuals have spouses who also experienced loss of employment. Indeed, when we consider these possibilities, some very striking findings emerge. Our results indicate that the percentage of women suffering from a mental health problem increases dramatically if their husbands had experienced job loss in the last four years. Among stably employed women with employed spouses, 19.7 percent had experienced a mental health problem in the last year; for stably employed women whose husbands had experienced job loss, this figure rises to 29.6 percent. Among women who are housewives, these figures are 19.4 percent and 39.1 percent. Of those women who had themselves experienced unemployment but whose husbands remained steadily employed, 30.8 percent experienced a psychological disorder. Among women who experienced job loss and whose husbands were also unemployed, almost half (46.8 percent) reported an emotional problem within the last 12 months.

By contrast, men's rates of disorder are largely unaffected by their wives' employment experience. In all likelihood, the major explanation for this pattern is found in the relative contribution of husbands' and wives' earnings to their total household incomes. Despite the increasing proportion of family incomes contributed by wives, on average, husbands' earnings still constitute the greater portion. Accordingly, loss of a husband's income because of unemployment may generate more severe economic and financial stressors in the household. These, in turn, may account for higher rates of mental health problems among women whose husbands have lost their jobs than when the reverse is the case.

Our preliminary analyses of the impact of job loss in the family on children reveal age-specific effects. In our surveys, both parents independently rated their oldest child on the Child Behaviour Checklist, a comprehensive measure of children's behavioural and emotional problems. Among children who are 10 or younger, we find no indication that parental unemployment has any substantial effect on their levels of behavioural or emotional problems. By contrast, for children who are 11 or older, family unemployment is associated with both more internalizing behaviours (symptoms of depression, anxiety, emotional withdrawal) and more externalizing behaviour (conduct problems, delinquency) as reported by their parents. Interestingly, these differences are not corroborated by children's own reports. When we examine children's self-reports, family unemployment is unrelated to either internalizing or externalizing problems.

The finding that older but not younger children may be affected by family unemployment is expected. Older children are more likely to be aware of the economic hardships that occur in their families. They may also find themselves to be more directly involved in any family conflicts that may emerge as a result of the stress of unemployment.

Reemployment and the Recovery of Health

For most Canadians, unemployment is a temporary status rather than a chronic experience: on average, individuals who lose their jobs are unemployed for approximately 20 weeks. Given that unemployment is a transitional status, it is surprising how little research has examined whether reemployment results in a relatively rapid recovery of health or whether the health costs of job loss are not immediately recouped by reentry into the labour force. Research findings suggest that recovery of good health is by no means immediate once individuals are reemployed. In their community study of unemployment, Kessler et al. (1987, 1988) compare currently unemployed and previously unemployed individuals on a range of health outcomes. While they find higher levels of health problems among the currently unemployed, previously unemployed individuals still have significant numbers of symptoms. Kessler et al. (1987, 954) conclude that "...job loss creates risks to mental and physical health and that these risks are not entirely removed by reemployment."

In our own study of unemployment in London, Ontario, we find similar patterns indicating that recovery after reemployment is by no means immediate or complete. Among both men and women in our survey, we find rates of mental health problems for the currently unemployed to be only somewhat higher than those for the previously unemployed. One interpretation of this pattern is that the experience of job loss results in emotional difficulties that persist even after reemployment.

Clearly, more research is needed on this issue. If, as it appears, job loss is a particularly stressful experience that produces long-lasting emotional injury to individuals, this will have important implications for the kinds of intervention programs that are likely to be effective.

Mediating and Moderating Factors

Researchers interested in understanding how stress manifests itself in an array of health problems have developed stress process models to address these issues (Pearlin et al. 1981; Billings and Moos 1981; Cronkite and Moos 1984; Lazarus and Folkman 1984). These perspectives contend that social resources, social supports, coping resources, and psychosocial resources are mediating factors that either intervene between stress and illness or have interactive or buffering effects. In addition, stress process models postulate that the impact of specific stressors on health outcomes is magnified when other stressful circumstances are experienced. Although various authors have modified it, the stress model in figure 1 is generally accepted as a depiction of this process.

The application of this model to the study of unemployment and health outcomes has a number of advantages. First, the model is a dynamic one that considers change over time. Second, it can be generalized to a wide array of health outcomes. While its major applications have been to the study of psychological distress and depressive symptomatology, it has also been successfully used to explore the factors associated with physical health and to examine determinants of alcohol consumption. Third, this model recognizes that individuals' levels of health are importantly influenced by others in their social world and by their own involvement in a variety of roles. Finally, the stress process model depicted in figure 1 can also assist service providers and policymakers in identifying important points of intervention in the chain of events that connect job loss or unemployment with its health consequences, a topic that we consider in the final section of this paper.

Figure 1
Unemployment and the stress process

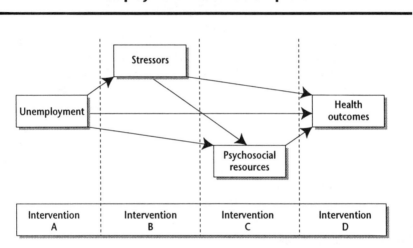

In the present context, the search for *mediators* in the stress process involves identifying the pathways or intervening variables that link job loss with various health outcomes. Given the apparent effects of job loss on the individual and other family members, it is important to understand the pathways along which this process operates. Studies of the factors that intervene between individuals' job losses and their health problems have focused on four potential mediators. Some researchers have argued that unemployment results in a loss of *self-esteem* and *personal efficacy* that, in turn, result in symptoms of mental health problems (cf. Fryer and Payne 1986; Pearlin et al. 1981). Others have suggested that job loss results in substantially altered *social support networks* where the absence of support increases psychological distress (Atkinson, Liem, and Liem 1986; Banks and Ullah 1987; Bolton and Oatley 1987; Gore 1978; Warr et al. 1988).

A third line of inquiry has focused on the process by which job loss and unemployment create *financial strains* that lead to mental health problems (Kessler et al. 1988; Voydanoff and Donnelly 1989). Finally, some researchers have examined the mediating role of *marital and family conflict*. These studies report that unemployment leads to increasing conflicts between the unemployed worker and other family members (Liker and Elder 1983; Voydanoff 1990) and that these changes in the family environment are not conducive to good health (Conger, Elder, Lorenz, Conger, Simons, Whitbeck, Huck, and Melby 1990; Fryer and Payne 1986; Liem and Liem 1990). However, while there is ample research documenting the relationship between economic distress and marital/family conflict and the association between family conflict and psychological distress, only a few studies have examined this entire process.

Those few studies of the effects of job loss on other family members tend also to focus on these same mediating factors (cf. Liem and Liem 1990). There is also evidence that the unemployed experience problems in parenting that may have a negative effect on their children's behaviour (Elder et al. 1985; Rutter 1985). In addition, Voydanoff and Donnelly (1989) present results indicating that family coping strategies may have a modest role in mediating the effects of economic hardships on family life.

Recently, a richer line of inquiry has examined the ways in which personal resources of the unemployed, family interactional patterns, and other social factors either exacerbate or attenuate the effects of job loss on health outcomes. These are commonly referred to as *moderators*. For example, Kessler et al. (1988) have demonstrated that the negative effects of unemployment on poor health outcomes are substantially less among individuals with higher levels of self-esteem than among those with lower self-esteem. Moreover, these moderating or "buffering" effects of self-esteem were significant for anxiety, depression, somatization, and physical health measures. In examining the effects of social support in attenuating the unemployment-distress relationship, such buffering effects were found only among the unmarried. Liem and Liem (1990) have also argued that marital satisfaction prior to unemployment also has a critical role to play in moderating the effects of job loss on both worker and spouse. Perhaps the most compelling evidence for moderating effects comes from studies of the effects of additional stressors on the unemployed and their families. Wheaton (1990) has argued persuasively that work and family are inextricably related and that we ought to expect stress in one role domain to exert influences in the other: "When someone gets a divorce, we think of it as a family problem. When someone loses a job, we look to the work situation or the economy for an explanation... But roles are related, although not always in obvious fashion, suggesting in general that the occurrence of stress in one role will have implications for the meaning of stress in other roles" (153). Other researchers have made similar arguments. In her comprehensive review of the literature on the interplay between work and family, Menaghan (1991) argues for research designs that more completely examine the effects of work-related stressors on the mental health of family members. She also suggests that other stressors are likely to further exacerbate the effects of work stress on individual and family functioning.

This attempt to examine how work and family life intersect and have implications for the health of family members is a relatively new direction for health research (cf. Eckenrode and Gore 1990). Wheaton (1990) has documented how the relationship between job loss and distress is further aggravated by marital difficulties. In addition, Kessler et al. (1988) have described how additional life stress magnifies the effects of unemployment on health problems.

Summary of Key Findings

There is remarkable consistency in the results of these studies: *unemployment has a pernicious effect on individuals' health.* Across an array of studies in different countries, it seems clear that job loss is a significant risk factor for physical and mental health problems.

Taken together, there is overwhelming evidence that unemployment is a significant risk factor for mortality. Whether aggregate data or individual data are examined, this association appears to emerge with remarkable consistency. Moreover, the observations that duration of unemployment appears to increase the risk of mortality and that unemployment is specifically associated with suicide and cardiovascular deaths are both consistent with the conclusion that job loss may significantly contribute to premature mortality.

Similarly, there is no doubt that involuntary job loss results in elevated levels of mental health problems. Unemployed individuals experience higher levels of psychological distress than do their stably employed counterparts. They also suffer from higher rates of diagnosable disorders such as depression, panic, and substance abuse.

Somewhat surprisingly, these elevated rates of illness do not uniformly produce higher levels of health care utilization. However, a difficulty in drawing any conclusions about the link between unemployment and the use of health care services is the variation in accessibility to services imposed by different health care systems around the world. In some societies, job loss is likely to reduce access to services even though need may increase. In others with more universal access, unemployment seems clearly related to greater health services utilization.

It also appears that the health costs of job loss are not immediately reversed by reemployment. Physical and mental health problems that are the consequences of unemployment persist for some years after reemployment.

While the evidence is somewhat fragmentary, *recent research clearly suggests that job loss has detrimental effects on the health of other family members.* Spouses of unemployed workers experience increased emotional problems. As well, there is some indication that children, especially teens, whose parents are unemployed are at higher risk of emotional and behavioural problems than are children whose parents are stably employed.

Finally, our review has highlighted some of the pathways that link unemployment to health problems. *It appears that job loss simultaneously results in increases in stressors (principally, experiences of financial strain and family conflict) and the erosion of self-esteem, self-efficacy, and feelings of social support.* These experiences contribute directly to emotional and physical health problems.

SUCCESS STORIES

Despite the substantial number of efforts to assist individuals in coping with job loss and unemployment, a review of the literature reveals few well-documented, carefully evaluated programs that explicitly address the health of unemployed individuals. There appear to be several reasons for this. First, until recently, those who conduct intervention programs have seldom been charged with the responsibility of formally evaluating their efforts. Second, intervention initiatives rarely receive sufficient funding to undertake broad-ranging evaluations that assess outcomes such as health. Third, it is exceedingly difficult to coordinate the delivery of an intervention and its evaluation in a manner that is mutually satisfactory to clients, service providers, and researchers.

Given these obstacles, it may not be surprising that a review of the literature uncovered only one major initiative where the program has been well documented, the evaluation has been rigorously conducted, and the results on health outcomes have been positive. This section reviews the Michigan JOBS Program, a preventive intervention designed to support individuals who have experienced job loss. Brief commentary is also provided on Job Clubs and on local community initiatives that may have promise but which have not been formally evaluated for their impact on individuals' health.

The Michigan JOBS Program

Over the last decade, the Michigan Prevention Research Center has developed a preventive intervention to assist unemployed individuals in gaining new employment and in reducing the psychological distress associated with job loss and reemployment. This program has had demonstrable success in addressing both the employment and mental health needs of its clients.

Actions on Nonmedical Determinants of Health

The Michigan JOBS Program has three major components: a) it employs active learning techniques to reinforce the job seeker's coping resources and motivation; b) it assists the job seeker in developing a job-seeking script; and c) it teaches actual job-seeking skills.

The JOBS Program is designed to simultaneously address two major needs of job seekers. It provides assistance in strengthening job seekers' motivational and coping processes and it also offers these individuals concrete skills in job hunting. Thus, it offers clients a combination of psychosocial support and skills training in job seeking. The psychosocial component of the program has been described in detail by Caplan, Vinokur, Price, and van Ryn (1989). Briefly, the underlying model on which the intervention is based closely resembles the stress process formulation described earlier. The model assumes that individuals who have suffered job loss have undergone a period of high uncertainty during which their self-esteem and self-efficacy may have been seriously challenged. In turn, these threats to self-esteem and self-efficacy result in feelings of depression.

The JOBS Program focuses on four psychosocial components. First, a set of *motivations and expectancies* must be stimulated. These involve the activation of a set of beliefs in the expertise of the JOBS Program trainers, the acceptance of assistance from an expert, and the belief that effort will lead to success. Second, the job seeker is encouraged to engage in *problem appraisal*, an assessment of the barriers that will stand in the way of reemployment. The third component emphasizes *skill and efficacy enhancement*. This includes the enhancement of job-seeking skills and the reinforcement of the job seeker's sense of control. A fourth, important aspect of this program is *inoculation against setbacks*. Given the high probability that the job seeker may not succeed immediately in gaining reemployment, it is critical that they anticipate setbacks and rehearse alternative coping strategies. Finally, a fifth set of processes that are emphasized by the JOBS Program involve *support mobilization*, the enhancement of emotional and instrumental support from family and friends, as well as from more formal sources.

At the same time that these psychosocial skills and resources are bolstered by the JOBS Program, a set of pragmatic skills are also provided to the job seeker. Participants in the intervention are provided with *self-appraisal and market appraisal skills* that assist them in objectively assessing their own job skills vis-à-vis the market opportunities in the employment sector. In addition, job seekers learn to *enlarge the job market* by enhancing their networking skills, learning to broaden their job contacts, and honing their self-presentation skills. Last, participants in the program receive training in *job search outcome management*. Again, this involves inoculation against setbacks and provides the job seeker with skills in choosing among competing job options.

Price and Vinokur (1995) make a very compelling argument that the utility of any program ultimately depends upon organizations' readiness to accept it and the assurance that the program can be delivered with fidelity. Organizational readiness refers to a set of values and beliefs that facilitate the acceptance of an intervention program and encourage the organization's full participation in it. Price and Vinokur (1995) and Price and Lorion (1989) argue that a successful preventive program can be launched if organizations both recognize the need for the intervention and facilitate its adoption by providing appropriate incentives. Moreover, key staff in these organizations must have attitudes and beliefs that support such interventions and they must have opportunities to participate in the delivery of the intervention. Where organization readiness is not optimal, the successful implementation of interventions such as the JOBS Program may be compromised.

The Actors

The JOBS Program has been designed for delivery in both public and private sector settings. Participants can be recruited from a variety of sources including government unemployment offices, outplacement programs in corporate settings, or other counselling services. The program consists of 20 hours delivered in five four-hour segments over one or two weeks. Usually, groups of 15 to 20 individuals are assigned to a pair of trainers, one female and one male, who guide the group process sessions. These sessions involve dramatizations, modelling, and role playing. Over the course of the intervention, trainers present structured training problems for the group to address. These problems require active learning and participation by job seekers as well as the provision of support and feedback to others in the group. A more detailed account of the actual process has been provided by Price and Vinokur (1995) and a manual for the JOBS Program is available (Curran 1992).

The challenge of providing high-fidelity intervention programs requires a standardized delivery and regular monitoring of the program and trainers. The detailed JOBS Program Manual (Curran 1992) provides a wealth of information on recruitment and training of staff as well as in-depth discussions of the five-session program. Monitoring of trainers has also been described by Price and Vinokur (1995).

Analysis of Results

Results clearly show that participants in the JOBS Program achieved higher rates of reemployment than did members of the control group. They also found jobs sooner than did job seekers in the control group and there is evidence that they also found better paying jobs. Moreover, there is no indication that these initial advantages in reemployment dissipated over the two and one-half year course of the evaluation (Vinokur, van Ryn, Gramlich, and Price 1991).

In terms of mental health benefits, participants in the JOBS Program had lower scores on measures of psychological distress than did control group members. This was the case even among those who initially did not find reemployment.

One other feature of the evaluation of the JOBS Program is especially noteworthy. Vinokur et al. (1991) have also presented a cost-benefit analysis of this intervention—a rare but extremely useful evaluation tool. They demonstrate that the higher incomes earned by participants in the JOBS Program generated higher state and federal tax revenues. Indeed, they assert that a government-run JOBS Program would pay for itself within 12 months.

There are at least three reasons that account for the success of this program. First, the intervention has been designed on the basis of sound psychosocial research applied to the problem at hand; that is, it is based on rigorous scientific research. Second, the program has been carefully standardized and the fidelity of its delivery has been assured. Third, the program addresses multiple needs of its clients; it simultaneously provides both practical job-seeking skills and psychosocial education.

Replicability

The Michigan JOBS Program appears to be unique insofar as it combines a sophisticated intervention program with a comprehensive outcome evaluation. There are several advantages of this intervention program that recommend it for wider adoption. First, the intervention does not require large commitments of time by job seekers nor does it require intensive commitments of capital or staff by organizations that wish to offer the program. Second, there is evidence that JOBS is especially effective as an intervention among higher risk individuals—those job seekers who are particularly vulnerable to the mental health costs of unemployment because of low self-esteem or low mastery. This is encouraging because many interventions prove to be successful only for lower-risk individuals. Third, it seems clear that the JOBS Program can be delivered in a variety of organizational milieux—private or public, large or small organizations. Finally, participants can be recruited from a variety of sites including outplacement services and government employment offices. All of these advantages make the Michigan JOBS Program a success story that deserves serious consideration by those who wish to address the needs of unemployed individuals.

Funding

To date, this program appears to have been funded by federal demonstration and evaluation grants. Whether corporate partnerships can be developed to sustain such initiatives is an important question at this point.

Evaluation

To date, the results of the JOBS intervention have been very promising (cf. Caplan et al. 1989; Vinokur, Price, and Schul 1995). In these two evaluations, participants in JOBS were compared to control groups of individuals who were offered take-home materials that contained the written component of the JOBS Program. This program is one of the most rigorously evaluated employment interventions ever conducted.

Local Success Stories

Virtually every urban centre in Canada can point to at least one community-based program that attempts to assist unemployed individuals in reentering the workforce. Unfortunately, much of the information that is available about these programs is anecdotal and descriptive rather than analytical and evaluative. Nevertheless, there are three such local programs that appear to have considerable potential to address the health needs of unemployed persons.

Women Immigrants of London (WIL)

Women Immigrants of London (WIL) was established in London, Ontario, in 1984 to provide counselling and support services to immigrant and visible minority women. In 1986, it began to offer employment skills training (WILEST) in response to the unique barriers that confront these women.

Actions on nonmedical determinants of health – Participants in WILEST take part in an integrated program that includes a 20-hour group assessment where barriers to training or employment are examined. As well, language and technical skills are evaluated and level of preparedness for the Canadian workplace are assessed. When this process is completed, individual training plans are developed that may include external referrals to other programs, direct referral to the WILEST Placement Coordinator, or internal referral to one of three on-site training streams: customer/food service, office skills, or a generic training program. Each training stream involves 20.8 weeks of training that includes life skills and work skills training, language and communications, and instruction and training in techniques and skills specific to the particular work stream. On-site training accounts for 12.8 weeks and an off-site training placement is provided for 8 weeks.

Reasons for the initiative – London, Ontario, is the third most popular settlement choice of metropolitan areas in Ontario. In recent years, over 3,000 immigrants to Canada have settled in this community. One of the first priorities of new immigrants to Canada is to find work. WILEST provides an integrated training program that addresses the multiple needs of immigrant women in their new environment.

Actors – The program's eligibility criteria for immigrant women include: possessing legal entitlement to work in Canada; speaking a language other than English as a first language; belonging to a visible minority; being economically disadvantaged and/or socially isolated; having a lack of Canadian work experience; possessing the ability to read, write, and speak English at a level allowing participation in the program; and having experienced barriers to employment.

The WIL Counselling Unit has been providing assistance to over 700 women per year, much of which relates to employment issues. Waiting lists for employment programs are as long as one year. Since its inception, 590 women have graduated from WILEST.

Training plan instructors include a training coordinator and instructors in life/work skills and job search/language and communications. These individuals have university degrees and/or are certified as teachers. In addition, trainers with management experience in office skills, customer service, and food service provide training expertise.

Analysis of results – To date, 590 women have graduated from WILEST. The program reports a 92 percent success rate in placing graduates at a cost of only $6,552 per placement. This is a remarkable record at a most reasonable cost.

A key element in the success of this program is its integrated format. WILEST combines life skills and work skills programs with job training and the development of language and communications skills. This on-site education is supplemented with job placements that provide participants with valuable work experience.

Another contributor to the success of this program is its visibility in the London community. WIL plays an important role in London on coordinating committees and boards. In addition, its own Board is comprised of visible and vibrant members of the community.

Replicability – In the 12 years since its inception, WIL has become a key player among agencies in London that deal with training and employment. Moreover, WILEST continues into its tenth year with steady demand for its services. This program might well serve as a model for other communities where large numbers of immigrants choose to live.

Funding – WIL continues to receive funding from a variety of government sources. Support from the Secretary of State and Human Resources Development Canada appear to be important sources that sustain this program.

Evaluation – While the evaluation of WILEST tends to be limited to placement rates and costs per placements, the program's administration maintains ongoing records that would make a more formal evaluation relatively simple to conduct. Annual reports have provided information that has maintained ongoing funding from a variety of sources.

The Learning Enrichment Foundation

The Learning Enrichment Foundation is located in the City of York in the Metropolitan Toronto area. It is the largest not-for-profit training and employment centre in the Metro region. Recent newspaper accounts suggest that this initiative has been a resounding success.

Actions on nonmedical determinants of health – A major thrust of the program is to provide an integrated spectrum of services that contribute to assisting individuals in finding work. These programs include the operation of 13 daycare centres and an industrial kitchen to provide meals to the staff and clients of these centres. In addition, programs are provided for training in microcomputer skills, English as a second language, and job training in a variety of skilled trades. The Foundation also supports clients in venture programs to start small businesses. As well, there is an action centre for employment in which clients make cold calls to identify potential employers. Any possibilities are then passed on to a coordinator who contacts the potential employer and recommends clients for any available jobs.

Actors – Given the wide range of programs, participants in Foundation activities come from all segments of the community. One of the key aspects of this program appears to be the high level of commitment and enthusiasm of staff who provide assistance and mentoring to program participants.

Analysis of results – One of the successes of the Learning Enrichment Foundation is that it reports that 85 percent of its graduating clients find jobs.

Replicability – The Foundation has been in operation for a substantial length of time. This suggests that integrated programs of this type are sustainable despite the erosion of government funds that support such work. It is difficult to determine whether such a large-scale initiative could be successfully developed in other locations. Indeed, an interesting project would be the development of a manual or training document describing the process leading up to the creation of the Learning Enrichment Foundation. Such a handbook might enable other communities to develop similar initiatives.

Funding – The Learning Enrichment Foundation administers a budget approaching $16 million and operates 22 programs serving approximately 7,000 persons per year. Funding comes from a variety of public and corporate sources. Additionally, many of the programs generate income to support the operation of the Foundation.

Evaluation – Integrated programs of this nature deserve closer study and evaluation to determine whether the successes that have been achieved in one community can be exported to other communities across Canada. Moreover, such evaluations need to assess changes in health outcomes among program participants.

Niigwin Skills Development and Placement Centre

Niigwin Skills Development and Placement Centre is a community-based training program that was established in London, Ontario, in 1989. Niigwin (Ojibway name for "New Beginning") provides job skills and life skills training to long-term recipients of social assistance who have been classified by the London Department of Social Services as "employment challenged." This program has had considerable success in placing its participants in jobs in the greater London area.

Actions on nonmedical determinants of health – Niigwin's training program includes a component that provides participants with the skills to achieve self-sufficiency. Workshops are provided on self-esteem, anger management, problem solving, addictions, résumé preparation, and job search strategies. To overcome participants' lack of specific job training, they are provided with custodial maintenance training. As well, they receive training in marble/stone maintenance and certificates for First Aid, Heart Saver, and the Workplace Hazardous Materials Information System. After completing the life skills and custodial maintenance modules, participants are placed in jobs and are monitored on a regular basis by Niigwin staff.

Reasons for the initiative – According to an earlier assessment by the London Department of Social Services, personal barriers to employment confront large numbers of clients who are on General Welfare Assistance. Only 16.5 percent of participants were judged to be "job ready" upon enrolment in the program; another 55.3 percent were rated as "moderately employable"; the remaining 28.3 percent were severely employment disadvantaged individuals. This last group represent the target group for Niigwin's program. Almost one-third of participants in Niigwin's program report that previous incarceration or institutionalization interferes with their ability to find work. As well, one-third of participants report problems with substance abuse that interfere with their work records.

Actors – Participants in Niigwin are employment disadvantaged men and women over the age of 25 who are on General Welfare Assistance. Almost two-thirds of Niigwin's clients are over age 35. Over 40 percent do not have a high school diploma.

Analysis of results – Niigwin reports that 500 participants have completed the training program since June 1989. In an analysis of ques-tionnaires administered to 416 graduates of this program, over 80 percent had returned to the workforce. Of those who found work, 3.9 percent held positions as managers, 10.4 percent held supervisory positions, 14.3 percent owned their own businesses, and 79.0 percent working in the custodial field.

The evaluation of this project also contains a detailed social accounting section. The report asserts that for every dollar spent in the Niigwin program, there is a societal return of over $30.

Replicability – Given the nature of the program and the need for custodial services in every community, it seems likely that integrated training programs such as Niigwin could be established in many locations across Canada.

Funding – Since its inception, Niigwin has been funded by Human Resources Development Canada.

Evaluation – The program provided by Niigwin has been the subject of a very detailed outcome evaluation (Kellie 1995). Data have been systematically collected from over 80 percent of all participants in the custodial maintenance program. Moreover, this information has been analyzed carefully. In addition, the evaluation contains one of the more sophisticated economic analyses of an employment program. The social accounting approach provides very clear evidence that Niigwin is a value-added program.

Job Clubs

For some years, various attempts have been made to test the impact of job-finding clubs as vehicles to assist individuals in gaining employment. These programs have tended to involve the creation of small groups of job seekers who assist each other in looking for work. The major components of these programs have been to expand job seekers' social networks to increase the number of job contacts available to each club member. Such voluntary associations also bolster participants' levels of perceived social support.

Despite the popularity of job clubs, relatively few attempts have been made to evaluate their effectiveness. Those evaluations that have been conducted have usually reported impressive rates of reemployment. Few of these studies, however, have estimated the impact of job clubs on health outcomes.

While there is good reason to believe that job clubs fulfill an important function, some caution seems warranted before recommending that such programs be widely instituted. First, many job club have recruited their participants with specific inclusion criteria in mind. For example, some have been directed toward supporting the employment of handicapped individuals (Azrin and Philip 1979) while others have recruited individuals who are searching for a first job rather than for reemployment (Azrin, Flores, and Kaplan 1975). Second, most of the published reports that evaluated job clubs appeared in the 1970s when the structure of the economy was considerable different from today's circumstance. In particular, opportunities for reemployment were clearly more available then than now. Accordingly, it is difficult to assess whether job clubs in today's economic situation are effective interventions.

POLICY IMPLICATIONS

The review of the literature in this paper clearly demonstrates that unemployment has a pervasive impact on individuals' health. The stresses and strains that accompany the loss of a job clearly erode individuals' physical and mental health. Moreover, there is a kind of multiplier effect that also has consequences for the health of the unemployed person's spouse and children. Given these widespread health costs of unemployment, what actions can we recommend to policymakers and program providers?

Any suggestions of this type must take into account that there are several levels at which policy operates. At the individual level, we can recommend programs and policies that directly affect individuals' lives. Frequently, these are recommendations for preventive interventions or treatment programs. At the organizational level, recommendations tend to focus on policies and initiatives that corporations and larger organizations can implement. At the community level, such recommendations may focus on economic or fiscal policies that governments may adopt.

Figure 1's depiction of the stress process model provides a number of potential points of intervention where programs could be designed to alleviate the health costs of unemployment. Interventions at Point A in the process focus on reducing the numbers of individuals who will experience unemployment. At Point B, the emphasis is on reducing the stressful consequences of unemployment or involuntary job loss. Interventions at Point C focus on strengthening individuals' life skills and psychosocial resources. At Point D, interventions tend to be limited to counselling and clinical interventions.

Given the pressure on governments to stem the growth of health care costs, it seems unlikely that health care and counselling services will be expanded specifically to meet the needs of unemployed workers and their families. Rather, a potentially more cost-effective strategy is to deliver health promotion and primary prevention interventions that can limit the negative health consequences of unemployment. In the context of figure 1, this means placing greater emphasis on interventions at Points A, B, or C rather than at Point D.

Reducing Unemployment

Policy advisors and analysts have generated a great variety of suggestions to reduce rates of unemployment in our society. These can roughly be divided into those that encourage change at the individual level, those that call for change at the organizational or corporate level, and those that require change at the societal level.

The Individual Level

Programs and policies that remove barriers to employment and provide incentives to work hold the greatest promise for protecting individuals from unemployment. *While it seems self-evident, education still remains the most effective weapon against unemployment.* There are at least three principles that ought to guide policymaking and program development in this area.

First, *Canada's youth must be provided greater incentives to further their education and training.* A number of policies could be implemented to achieve this objective. A controversial approach might involve reduction of the minimum wage for young people. This may have the dual effect of reducing the incentive for high school students to leave school early or to engage in part-time work that often interferes with their academic progress while providing more minimum wage positions for adults with few work skills.

With increases in tuition costs at colleges and universities across Canada, federal and provincial tax credits for continuing postsecondary education could be enhanced. For younger college and university students, this could assist their parents in supporting their education.

Second, *we need to further develop the notion that adult education and training is an effective strategy for reemployment.* At the very least, this means that provincial governments must be encouraged to continue to fund adult education programs and that universities and colleges should continue to develop their part-time and continuing education programs. It also suggests the need for a more rewarding set of tax incentives for adult learners to alleviate the costs of returning to school.

Third, *educational institutions must be provided with the resources to facilitate students' transitions from the classroom to the workplace.* Traditionally, our schools, colleges and universities provide only nominal support for students in finding employment. Partnerships among these institutions, the corporate sector, and the appropriate federal and provincial ministries need to be established. In this way, cooperative programs that are sufficiently resourced can be offered to graduating students.

The Organizational or Corporate Level

There are a large number of policies that corporations could adopt which might well reduce unemployment in this country. First, wider acceptance of job sharing might increase the numbers of employed individuals. Second, movement to a shorter work week with a larger workforce might also create more employment with relatively little increase in cost. Indeed, many economists argue that there is already a shift in this direction and that many businesses have already recognized the benefits of shorter work weeks in terms of greater productivity and lower absenteeism.

A more controversial suggestion is that corporations might encourage early retirement and reduced responsibility as a means of creating opportunities for younger workers. Such arrangements will require the commitment of both management and collective bargaining units in developing mutually acceptable programs.

The Community and Societal Level

Ultimately, the problem of widespread unemployment is a problem for communities and their governments. High rates of unemployment threaten the well-being of our neighbourhoods and strain the fabric of society. In a recent analysis of the impact of economic change on community services utilization in London, Ontario, Baer, Leshied, Avison, and Liston (1995) have documented how increases in unemployment are associated with subsequent increases in demands for protective services for children, increases in sexualized violence, and increases in teenage violent crime. *These considerations suggest that a useful response to widespread unemployment in communities may be the development of ecological or community-based programs.* In recent years, there have been a number of reviews of a variety of ecological or community-based primary prevention initiatives (Institute of Medicine 1994; Yoshikawa 1994). These reviews clearly reveal that primary prevention interventions have considerable promise if they address multiple risk factors, focus on multiple settings (including the school, the family, and the neighbourhood), and target neighbourhoods or communities with high needs (areas with high proportions of unemployed families, single-parent families, low-income families, or cultural minorities). Such interventions encourage families and neighbours to work together to reduce their exposure to the more stressful aspects of their lives, especially those that occur to children and which appear to have long-term effects on their lives. They also assist individuals and families in building stronger social relationships that may enhance their feelings of social support and sense of self. In short, the promise of ecological prevention programs is based primarily on the programs' ability to intervene at multiple points in the stress process.

There is another potential advantage of constructing community-based interventions. Programs that enhance social networks in a community are also likely to include businesses in those networks. Given that small businesses are still largely responsible for job creation in Canada, it seems likely that their participation in ecological interventions may expose job seekers to more employment opportunities. Small businesses in Canada have an important role to play in assisting in the development of healthier communities that can withstand the pressures of economic difficulty.

There are also several economic policies that directly influence the unemployment rate in this country. In recent years, virtually every federal and provincial strategy in Canada has focused on balancing budgets and reducing deficits. While few people would argue that deficit spending by government is fiscally responsible or healthy for the economy, a growing number of social commentators, policy analysts, and economists have raised doubts about the merits of massive downsizing of government via layoffs as the sole means of expenditure reduction. By plunging thousands of Canadians into unemployment, balanced budgets may be achievable but at a horrendous health cost. *Moreover, it is a largely untested assumption that balanced budgets will lead to economic renewal sufficient to absorb all the excess labour in the marketplace.* It is by no means a given that balanced provincial or federal budgets will necessarily stimulate the economy. Indeed, when deficit reduction is accompanied by an aggressive policy of inflation control, little growth in the economy can be expected.

An alternative policy that deserves consideration and debate is the lowering of interest rates in this country. While interest rates have dropped considerably in recent years, real rates of interest are still high. Many economists argue that further reductions in interest rates will stimulate economic growth and create jobs.

Altering the Consequences of Unemployment

Many scientists have argued for health promotion and primary prevention programs as the most appropriate approach to reducing the stressful effects of contemporary social disadvantages (Institute of Medicine 1994; Price, Cozen, Lorion, and Ramos-McKay 1988; Rapoport 1985). Indeed, given recent epidemiologic estimates of the prevalence of mental health problems among adults (Kessler et al. 1994; Robins and Regier 1991) and children (Offord et al. 1987) and the extremely large numbers of cases that go untreated, it seems clear that any attempt to deal with this substantial problem by means of traditional treatment approaches is likely to fail for lack of sufficient resources.

It is clear that the effects of unemployment on the lives of family members are wide ranging. Economic disadvantage increases families' exposure to stresses and strains, threatens parents' sense of self, and ultimately engenders distress among parents and mental health problems among children. Prevention programs that intervene soon after job loss are likely to be particularly helpful in limiting the kinds of health problems documented in this position paper.

While the Michigan JOBS Program appears to hold particular promise because it simultaneously addresses the psychosocial and employment needs of individuals, it may be feasible to consider importing other prevention models that have been applied to other social difficulties. For example, many schools have instituted prevention interventions for children whose parents have recently separated or divorced or for those whose parent(s) suffer from substance abuse problems. Similar early intervention initiatives could be developed for children whose family has recently experienced job loss.

Clearly, if individuals are to be assisted in coping with the stressors that arise out of job loss and unemployment, individual treatment and counselling programs are likely to be too inefficient to deal with the volume of need that is being generated by unemployment in Canada. Health promotion and primary prevention interventions hold considerable promise for reducing the health burden resulting from unemployment.

As the Canadian economy continues to undergo unprecedented restructuring, large corporations will continue to reorganize their workforces to maximize their competitiveness. It is probable that this will manifest itself in fewer full-time, permanent jobs and more contractually limited, part-time positions where individuals are likely to experience more frequent layoffs or outright job loss. If, indeed, a pattern of initial employment, followed by job loss, followed by reemployment, followed again by job loss is a potential occupational scenario for many Canadians, professional associations and collective bargaining units that represent employees should consider negotiations for benefits that include access to preventive programs that both protect the health of laid-off workers and increase their likelihood of reemployment. For their part, corporations may be willing to contribute to such programs because they will ultimately be the beneficiaries of a more motivated and healthier workforce.

In the final analysis, the solutions to the problem of high unemployment are to be found in our governments' economic and fiscal policies. Canadians must begin to debate policies that tolerate high rates of interest and substantial unemployment rates in exchange for deficit reduction, low inflation, and only modest economic growth. As has been shown, the negative health consequences of unemployment are substantial. If Canadians and their governments are to engage in truly rational policymaking, they ignore these debates at their peril.

William Avison *is a professor of sociology, psychiatry, and epidemiology and biostatistics and director of the Centre for Health and Well-Being at the University of Western Ontario. He is also an Ontario Mental Health Foundation senior research fellow. His research examines the impact of socioeconomic disadvantages such as unemployment and single parenthood on family mental health issues.*

BIBLIOGRAPHY

ADAMS, O. B. 1981. *Health and Economic Activity: A Time-Series Analysis of Canadian Mortality and Unemployment Rates*. Ottawa: Health Division, Statistics Canada.

ANESHENSEL, C. S., C. M. RUTTER, and P. A. LACHENBRUCH. 1991. Social structure, stress, and mental health. *Am. Sociol. Rev.* 56: 166–178.

ATKINSON, T., R. LIEM, and J. H. LIEM. 1986. The social costs of unemployment: Implications for social support. *J. Health Soc. Behav.* 27: 317–331.

AZRIN, N. H., and R. A. PHILIP. 1979. The job club method vs. a lecture-discussion-role play method of obtaining employment for clients with job-finding handicaps. *Rehab. Counsel. Bull.* 23: 144–155.

AZRIN, N. H., T. FLORES, and S. J. KAPLAN. 1975. Job-finding club: A group-assisted program for obtaining employment. *Behav. Res. and Therapy* 13: 17–27.

BAER, D., A. LESHIED, W. R. AVISON, and J. LISTON. 1995. The impact of economic change on some of London's community services: Critical issues for service planning and co-ordination. *J. Ontario Assoc. Children's Aid Societies* 39: 18–24.

BAKKE, E. W. 1940. *Citizens Without Work*. New Haven: Yale University Press.

BANKS, M. H., and P. R. JACKSON. 1982. Unemployment and risk of minor psychiatric disorder in young people: Cross-sectional and longitudinal evidence. *Psychol. Med.* 12: 789–798.

BANKS, M. H., and P. ULLAH. 1987. *Youth Unemployment: Social and Psychological Perspectives*. (Department of Employment Research Paper No. 61). London: HMSO.

BEALE, N., and S. NETHERCOTT. 1985. Job loss and family morbidity: A study of a factory closure. *J. R. Coll. General Practitioners* 35: 510–514.

BILLINGS, A. G., and R. H. MOOS. 1981. The role of coping responses and social resources in attenuating the stress of life events. *J. Behav. Med.* 4: 139–157.

BOLTON, W., and K. OATLEY. 1987. A longitudinal study of social support and depression in unemployed men. *Psychol. Med.* 17: 453–460.

BREAKWELL, G. M., B. HARRISON, and C. PROPPER. 1984. Explaining the psychological effects of unemployment for young people: The importance of specific situational factors. *Br. J. Guidance Counsel.* 21: 132–140.

BRENNER, M. H. 1973. *Mental illness and the economy*. Cambridge, MA: Harvard University Press.

_____. 1979. Mortality and the national economy: A review, and the experience of England and Wales, 1936–1976. *Lancet* 2: 568–573.

_____. 1984. *Estimating the Effects of Economic Change on National Health and Social Well-Being*. Washington (DC): Joint Economic Committee of the U.S. Congress.

_____. 1987a. Economic change, alcohol consumption and heart disease mortality in nine industrialized countries. *Soc. Sci. Med.* 25: 119–132.

_____. 1987b. Economic instability, unemployment rates, behavioural risks, and mortality rates in Scotland, 1952–1983. *Int. J. Health Services* 17: 475–487.

_____. 1987c. Relation of economic change to Swedish health and social well-being. *Soc. Sci. Med.* 25: 183–195.

BRENNER, M. H. and A. MOONEY. 1983. Economic change and sex-specific cardiovascular mortality in Britain, 1955–1976. *Soc. Sci. Med.* 16: 431–436.

BUSS, T., and F. REDBURN. 1983. *Mass Unemployment: Plant Closings and Community Health*. Beverly Hills (CA): Sage.

CAPLAN, R. D., A. D. VINOKUR, R. H. PRICE, and M. VAN RYN. 1989. Job seeking, reemployment, and mental health: A randomized field experiment in coping with job loss. *J. Applied Psychol.* 74: 759–769.

CATALANO, R. 1991. The health effects of economic insecurity: An analytic review. *Am. J. Pub. Health* 81: 1148–1152.

_____. 1995. The effect of economic contraction on the prevalence of psychiatric disorder. Paper presented to NIMH Workshop on Social Stressors, Personal and Social Resources, and Their Health Consequences, Bethesda (MD).

CATALANO, R., K. ROOK, and D. DOOLEY. 1986. Labor markets and help-seeking: A test of the employment security hypothesis. *J. Health Soc. Behav.* 27: 277–287.

CATALANO, R., D. DOOLEY, G. WILSON, and R. HOUGH. 1993. Job loss and alcohol abuse: A test using data from the epidemiologic catchment area project. *J. Health Soc. Behav.* 34: 215-226.

CATALANO, R., D. DOOLEY, R. NOVACO, G. WILSON, and R. HOUGH. 1993. Using ECA survey data to examine the effect of job layoffs on violent behavior. *Hosp. Commun. Psychiatry* 44: 874–878.

COCHRANE, R. and M. STOPES-ROE. 1981. Women, marriage, employment and mental health. *Br. J. Psychiatry* 139: 373–381.

COHN, R. M. 1978. The effect of employment status change on self attitudes. *Soc. Psychology* 41:81–93.

CONGER, R. D., X. GE, G. H. ELDER, JR., F. O. LORENZ, and R. L. SIMONS. 1994. Economic stress, coercive family process, and developmental problems of adolescents. *Child Dev.* 65: 541–561.

CONGER, R. D., G. H. ELDER, JR., F. O. LORENZ, K. J. CONGER, R. L. SIMONS, L. B. WHITBECK, S. HUCK, and J. N. MELBY. 1990. Linking economic hardship to marital quality and instability. *J. Marriage Fam.* 52: 643–656.

COSTA, G., and N. SEGMAN. 1987. Unemployment and mortality. *Br. Med. J.* 294: 1550–1551.

COYNE, J. C., C. ALDWIN, and R. S. LAZARUS. 1981. Depression and coping in stressful episodes. *J. Abnorm. Psychol.* 90: 439–447.

CRONKITE, R. C., and R. H. MOOS. 1984. The role of predisposing and moderating factors in the stress-illness relationship. *J. Health Soc. Behav.* 25: 372.

CURRAN, J. 1992. *JOBS: A Manual for Teaching People Successful Job Search Strategies.* Ann Arbor (MI): Michigan Prevention Research Center, University of Michigan.

D'ARCY, C. 1986. Unemployment and health: Data and implications. *Can. J. Pub. Health* 77: 124–131.

D'ARCY, C., and C. M. SIDDIQUE. 1984. Psychological distress among Canadian adolescents. *Psychol. Med.* 14: 615–625.

DEW, M. A., E. J. BROMET, and H. C. SCHULBERG. 1987. A comparative analysis of two community stressors' long-term mental health effects. *Am. J. Commun. Psychol.* 15: 167–184.

DOOLEY, D., R. CATALANO, and R. HOUGH. 1992. Unemployment and alcoholism in 1910 and 1990: Drift versus social causation. *J. Occup. Org. Psychiatry* 65: 277–290.

DOOLEY, D., R. CATALANO, and K. S. ROOK. 1988. Personal and aggregate unemployment and psychological symptoms. *J. Soc. Issues* 44: 107–123.

ECKENRODE, J., and S. GORE (Eds.). 1990. *Stress Between Work and Family.* New York: Plenum Press.

ELDER, G. H., Jr. 1974. *Children of the Great Depression.* Chicago: University of Chicago Press.

ELDER, G. H., Jr., and A. CASPI. 1988. Economic stress in lives: Developmental perspectives. *J. Soc. Issues* 44: 25–45.

ELDER, G. H., Jr., T. V. NGUYEN, and A. CASPI. 1985. Linking family hardship to children's lives. *Child Dev.* 56: 361–375.

FREEMAN, A. 1992. Unemployed are giving up, economists fear. *The Globe and Mail,* Toronto, May 9, sec. B.

FRYER, D., and R. PAYNE. 1986. Being unemployed: A review of the literature on the psychological experience of unemployment. In *International Review of Industrial and Organizational Psychology,* eds. C. L. COOPER and I. ROBERTSON. New York: Wiley. pp. 235–278.

GE, X., R. D. CONGER, F. O. LORENZ, F. O., and R. L. SIMONS. 1994. Parents' stressful life events and adolescent depressed mood. *J. Health Soc. Behav.* 35: 28–44.

GIESBRECHT, N., S. MARKELE, and S. MACDONALD. 1982. The 1978–1979 Inco worker's strike in the Sudbury Basin and its impact on alcohol consumption and drinking patterns. *J. Public Health Policy* 3: 22–28.

GORE, S. 1978. The effect of social support in moderating the health consequences of unemployment. *J. Health Soc. Behav.* 19: 157–165.

GRAYSON, J. P. 1985. The closure of a factory (SKF) and its impact on health. *Int. J. Health Services* 15: 69–93.

———. 1989. Reported illness from a CGE closure. *Can. J. Public Health* 80: 16–19.

INSTITUTE OF MEDICINE. 1994. *Reducing Risks for Mental Disorders.* Washington (DC): National Academy Press.

IVERSEN, L., and H. KLAUSEN. 1986. Alcohol consumption among laid-off workers before and after closure of a Danish shipyard: A 2-year follow-up study. *Soc. Sci. Med.* 22: 107–119.

IVERSEN, L., O. ANDERSEN, P. K. ANDERSEN, K. CHRISTOFFERSEN, and N. KEIDING. 1987. Unemployment and mortality in Denmark, 1970–1980. *Br. Med. J.* 295: 879–884.

JACKSON, P. R., E. M. STAFFORD, M. H. BANKS, and P. B. WARR. 1983. Unemployment and psychological distress in young people: The moderating role of employment commitment. *J. Appl. Psychology* 68: 525–535.

JAHODA, M., P. F. LAZARSFELD, and H. ZEISEL. 1933. *Marienthal: The Sociography of an Unemployed Community.* (English translation, 1971). New York: Aldine-Atherton.

KASL, S. V., and S. COBB. 1980. The experience of losing a job: Some effects on cardiovascular functioning. *Psychotherapy and Psychsom.* 34: 88–109.

———. 1982. Variability of stress effects among men experiencing job loss. In *Handbook of Stress*, eds. L. GOLDBERGER and S. BRESNITZ. New York: Free Press. pp. 445–465.

KASL, S. V., S. GORE, and S. COBB. 1975. The experience of losing a job: Reported changes in health, symptoms and illness behavior. *Psychosom. Med.* 37: 106–122.

KELLIE, J. 1995. *An Analysis of the Social and Economic Impact of Niigwin Skills Development and Placement Centre through a Study of the Agency's Participants 1989–1994.* London, Ontario: Niigwin Skills Development and Placement Centre.

KESSLER, R. C., and M. ESSEX. 1982. Marital status and depression: The importance of coping resources. *Soc. Forces* 61: 484–506.

KESSLER, R. C., J. S. HOUSE, and J. B. TURNER. 1987. Unemployment and health in a community sample. *J. Health Soc. Behav.* 28: 51–59.

KESSLER, R. C., J. B. TURNER, and J. S. HOUSE. 1988. Effects of unemployment on health in a community survey. *J. Soc. Issues* 44: 69–85.

KESSLER, R. C., K. A. MCGONAGLE, S. ZHAO, C. B. NELSON, M. HUGHES, S. ESHELMAN, H. U. WITTCHEN, and K. S. KENDLER. 1994. Lifetime and 12-month prevalence of DSM-III-R psychiatric disorders in the United States: Results from the National Comorbidity Survey. *Arch. Gen. Psychiatr.* 51: 8–19.

KRAUSE, N., and S. STRYKER. 1980. Job-related stress, economic stress, and psychological well-being. Paper presented at the annual meeting of the North Central Sociological Association, Dayton (OH).

LAZARUS, R. S., and S. FOLKMAN. 1984. *Stress, Appraisal and Coping.* New York: Springer Publishing Co.

LIEM, J. H., and G. R. LIEM. 1990. Understanding the individual and family effects of unemployment. In *Stress Between Work and Family*, eds. J. ECKENRODE and S. GORE. New York: Plenum Press. pp. 175–204.

LIEM, R., and J. H. LIEM. 1988. Psychological effects of unemployment on workers and their families. *J. Soc. Issues* 44: 87–105.

LIKER, J. K., and G. H. ELDER, Jr. 1983. Economic hardship and marital relations in the 1930s. *Am. Sociol. Rev.* 48: 343–359.

LINN, M. W., R. SANDIFER, and S. STEIN. 1985. Effects of unemployment on mental and physical health. *Am. J. Phys. Health* 75: 502–506.

MARTIKAINEN, P. T. 1990. Unemployment and mortality among Finnish men, 1981–1985. *Br. Med. J.* 301: 407–411.

MCLANAHAN, S., and J. L. GLASS. 1985. A note on the trend in sex differences in psychological distress. *J. Health Soc. Behav.* 26: 328–336.

MENAGHAN, E. G. 1989. Role changes and psychological well-being: Variations in effects by gender and role repertoire. *Soc. Forces* 67: 693–714.

_____. 1991. Work experiences and family interaction processes: The long reach of the job? *Ann. Rev. Sociol.* 17: 419–444.

MORRELL, S., R. TAYLOR, and S. QUINE. 1993. Suicide and unemployment in Australia. *Soc. Sci. Med.* 36: 749–756.

MOSER, K. A., A. J. FOX, and D. JONES. 1984. Unemployment and mortality in the PPCS longitudinal study. *Lancet* 1324–1329.

MOSER, K. A., P. O. GOLDBLATT, A. J. FOX, and D. JONES. 1987. Unemployment and mortality: Comparison of the 1971 and 1981 longitudinal study census samples. *Br. Med. J.* 294: 85–90.

OFFORD, D.R., and M.H. BOYLE. 1988. The Epidemiology of antisocial behavior in early adolescents, aged 12 to 14. In *Early adolescent transitions,* eds. M. D. LEVINE and E. R. MCANARNEY. Lexington (MA): Lexington Books. pp. 245–259.

OFFORD, D. R., M. H. BOYLE, and B. R. JONES. 1987. Psychiatric disorder and poor school performance among welfare children in Ontario. *Can. J. Psychiatry* 32: 518–525.

OFFORD, D. R., M. H. BOYLE, and Y. RACINE. 1989. Ontario Child Health Study: Correlates of disorder. *J. Am. Acad. Child Adol. Psychiatry* 28: 856–860.

PEARLIN, L. I., M. A. LIEBERMAN, E. G. MENAGHAN, and J. T. MULLAN. 1981. The stress process. *J. Health Soc. Behav.* 22: 337–356.

PERRUCCI, C. C., R. PERRUCCI, D. B. TARG, and H. R. TARG. 1985. Impact of a plant closing on workers and the community. In *Research in the Sociology of Work: A Research Annual (Vol. 3),* eds. I. H. SIMPSON and R. L. SIMPSON. Greenwich (CT): JAI Press. pp. 231–260.

PLATT, S. 1984. Unemployment and suicidal behaviour: A review of the literature. *Soc. Sci. Med.* 19: 93–115.

PRICE, R. H., E. L. COWEN, R. P. LORION, and J. RAMOS-MCKAY (Eds.). 1988. *14 Ounces of Prevention: A Casebook for Practitioners.* Washington (DC): American Psychological Association.

PRICE, R. H., and R. P. LORION. 1989. Prevention programming as organizational reinvention: From research to intervention. In *Prevention of Mental Disorders, Alcohol and Drug Use in Children and Adolescents,* eds. D. SCHAFFER, I. PHILLIPS, and N. B. ENZER. Rockville (MD): Office of Substance Abuse Prevention/American Academy of Child and Adolescent Psychiatry. pp. 97–71.

PRICE, R. H., and A. D. VINOKUR. 1995. Supporting career transitions in a time of organizational downsizing. In *Employees, Careers and Job Creation,* eds. M. LONDON. San Francisco: Jossey-Bass. pp. 191–209.

PRITCHARD, C. 1992. Is there a link between suicide in young men and unemployment? *Br. J. Psychiatry* 160: 750–756.

RAPOPORT, R.N. (Ed.). 1985. *Children, Youth, and Families: The Action-Research Relationship.* New York: Cambridge University Press.

ROBINS, L. N., and D. A. REGIER. 1991. *Psychiatric Disorders in America.* New York: Free Press.

RUTTER, M. 1985. Family and school influences on behavioral development. *J. Child Psychol. Psychiatry* 26: 349–368.

RUTTER, M., and N. MADGE. 1976. *Cycles of Disadvantage.* London: Heinemann.

SHAMIR, B. 1985. Sex differences in psychological adjustment to unemployment and reemployment: A question of commitment, alternatives, or finance? *Soc. Problems* 33: 67–79.

STATISTICS CANADA. 1990. *Income Distributions by Size in Canada.* Ottawa: Ministry of Supply and Services Canada.

SZATMARI, P., D. R. OFFORD, and M. BOYLE. 1989. Ontario Child Health Study: Prevalence of attention deficit disorder with hyperactivity. *J. Child Psychol. Psychiatry* 30: 219–230.

VERBRUGGE, L.M. 1983. Multiple roles and physical health for women and men. *J. Health Soc. Behav.* 24: 16–30.

VINOKUR, A., R. H. PRICE, and Y. SCHUL. 1995. Impact of JOBS intervention on unemployed workers varying in risk for depression. *Am. J. Comm. Psychol.* 23: 39–74.

VINOKUR, A. D., M. VAN RYN, E. M. GRAMLICH, and R. H. PRICE. 1991. Long-term follow-up and benefit-cost analysis of the jobs program: A preventive intervention for the unemployed. *J. Appl. Psychol.* 76: 213–219.

VOYDANOFF, P. 1990. Economic distress and family relations: A review of the eighties. *J. Marriage Fam.* 52: 1099–1115.

VOYDANOFF, P., and B. W. DONNELLY. 1989. Economic distress and mental health. *Lifestyles* 10: 139–162.

WARR, P. 1987. *Work, Unemployment and Mental Health.* New York: Oxford University Press.

WARR, P., P. JACKSON, and M. BANKS. 1988. Unemployment and mental health: Some British studies. *J. Soc. Issues* 44: 47–68.

WARR, P. B., and P. R. JACKSON. 1983. Self-esteem and unemployment among young workers. *Le Travail Humain* 46: 355–366.

WEISSMAN, M. M., and G. L. KLERMAN. 1977. Sex differences in the epidemiology of depression. *Arch. Gen. Psychiatry* 34: 98–111.

WEISSMAN, M. M., M. L. BRUCE, P. J. LEAF, L. P. FLORIO, and C. HOLZER, III. 1991. Affective disorders. In *Psychiatric Disorders in America*, eds. L. N. ROBINS and D. A. REGIER. New York: Free Press. pp. 53–80.

WHEATON, B. 1990. Where work and family meet: Stress across social roles. In *Stress between Work and Family*, eds. J. ECKENRODE and S. GORE. New York: Plenum Press. pp. 153–174.

_____. 1991. Chronic stress: Specification, measurement, and estimation issues. Paper presented at the annual meeting of the Society for the Study of Social Problems, Cincinnatti (OH).

_____. 1994. Sampling the stress universe: A multi-dimensional assessment of stress effects. In *Stress and Mental Health: Contemporary Issues and Prospects for the Future*, eds. W. R. AVISON and I. H. GOTLIB. New York: Plenum. pp. 77–114.

YOSHIKAWA, H. 1994. Prevention as cumulative protection: Effects of early family support and education on chronic delinquency and its risks. *Psychol. Bull.* 115: 28–54.

Promoting Literacy, Improving Health

MARY J. BREEN, B.SC., M.ED.

Writer and Specialist in the Effect of Literacy on Health

SUMMARY

In 1990, Statistics Canada released the results of a study, Literacy Skills Used in Daily Activities, *that found that one-third of all adult Canadians had limited literacy skills, and about half of this third had very restricted skills.* Promoting Literacy, Improving Health *begins with the key findings from that study, showing that seniors, Aboriginal peoples, prison inmates, the poor, the developmentally challenged and the learning disabled are most likely to have literacy limitations. It also examines the role of both personal factors, such as health problems, and social factors, such as poverty, that significantly contribute to literacy limitations. The report provides an overview of the personal costs of literacy limitations, in particular, restricted access to information and reduced employment opportunities, as well as the broader social costs, which include poverty and higher health care costs. It briefly examines the assumption that schools alone are responsible for literacy limitations and concludes that the causes are much broader.*

The purposes of literacy work are discussed, and the three principal literacy programming models in Canada are described—programs based in educational institutions, community-based programs and workplace programs. Research on the effectiveness of literacy programming is provided, concluding that, with the popularity of community-based programs, better methodologies are required to assess their effectiveness. The role of communication technologies in literacy work is discussed, and concludes that while their potential may be great, more research is also needed in this area.

Four key program groups are briefly highlighted: Aboriginal peoples, Francophones, inmates and women. Literacy work with both Francophones and Aboriginal peoples is described in terms of the efforts towards retaining mother tongue literacy as a means of ensuring cultural survival. The section on literacy work with women identifies barriers experienced by women in literacy programs.

Regarding the impact on health, the report details how literacy limitations can negatively influence health status. It describes the direct impacts that result from restricted access to printed health materials, particularly health and safety information in the workplace. It also describes the significant indirect negative effects on health that are the result of barriers to employment and economic security. The report examines how health workers are addressing this issue by supporting social policy changes that would address the broader nonmedical aspects of the issue; raising awareness of the issue among health workers; developing collaborations between health and literacy workers in order to build better community responses to the issue; and increasing access to health information through reduced reliance on print, clear language policies and, when appropriate, easy-to-read print resources.

The report provides descriptions of four key innovative literacy programs with different target groups: youth, workers, parents and seniors. Information about the rationale, goals and outcomes of each is provided along with the issues pertinent to literacy programming for each group. Each attests to the value of programs that respond to the needs and interests of their participants.

- Beat the Street *is a successful literacy program of Frontier College for homeless youth in Toronto. Its goal is to provide street youth with opportunities to improve their literacy skills as another form of social support.*

- *The* BEST *program is a highly successful labour education project of the Ontario Federation of Labour. Its goals are to help workers improve their self-identified individual literacy skills, and to help them become more involved in their union and/or their community.*

- *The* Intergenerational Literacy Program *was a literacy program for parents and children at the Invergarry Learning Centre, Surrey, B.C. Its goal was to provide opportunities for adults to learn more about child development and improve their literacy skills, and to provide activities for the children to foster their linguistic development.*

- Something Special for Seniors *is a successful literacy program for seniors in Medicine Hat, Alberta that is designed to help older adults live more independently by improving their literacy and numeracy skills.*

The report closes with recommendations regarding key policy implications in three areas—health, literacy and social equity—and concludes that coordinated policy responses are needed to address these issues.

Promoting Literacy, Improving Health *concludes that literacy problems must be both understood and resolved in the context of the disadvantages that cause and perpetuate them.*

TABLE OF CONTENTS

OVERVIEW OF LITERACY WORK

Literacy and the "literacy problem" in our society have become the focus of considerable interest and debate among social scientists, politicians, health workers and educators. Most of the arguments focus on literacy as a universal basic human right essential for active participation in society. More recently a new set of arguments has joined the debate, focusing more on the collective economic benefits of a literate population. Each of these positions has some merit and each leads to different programming/solutions.

Until the *Southam Literacy Report* (Calamai 1987), literacy and numeracy were measured by self-assessment or by grade level achievement. However, grade level achievement is a somewhat inaccurate measure as it does not take into account those who graduate from high school with inadequate reading skills, those who lose their literacy skills after leaving school, or those who are literate despite little formal education. It is also a problematic definition as it suggests that literacy is a static condition rather than a set of skills that decreases or increases over a person's lifetime, depending on many factors, including practice.

The more common definitions currently used in Canada are much broader and refer to the capacity to acquire and convey information using the written word. The definition used by the 1990 Statistics Canada study *Literacy Skills Used in Daily Activities* (*LSUDA*) was: "the information processing skills necessary to use the printed materials commonly encountered at work, at home and in the community" (Statistics Canada 1990). The definition used in the 1995 *International Adult Literacy Survey* (*IALS*) is similar: "the ability to understand and employ printed information in daily activities at home, at work, and in the community—to achieve one's goals and to develop one's knowledge and potential" (Fellegi 1995). These definitions recognize that reading is much more than the ability to decode the alphabet; rather it is a means whereby people use written information in their lives. The teaching of literacy has changed from a focus on discrete skills out of context, to a focus on skills in social, political and personal contexts. The definition in which literacy is seen as an intimate indicator of a set of social, political and economic issues, also leads to the fullest understanding of the causes and impacts of literacy problems[1] (Burnaby 1992).

---

1. This paper does not use the term "illiterate" to describe literacy students because they find the term derogatory and prefer to be called "learners" or "students." The term is also inaccurate since very few people in our culture are absolutely without any reading skills.

Statistics

The 1990 Statistics Canada study *LSUDA* set out to determine the literacy skill levels among Canadians aged 16 to 69. The survey only assessed reading skills in French or English, and did not include Aboriginal peoples on reserves, residents of institutions such as prisons, residents of the Yukon and NWT, and members of the armed forces. The results were as follows (Statistics Canada 1990):

- Level 1: extremely limited readers (7 percent)
- Level 2: difficulty with common reading materials (9 percent)
- Level 3: can read uncomplicated print materials (22 percent)
- Level 4: skilled readers (62 percent)

In summary, only three in five adults (62 percent) have the range of skills necessary to read most materials they encounter in their everyday lives. Of the remainder, 16 percent are essentially nonreaders. The other 22 percent *can* read in a variety of situations, if the material is simple and clearly laid out, and if the task is not too complicated. They are "narrow readers" (Jones 1993) who can read competently when these conditions are met, consequently, the reading requirements of a new work situation, for example, could pose difficulties for them. Although this group would not identify themselves as having significant reading difficulties, they might avoid certain reading situations. The restrictions due to their lack of reading skills are not nearly as severe as for more limited readers.

Of course, literacy rates vary across the population. The highest rates of literacy are in the western provinces, and the lowest in the east. Literacy rates are considerably lower among seniors, with only one-third reading at level 4, one-third at level 3, and one-third at levels 1 and 2 combined. In contrast, among people under 25, only 6 to 9 percent are at levels 1 and 2 (Statistics Canada 1992).

The rates for men and women born in Canada are almost identical, although worldwide, women make up about two-thirds of all adults with low literacy skills (International Council for Adult Education 1995). Immigrant women in Canada are much more likely to read at levels 1 or 2 (Boyd 1991), and immigrants of both genders are less likely to have level 4 reading skills. Only 36 percent of those whose mother tongue is other than French or English are at level 4, versus 63 percent for those who speak French or English. Canadian-born children of immigrants, however, have the same rates as children of Canadian-born parents.

Limited literacy is higher for Francophones than for Anglophones. Limited literacy is also very high among Aboriginal peoples, the poor, people with disabilities, prison inmates and the unemployed.

The *International Adult Literacy Survey* (*IALS*) published its findings in late 1995, and detailed data for Canada will be published in 1996. Seven countries were involved in this study: Canada, Germany, the Netherlands,

Poland, Sweden, Switzerland and the United States. Sweden out-performed all countries, having more people at the higher levels; all the other countries, except for Poland, were found to have relatively similar levels of literacy proficiency (Statistics Canada 1995). In contrast to the *LSUDA*, the data from this study shows an even higher incidence of literacy problems among adult Canadians, finding only 58 percent to be skilled readers, as opposed to 62 percent. It is unclear if the drop is because skill levels have declined, or whether a different population was surveyed or the methodology was significantly different.

Causes of Limited Literacy

A cluster of personal, social and cultural factors influence both the acquisition and retention of literacy skills.

Personal Factors

Some people have reading problems because of personal factors such as perceptual or cognitive difficulties, and health problems such as sight or hearing disabilities. Sometimes reading difficulties are the result of learning disabilities; however, only about 10 percent of the adult population have some kind of learning disability, with men outnumbering women four to one (Ontario Association for Children and Adults with Learning Disabilities 1986). Other personal factors include family circumstances and geographical location that may require people to learn literacy skills in a language they do not speak well—a common situation for most Francophones outside of Quebec.

About one-third of participants in literacy programs have a learning disability (Ontario Association for Children and Adults with Learning Disabilities 1986). Learning disabilities, however, are often not identified, with the result that people often drop out of school, believing themselves to be failures. A learning disability need not lead to reading limitations if it is diagnosed, especially if it is diagnosed early. Diagnostic clinics and programs for children do exist, but the services for adults are expensive and much harder to access. Special education programs and services for people with learning disabilities are needed as well as further research into the efficacy of communication technologies for students with learning disabilities.

The developmentally challenged are more likely to have reading difficulties, and the acquisition of even basic literacy skills can be very useful to them. Since many are poor and many have serious reading limitations, it is all the more difficult for them to claim their basic human rights. Learner-centred literacy programs therefore can help to give developmentally challenged people more control over their lives (G. Allen Roeher Institute 1990). School boards and some community literacy groups across the country offer literacy programs for the developmentally challenged. These are especially important now that so many people are living independently in the community, and are required to cope with basic tasks such as shopping and paying the rent. This issue deserves the attention of anyone concerned with the effects of low reading skills. For further information, see publications from the G. Allen Roeher Institute.

Social and Economic Factors

The causes of literacy problems are social factors more often than personal factors, and are rooted in a complex of interrelated factors including inadequate educational opportunities (both as children and as adults), family background, unequal gender roles, abuse and poverty. Although it is difficult to separate these factors since they are not independent, this report briefly discusses the impact of gender and abuse on literacy skills in the section "Key Program Groups—Women." Family background and poverty are discussed below.

The role of the family is a subject of interest to literacy practitioners since evidence strongly indicates that children of parents with reading problems are more likely to have reading problems themselves (Puchner 1993). The Ontario Ministry of Skills Development (1988) estimated that one-third of children whose parents have less than eight years of education go no further than that grade themselves. This research suggests that attention must be paid to the linguistic development of children in their early years. There is less agreement on how this can be accomplished since the issue is intimately linked with poverty.

In 1992, the National Anti-Poverty Organization (NAPO) conducted the study *Literacy and Poverty: A View from the Inside* to examine the links between poverty and literacy. After talking with people with low literacy skills, and with literacy and community workers across the country, NAPO concluded: "It is poverty and other forms of inequality that create the barriers to good education for many Canadians" (1992, 1). NAPO identified the following barriers:

- hunger, which makes it harder to concentrate at school for children and adults. (There are 1.4 million poor children in Canada. One in five children under 18 lives in a poor family; among preschool children, the ratio is one in four [Canadian Council on Social Development 1996]);
- poor housing, which provides fewer good places to study, and affects a child's status in the school;
- disruptions in family life, which affect school life;
- inequality within schools, which results in children of poor families being more often put into lower academic streams;

— lower status for poor parents, which makes it harder to participate in school activities or to challenge the school system on behalf of their children.

People who are both poor and have lower reading skills are caught in a self-perpetuating cycle in which they are poor and unemployed in part because they have low reading skills, and they have lower reading skills in part because they are poor. Poverty, therefore, must be viewed as both a primary cause and a symptom of lower reading skills. The NAPO study concluded that although literacy problems may compound social problems, they are not the root cause of them, and poverty must be addressed before literacy problems can be tackled. They stress that reading, writing and numeracy skills alone do not create jobs nor make it easier to live on a low income, nor do they decrease discrimination (NAPO 1992). "Adult learners gain many benefits from literacy programs and achieve a wide range of personal goals, but the gains are largely non-economic. The new knowledge rarely helps them escape poverty" (NAPO 1992, 72–73).

Although issues connected to poverty do emerge in all literacy classes, very few classes have the will or the freedom to focus much on economic issues. One interesting model worth mentioning here is Ottawa's *also Works*, "an industrial cleaning company started by adult learners in a community-based literacy program" (Fyles 1995, 1). Run as a business, the goal of *also Works* is to provide both jobs and new skills to their workers, allowing them to earn wages and study literacy and numeracy at the same time. *Also Works* has been managed successfully as a nonprofit organization by its workers—without a boss—for 10 years.

The Role of Schools

Schools have traditionally played a central role in the development of reading skills in children. However, not everyone who graduates from high school is fully literate. The Ontario Ministry of Skills Development (1988) found that 25 percent of community college students have lower reading skills than they require. A Canadian Teachers' Federation survey also found that teachers believe 18 percent of their students have "basic" literacy difficulties (Darville 1992). In the face of statistics such as these, it has become commonplace to blame schools for the literacy problems in the country; hence it is important to examine some of the facts:

- Contrary to public opinion, literacy rates are improving. The *smallest* group in levels 1 and 2 is the 16–24–year-olds.
- The number of early dropouts is also decreasing: in 1991 only 14.2 percent of women and 13.6 percent of men had less than Grade 9—a drop of over 50 percent since 1971 (Meaghan and Casas 1994).
- To compare the reading skills of today's high school populations with those of even 25 years ago is not fruitful, as high schools today have

students with a much wider range of reading skills, especially in the higher grades. Until recent years, many students left school before they completed Grade 12 because they had several viable options: they could work on farms or in factories, or they could enter technical courses. None of these options required higher-level reading skills, so any limitations in literacy skills were not a drawback in terms of employment. However, the work world has changed: 98 percent of jobs require good reading skills, and there are extremely few jobs requiring no reading skills (Frontier College 1989). Therefore, with many fewer options, many more students stay in high school through Grade 12. Students at advanced, general and basic levels of academic achievement now have the option of graduating from Grade 12, making the *average* reading level for the schools much lower.

- Streaming into academic levels is a cause of considerable concern among school critics. In his 1987 study of dropouts in Ontario schools, Radwanski found that only 12 percent of students in the advanced stream leave school before graduation in contrast to 62 percent of general students and 79 percent of basic students. Significantly, the level of placement and the socioeconomic status of their families are closely correlated; Aboriginal children, poor children, disabled children, and children from certain minority groups are more likely to end up in lower streams (Alden 1982). The 1992 NAPO study also confirms these findings. It is clear that, despite attempts to provide universal education to all children, schools still serve some better than others. Even the best of schools cannot make up for deep social and economic inequalities. These social problems must be addressed before the literacy problem can be resolved.

- Several solutions are being explored such as delayed streaming until Grade 10, the development of curricula that better meet the needs of minority students, greater focus on the very early grades, early identification of "at-risk" students, and meal programs for poor children. Some critics regard changes such as these as experimental and unnec- essarily costly and instead call for a move "back to basics," a form of pedagogy that is widely believed to be more beneficial to privileged students than to the marginalized.

- Lastly, the impact of schools must be viewed in light of the environments in which young people live. A commonly quoted estimate is that in the first 18 years of their lives, children and young people spend 50 percent more time watching television than attending school. Blaming schools for all literacy problems is inadequate and fails to take into account the breadth of the issue.

Research has *not* shown a marked fall in the ability of schools to teach literacy, but it has identified significant changes in the work world (Hirsch 1991). Educational requirements are now much higher for most working people, and predictions are that they will continue to rise (ABC Canada 1991). Therefore, although satisfying the need for labour is only one of their responsibilities, preparing students for the work world will be a key challenge for schools in the years ahead.

Impact of Limited Literacy

Levine summarized the impact of limited literacy as follows: "… substantial illiteracy is nearly always a grave social disadvantage, setting a low ceiling on educational achievement, and thereby barring entry … to a wide range of employment" (1986, 123). Indeed, literacy problems extract extensive personal and social costs. Clearly, it is more difficult for the lower-skilled reader to actively participate in a society so dependent on written materials. As a result, a wide range of activities from shopping to voting are much more difficult. Without strong reading skills, access to vital information on a wide variety of topics, including health issues, is also restricted and leads to further marginalization. Limited reading skills also exact a heavy cost in self-esteem in a culture that assumes reading and numeracy skills of everyone. Of course, limited reading skills also cut one off from the pleasures of the world of books, newspapers, study, letters, etc. Finally, it must be remembered that would-be literacy students face significant economic barriers to joining literacy classes; some courses charge tuition, and even those that are free may be expensive in terms of lost wages, child care and travel costs. The consequence of having low literacy skills, therefore, is restricted access to information and services, including the very literacy courses that might alleviate these constraints.

Limited literacy skills also severely restrict access to employment and economic security. Since reading skills are required for 98 percent of jobs in Canada (Frontier College 1989), most people who lack good reading skills are either unemployed or employed in jobs that are low paid, irregular and dangerous, for example, jobs in construction or primary resources. For the majority of lower-skilled readers, the result is poverty and its attendant health risks.

These costs are borne heavily by both the individual and by society that is deprived of participation by a significant segment of the population and bears the costs of income supplements, retraining and greater health care costs. The economy as a whole is also affected by literacy problems. When a significant number of workers are unskilled readers and when workplace information is provided primarily in print, production costs increase due to errors and industrial accidents. The Canadian Business Task Force on Literacy (Woods 1987) estimated that literacy problems account for costs of $4 billion per year. Although some people have challenged this figure due to the difficulties of computing such an estimate, and although these estimates can be used to blame lower-skilled readers rather than the forces that produce such high numbers of less skilled readers or the forces that allow workers to be unprotected in new work situations, calculations of this kind serve to illuminate the extent of the problem.[2]

While it is vital to understand the varied impacts of lower reading skills, it is also important to avoid creating a deficit model that focuses on what people with limited literacy lack, rather than on what strengths they possess. Portrayals in the popular media often make this error, stressing lack of self-esteem, fear of failure and limited life experiences. However, as literacy workers can attest, literacy students are often people with remarkable memory, ingenuity and intelligence. They are competent workers, loving parents and good neighbours who depend on sources of information other than the printed word. Their survival in a print-based culture is testament to this. Not only does a portrayal of literacy learners as deficit lead to efforts at "rehabilitation"—helping the unfortunate lower-skilled adults to be more middle class—but it prevents literacy workers from listening to learners and helping them to articulate their literacy needs.

Literacy Programming

Under the Constitution, literacy (as an aspect of education) is the responsibility of the provinces and territories. Literacy programs are funded through a variety of provincial or territorial ministries—Education, Culture, Social Services and Labour—with the additional involvement of other ministries. To support and strengthen the work being done by literacy organizations, the National Literacy Secretariat provides funds to support outreach, research, materials development and information sharing among literacy workers (Canada, Department of the Secretary of State 1988).

Funding for literacy is far from adequate in any jurisdiction of the country; there is also great variation between the provinces regarding the kinds of programs, where they are offered, and how well they are funded.[3] According to the Movement for Canadian Literacy (1994), there is only about one literacy program for every 3,000 learners in Canada. Darville (1992) estimates that at most 3.5 percent of the 2.8 million adults at skill levels 1 and 2 are enrolled in literacy programs. (But it must be kept in mind that the Statistics Canada *LSUDA* survey found that even though 16 percent were at levels 1 and 2, only 5 percent stated that they thought their skills were inadequate (Jones 1991).) With the decrease in transfer payments to the provinces and thereby to Education ministries, literacy programs may

---

2. The section titled "Health Care and Literacy" provides a further examination of the specific impact of limited literacy on health status.

3. For an excellent detailed overview of literacy work in each province, see Darville (1992).

be put in further jeopardy. In addition, Human Resources Development Canada, which has provided considerable funding for upgrading, is planning yet-to-be-announced changes to its provision of training dollars.

The Movement for Canadian Literacy and the Federation francophone pour l'alphabétisation en français are national nonprofit organizations representing literacy coalitions, organizations and workers. They work at a policy level to achieve equitable access to literacy education for all adults. There are also provincial Francophone and Anglophone literacy workers' associations. Because underfunding is chronic, few resources are available for coordinating programs beyond the local level. The result is an uncoordinated but remarkably vital array of programs.

Literacy programs are provided by educational institutions, community-based groups and employers and/or unions in workplaces. Many of these programs also work with other groups such as community centres, libraries, women's centres, unions, ex-offenders' organizations and Native groups. The programs are offered in a wide variety of locations, in both official languages, and are taught by both trained, experienced literacy teachers and volunteer tutors. Learners study from one to 20 hours a week, depending on the program.

It is useful to consider the reasons people give for wanting to improve their literacy skills. In its *Brief to the Standing Committee on Human Resources* (1994), the Movement for Canadian Literacy (MCL) stressed that jobs are only one reason people attend literacy classes; family and personal reasons are equally important. A recent report from the United States reflected the same priorities: "Adult learners seek the knowledge and skills to orient themselves in a rapidly changing world, to find their own voices and make them heard, and to act independently as parents, citizens and workers for the good of their families, communities and nation" (National Institute for Literacy 1995, 3). Similar to the findings of the MCL report, these learners see literacy as giving them opportunities to better control their lives.

It is very important to understand that when adults join literacy programs, learning to read is often a slow process. A frequently mentioned estimate is that on average, it takes 100 hours of literacy classes to raise a person's literacy skills by one grade level (Ontario Ministry of Skills Development 1988). Sticht (1992) looked at testing of literacy students in three different programs, and found similar slow rates of progress in learning to read. He discovered that learners make most of their gains in the first year, progressing on average one to one and a half grades, and then improve more slowly. For students who entered the programs reading below a grade seven and a half level, these improvements levelled off after the first year and progress was quite slow thereafter. Sticht's findings suggest a need for many years of education if very low skilled readers are to become literate. Pritchard and Yee (1989) found similar slow rates of progress. One of the reasons for these slow rates is that reading is a complex process, and a complex set of skills must be learned. Other reasons are part-time attendance, the demands of jobs and family, fear and anxiety in a formal education situation, low self-esteem, learning disabilities, and age (Thomas 1990).

The design of literacy programs reflect an important difference in how literacy workers perceive their work. Some literacy workers view literacy primarily as a personal issue and others see it as a social issue. The first group tends to view their students as needing a set of personal skills that may help them to achieve greater personal happiness, advancement and prosperity (which may in turn help the country achieve prosperity). The second group tends to see their students as part of a group of disenfranchised people for whom literacy would increase access to the information and power they are entitled to. They see literacy as more than the ability to read, write and work with numbers; they see it as the means by which people read and write and better their worlds. Of course there is some merging of these two streams, as literacy, like health, is very difficult to understand apart from the social factors it reflects. However, literacy teaching tends to avoid political issues, so that, except for individual teachers' interests in these issues, an analysis of the causes of a person's literacy problems is very seldom an official part of literacy lessons.

Both of these approaches have merit, the question for teachers is which works better for whom at what time.

Program Delivery

Programs in Educational Institutions

Literacy programs in educational institutions have been the backbone of literacy programming in Canada. In Ontario, for example, over three times as much funding goes to literacy programs in community colleges than is provided to community-based programs (Darville 1992). Programs are run through school boards and community colleges with paid, trained staff, and focus on upgrading and preparation for the job market. These programs cannot follow a learner-centred model as they are based on relatively strict upgrading curricula, and the students are usually enrolled in order to qualify to enter diploma courses within the college.

Community-Based Programs

Although the term is not used consistently, "community-based" programs are usually nonprofit independent programs that use volunteers and have a separate board of directors, which may include some learners. These programs receive some money from provincial governments along with support from educational institutions in the form of training or materials. They tend to run on a small budget and depend on volunteer tutors to carry out a significant portion of their work. They usually offer free or very low cost one-to-one tutoring and classes.

By using literacy teachers who are often paid below par, and by making extensive use of volunteers, community groups are a less expensive way for the government to fund literacy. For example, in 1995, according to the Ontario Training and Adjustment Board, 6,912 people worked as volunteer tutors in English community-based literacy programs in Ontario, contributing on average two to three hours a week. With this level of volunteer work, this aspect of literacy programming deserves much further research.

A very common characteristic of community-based programs is the commitment to "learner-centred" programs. Since community-based programs are seldom under the restraint of colleges or school boards that often need to follow prescribed curricula, teachers are more free to base their lessons on the students' interests, knowledge and experiences. The result is a wide variety of innovative programs across the country. Learner-centred materials form an important part of community-based programs. For example, these might be banking forms, job application forms, prescription information, stories about sports stars and/or materials produced by the students themselves based on their own stories. Many programs also produce materials for local use, and some, like East End Literacy Press in Toronto, have established publishing companies to produce and sell relevant and readable materials for and by learners. They publish a range of easy-to-read adult books of excellent quality about people like their students—Native people, immigrants, women, and people with disabilities. Learners are actively involved in the whole process, and their publications have been a great success. Another excellent example of learner-written material is *VOICES: New Writers for New Readers. VOICES* is a magazine produced by the Canadian Centre for Educational Development in British Columbia, containing learner-written materials contributed by learners from Canada and the United States. Community-based programs are a well-established and vigorous form of literacy work in Canada.[4] In order to retain these kinds of programs, better methodologies must be developed to assess their effectiveness.

Workplace Programs

There is general agreement throughout the literature that those organizations and companies that have adjusted well to technological developments over the last decade are those that have changed how they organize work. These changes require workers with strong basic skills and high cognitive and problem-solving abilities. They require workers who can work in teams, conduct research, use computers and adapt well to change (Jurmo 1996).

---

4. See also Gaber-Katz and Watson (1991).

According to ABC Canada (1991), these demands are not going to diminish; they predict that of all the jobs created from now until the year 2000, 40 percent will require more than 16 years of training.

As a result, many workers—both highly skilled readers and not—need some form of retraining to adjust to these changes. In this climate, workers with limited literacy are at a greater disadvantage. For example, the Conference Board of Canada found that at least one-third of employers had problems in their workforces attributable to an absence of basic skills (Darville 1992, 75). Because, the abilities required in the new world of work are directly connected to literacy skills, workplace literacy programs are an important and growing aspect of literacy work in Canada.

Workplace education programs can benefit employers by providing them with the possibility of a more efficient operation—fewer errors and greater productivity, especially with the introduction of new technologies. The potential benefits to workers include: improved health and safety, especially with new technologies; improved efficiency leading to job satisfaction and company prosperity; opportunities for promotions and/or retraining; improved literacy skills that could help workers in their work and private worlds; and assistance with managing the radical changes some workplaces are facing.

The contentious issue regarding workplace education is the purpose of the training (Belfiore 1995). Unions tend to argue for worker "education" such as literacy classes, in addition to training in job-related skills, in order to provide their workers with training that is focused on generic, transferable skills they could use in other job situations. On the other hand, employers tend to speak in terms of worker "training" with the goal of producing a flexible, trainable, highly literate work force capable of performing certain job-specific or even machine-specific tasks. Groups such as the Canadian Business Task Force on Literacy (Woods 1987) argue for literacy training on economic grounds, contending that: (a) Canadian industries need to be more skilled to compete in the global market; (b) Canadian workers need to be better prepared for a changing work world; and (c) literacy skills are essential to allow workers to meet these challenges. While literacy programs of this kind may benefit workers, the focus on economic benefits can potentially lead to a greater interest in producing productive workers than educated workers.

However, it may be that both of these differing interests can be met. ABC Canada (1991) believes that successful workplace programs are those that consider both the needs of the company and those of the workers. Workplace education appears to be an excellent way for labour and business to support workers and help their business at the same time.

Teaching options for workplace education include bringing in an adult educator/teacher, peer tutoring by workers or volunteers, and/or integrating literacy training into existing training. Workplace education programs are slowly growing in popularity in Canada, but compared with other industrialized countries, Canadian businesses still offer very little. Commitment to worker education will be crucial in the years ahead.[5]

Effectiveness of Literacy Programs

"Compared to reading in school-aged children, the research literature on adult literacy acquisition is only just beginning" (Wagner 1993, 6). Key questions centre around the effectiveness of literacy programs and the methodologies needed to assess these programs. One of the difficulties in measuring the effectiveness of literacy teaching is the inadequacy of testing mechanisms developed to date. Although the standard school method of evaluation using tests has some merit in terms of assessing and placing students, testing is little used outside of programs within institutions. Many teachers feel that tests are both intimidating and disruptive, and students often react badly to testing as they equate it with school tests that only served to reveal and detail their deficiencies in the past. In learner-centred programs, learners set their own learning goals, hence it is impossible to set objective standards to measure against. In addition, many teachers as well as some researchers such as Levine (1986) are unwilling to assess their students' life goals, and are much more in favour of self-evaluation by the learners.

Despite the difficulties of evaluation, some important outcomes have been identified. Albert and D'Amico-Samuels (1991), studying learners in a basic education program in New York, found that participation had a positive impact on many aspects of their lives. Learners reported positive changes both in how they performed in their jobs, and in their searches for work. They also reported positive changes when reading to their children, dealing with their children's schools, as well as in a variety of social settings. Desmoreaux (1994) also studied learners in a community-based program in Sudbury, Ontario and found that learners reported greater confidence, greater independence, higher literacy skills, improved lives and better relationships with their families. Of the group studied, 80 percent said they felt better about themselves after the program, and a third had gone on to a higher level of study.

Because of the difficulty of interpreting and particularly of comparing findings of this kind with other programs, Venezky, Bristow and Sabatini (1994) stress the need for a "multiple indicator system for evaluating adult literacy programs, a system that attends to the multiple goals of adult literacy classes and that is free of elementary- and secondary-level conventions such as grade-equivalent scores". With funding for literacy programming in

---

5. See "Success Stories" for a description of the *BEST* workplace education program.

jeopardy, strong evaluation techniques are all the more necessary and all the more difficult to achieve.

The Role of Communication Technologies in Literacy

The new communication technologies are playing an increasing role in the life of literacy students. Much further work is needed in this field to determine the optimal ways to use these technologies with literacy learners; to date, some benefits and drawbacks have become evident.

The benefits of self-directed, computer-based learning programs are several: privacy, individual control, immediate feedback, flexibility, as well as a form of computer literacy. These programs also make literacy instruction available to people unable to attend classes because of disabilities, family responsibilities or geographic isolation (Turner 1993). Assistive devices such as voice-activated computer programs can greatly help people with certain disabilities such as dyslexia, as well as people who cannot easily use a pen and paper or a keyboard.

While these programs are beneficial to many learners, key issues must be considered regarding their use in literacy teaching (National Literacy Secretariat 1995):

- Technologies do not replace people; teachers are vital to the fit between student and material. The social component of learning is too important to the learning process—especially for literacy students. These instructional programs are not 'stand alone' systems; they are one component of a literacy program that should include work with the teacher and classmates.
- Technologies can increase the burden on teachers. Teachers need training in how to use computers to their students' best advantage and in the wide range of distance education models. Even the good computer programs need to be made to fit with the needs, capabilities and goals of the students, which must remain paramount.
- Technologies are not ideal for all students. The multimedia quality may enhance learning for some, however many programs are complicated and require independent self-directed work, something which tends to be easier for more advanced students.
- Technologies can be expensive. Independent research is needed to assess the effectiveness of computer packages for learners at a variety of levels, and to explore cost sharing with business and employers.
- Technologies are seldom Canadian. Moreover, very few technological resources for literacy training are available in French or in Aboriginal languages.
- Technologies must reflect the learners' views and interests. To date, few connect well to adult needs, pre-employment issues and workplace training.

Communication technologies are being used, however, to the advantage of literacy teachers. Some example: STAPLE (Supplemental Training for Alberta Practitioners Literacy Education) is an innovative tutor training program that uses an interactive multimedia CD-ROM (Literacy Coordinators of Alberta 1996). It offers assistance to tutors and literacy coordinators as a supplement to tutor training workshops. ALPHA Ontario is a resource centre and information service for people involved in adult literacy and immigrant language training. Among other services, they offer dial-in access to their automated catalogue of thousands of resource materials, and a database about programs and organizations in Ontario. AlphaCom is a computer conferencing network for literacy workers in Ontario that greatly facilitates links between programs and practitioners. Through it, workers can get professional development, take part in electronic discussion groups and keep up on regular news about literacy work in Ontario. It is also a vehicle for learners to communicate with other learners across the province, and is the only one of its kind in Canada (George Brown College 1994).

At least one literacy program is focused on providing literacy and numeracy instruction to adults using computer technologies. *The Learning Centre* is an innovative storefront literacy program in Ottawa that has brought together business—computer companies, local merchants and the media—with both local and provincial governments. Besides teaching, *The Learning Centre* also conducts research on using computer software with literacy students (The Learning Centre 1996).

The new communication technologies have great potential; however, they will only be beneficial in literacy work if they are focused on the learning needs of students. Considerable research is needed in this area.

Key Program Groups

Aboriginal Peoples

Native literacy services recognize and affirm the unique cultures of Native peoples and the interconnectedness of all aspects of creation. As part of a life-long path of learning, Native literacy contributes to the development of self-knowledge and critical thinking. It is a continuum of skills that encompasses reading, writing, numeracy, speaking, good study habits, and communicating in other forms of language as needed. Based on the experience, abilities and goals of learners, Native literacy fosters and promotes achievement and a sense of purpose, which are both central to self-determination.

– The Ontario Native Literacy Coalition (Anderson 1995)

The importance that Aboriginal peoples place on language and control of education cannot be overstated. With rates for limited literacy more than double the national rates, literacy skills both in Aboriginal languages and in English or French are seen to be integral to achieving self-government and economic security. Literacy is seen as a key way to preserve language and culture and to record a fading way of life, for example, by producing texts in Aboriginal languages.

To this end, Native literacy workers believe that Native literacy work must be under Aboriginal control. They believe it must be delivered in a holistic way recognizing the physical, emotional, mental and spiritual aspects of the learning process. They also believe that literacy work must be done *within* Aboriginal culture, that is, instead of simply adding culture to literacy programs, literacy must be brought into Native issues such as self-government. Within this framework, literacy services are a part of all educational community work including training, healing, economic and cultural issues.

Francophones

Our mother tongue is usually the language of our major relationships; it frames the way we understand the world. Therefore, for Francophones (and Aboriginal peoples) language has come to be understood as a central means of survival and empowerment.

According to Statistics Canada (1992), the incidence of low literacy is highest in Quebec and in the Atlantic provinces, where only 57 percent of adults are level 4 readers compared to the national average of 62 percent. Among adults who only speak French, 17 percent are at reading levels 1 and 2, but among Anglophones the rate is only 9 percent (Darville 1992). Within Quebec, 8 percent more people whose mother tongue is English are at level 4 (the highest level) than those whose first language is French. A strong argument for these differences lies in the commonly held belief that we must become literate in our mother tongue *before* we can become literate in another (Boucher 1993). Illustrating this, there is a persistent and high incidence of literacy problems among Francophones outside of Quebec who have had very little access to education in French. Adult French speakers who were educated in English and spoke French at home are often unable to write well in either language (Boucher 1993). They "developed verbal skills in French which were not supported by written skills, and reading and writing skills in English [that] were not supported outside the classroom" (Ontario Ministry of Skills Development 1988, 20). This situation has clearly diminished the strength of the French language in Canada, and has serious consequences for the transmission of Francophone cultural values.

The core of the Francophone literacy movement is the right to French language literacy training sustained by, among other things, funding for

Francophone literacy training in every province, with special concern for people educated in English. It also involves training for Francophone literacy workers, the establishment of Francophone literacy networks, support for French language and Francophone cultural achievements, research and documentation of Francophone literacy projects, more Francophone resources, and literacy projects concerned with social issues such as community development (Boucher 1993).

Some progress has been made. A national coalition of Francophone literacy workers exists, and literacy programs are offered in French in every province. Also, Francophones in Ontario now have the right to receive literacy education in their first language (Ontario Training and Adjustment Board 1994). In addition, three new Francophone community colleges have been established in Ontario that will offer, among a range of courses, upgrading in French.

Inmates

Education (and within this, literacy work) has a long and mixed history within the prison system. The Correctional Service of Canada has a mandate to provide educational upgrading programs for inmates—a significant policy decision because, according to their findings, 65 percent of first-time inmates have low reading skills (Paul 1991). Statistics from the United States are almost identical (Lewin 1996). With the rate for literacy problems being this high among inmates, literacy classes are vital to prevent skills from diminishing even further.

Numerous studies have shown that literacy programs in prisons appear to do more than teach reading and writing. According to a National Center on Adult Literacy study of prison literacy, "the greater the literacy and the more extensive the education that inmates achieve, the lower will be their recidivism rate" (Newman et al. 1993, 35).

There is some consensus among people designing literacy programming in prisons. The principles they support are similar to those supporting programs for other disenfranchised groups. These include a wider focus than just reading and writing, the centrality of the needs of the learners, optional attendance and the importance of resources such as a good library. A strong theme is the importance of providing inmates with a constructive use of their time (Odell 1992).

Computer-assisted programs are growing in popularity within prisons and, although some educators doubt their efficacy, they do offer a degree of independence to the learner, as well as consistency if the inmate is moved from one institution to another. As in every program, relevant curriculum materials are scarce; prison programs need more materials about issues that inmates will encounter when they are released, such as housing and finding jobs.

Recognizing the link between literacy and crime, the National Associations Active in Criminal Justice have designed a kit called *Between the Lines/Entre les lignes.* The kit consists of 10 booklets, two brochures and an audio tape with a play and personal stories written by young offenders. The premise of the kit is that low literacy levels and high dropout rates, combined with unemployment and poverty, contribute to crime. Low literacy skills and low education reduce job choices and make it harder to escape poverty. The designers of the kit believe that if young people can upgrade their education and become more involved in their community, they will have more choices and thereby more control over their lives (National Associations Active in Criminal Justice 1995). The kit is intended to (a) inform community workers, including literacy workers, about the problems of juvenile crime and low literacy; and (b) direct them to think about practical, collaborative, community-based approaches to reduce both crime and low literacy rates.

Women

Some teachers view literacy classes as an ideal opportunity to explore women's issues as well as to learn literacy skills. The following is a summary of some of the issues considered important when developing literacy programs specifically for women.

One of the most common issues that emerges in women's literacy programs is violence. Women in literacy programs have identified men's violence (or its threat) as the *greatest* barrier to their learning (Davies 1995). Sometimes this violence takes the form of threats from male partners who fear that the women will acquire greater power (earning power, intellectual power) through literacy, or who fear the women will develop new relationships that will lead them away (Horsman 1990; Lloyd 1994). Violence during childhood can also deeply interfere with learning, and in fact, sexual abuse is one common reason that girls leave home and drop out of school. The complexity and implications of violence and its impact on women's learning are beyond the scope of this paper, but literacy workers would be well advised to be aware of these issues in their work.[6]

There is an urgent need for literacy materials that confirm the experiences of women's lives and address important issues such as health, poverty, violence and isolation. One response to the issue of violence and its effect on women's learning is a kit for teachers developed recently by the Canadian Congress for Learning Opportunities for Women (CCLOW) (1996). It presents the findings from four workshops addressing violence and its effects on women's education, and includes stories and curriculum materials.

---

6. See Horsman (1990) and Lloyd (1994) for further discussion.

Two interesting literacy programs specifically address gender issues, one for women and one for men. The Montreal YWCA (1996) has developed a new and innovative program, *Paroles de femmes/Words for Women*. This literacy program is unique, "woman-centred" and "woman positive." It uses tutors in one-to-one situations, is open to women of all ages, is bilingual and free. The goal of the program is to reach women with reading and writing instruction in order to increase their autonomy and personal strengths. They also offer literacy programs for immigrant women who can not take part in either English or Francophone programs. The program is also developing curriculum materials. In Nova Scotia, a project called *Men in Literacy against Sexism* is being developed to "assist men who are students and practitioners in literacy and upgrading programs to work together to understand the roots of sexism and men's violence and to find together ways to work toward positive social change" (Davies 1995).

Poverty is another key barrier that prevents women from attending literacy classes, hence literacy programs that want to reach women must provide supports such as very low tuition fees, child care and transportation. In addition, classes must be held at times and locations that are safe, accessible and compatible with women's schedules and their roles as parents, partners and workers. Feminist literacy workers also stress the importance of the social aspects of literacy work, seeing informal talking as an integral part of learning, especially if the class wants to respond to the real needs of the women attending.

The commitment to addressing these issues among women literacy workers has led to the establishment of a national Feminist Literacy Workers' Network (FLWN/RETRAFA) to, among other things, support feminist literacy work, share resources, promote nonsexist materials and support research regarding women and literacy.

HEALTH CARE AND LITERACY

Impact of Limited Literacy on Health

Several studies have shown unequivocally that literacy limitations have a major, negative impact on health (Ontario Public Health Association and Frontier College 1989; Jackson 1991; Weiss 1992). People with poor reading skills are at increased risk for health problems caused both directly and indirectly by their lack of reading skills. The mechanism whereby this relationship is established is complex and as yet understudied.

The direct impacts on health are attributable to the inability to access vital health information presented in print form. Printed health materials are widely used by health care workers as inexpensive and efficient means of conveying information to and gathering information from the public. They are used for hospital consent forms, preoperative instructions, birth control instructions, prescription information, self-care instructions, public health questionnaires and campaigns, and workplace health and safety information, to name but a few.[7] The use of print materials in health care is well established, and with widespread health care cutbacks, its use will most probably increase.

Most health materials are hard to read because they use terms, concepts and illustrations that are not familiar to lower-skilled readers, and because the ideas are often presented in unfamiliar ways (Breen and Catano 1987; LaPierre and Mallet 1987; Powers 1988; Doak, Doak, and Root 1995). Williams et al. (1995) found that about 40 percent of patients in a hospital setting were unable to read and comprehend directions for taking medication, and about 60 percent were unable to understand a standard consent form. Similarly, a study by Jackson et al. (1991) found that nearly all brochures used in their outpatient clinics were far above the reading skills of most of their patients. In situations such as these, when the health care professional thinks patients have received instructions but they have not, the results are often disastrous, due to errors, noncompliance, and the dangerous underuse or overuse of the health care system (Ontario Public Health Association 1989; Weiss 1992).

Not only do literacy problems lead to certain kinds of health problems, but they also make the resolution of these problems more difficult. Without adequate health information, people who are not strong readers are much less able to participate in critical decisions regarding their own and their family's health. Without the confidence that comes from education and income, people with lower reading skills may also be more reluctant to question their care, and less likely to receive information in terms they can understand.

People with lower reading skills are also at greater risk for injuries in the workplace (Industrial Accident Prevention Association 1989; Ontario Public Health Association 1989; Edwards 1995). The primary reasons are that people with lower reading skills tend to work in jobs in primary resources and construction where the rate of accidents is higher (Perrin 1989); they are often less aware of their rights regarding unsafe work; they often work in non-union jobs where they have less protection; and instructions regarding health and safety issues are routinely provided in print form. Although some of the above-mentioned jobs are unionized and do provide better wages and more health and safety protection, these jobs are diminishing in

---

7. Of course many other print materials also contain information pertinent to health and safety: instructions for baby formula, packaged food products and household chemicals; legal documents such as court orders and landlord-tenant agreements; and notices regarding school programs, community events, etc.

number, and people with lower reading skills tend to be overlooked for retraining.

Literacy is a critical factor in workplace health and safety, however few employers are aware of this. Many employers wrongly assume that their employees are both literate and English speakers, and believe they have adequately protected the safety of their workers by providing occupational health information in print and in English. WHMIS (Workplace Hazardous Materials Information System) materials, for example, are often written at a college level (Edwards 1995). The results of this false assumption are predictable: dangerous working conditions, costly errors and considerable lost time due to injuries. The Canadian Business Task Force on Literacy (Woods 1987) concurs, estimating that of the $4 billion lost to literacy problems mentioned above, $1.6 billion is attributable to workplace accidents. The cost in human suffering is incalculable. Employers must take literacy and language into account when they provide information regarding procedures and risks to their workers.

In addition to the direct causal links described above, reading problems also affect health in less direct ways by reducing access to well-paid employment and hence increasing the likelihood of poverty and its attendant stresses. Numerous studies have shown that income is a strong predictor of health status (Evans and Stoddart 1994). Morbidity and mortality rates are higher among the poor, and they have fewer disability-free years (Harding 1987). Because socioeconomic status is such a strong determinant, Winkleby et al. attempted to determine if one factor determining socioeconomic status could be isolated from the others. Their findings were very interesting: "higher education, rather than income or occupation, may be the strongest and most consistent predictor of good health" (Winkleby et al. 1992, 819). Weiss et al. also concluded that "illiteracy and poor health status are independently associated" (1992, 257). Marmot similarly concluded: "education is a powerful predictor of health status" (1994, 210), as did Leigh (1985): "years of schooling persists as a predictor of good health regardless of which other variables enter the equation" (cited in Perrin 1989, 11).

These findings regarding the importance of education as a vital determinant similar to the findings of Health and Welfare Canada's Health Promotion Survey (1988) which showed that years of schooling correlate positively with self-reported health status. This survey also showed that people with lower education have poorer nutrition, smoke more, are less active, and are under more stress. Although these factors no doubt predispose poor people to a higher incidence of health problems, these so-called negative health behaviours must also be understood as the result of an inability to purchase safe housing, healthy food and recreation, compounded by the restrictions imposed by literacy limitations. The obvious conclusion from these findings is that investment in early education could improve health.

Much more research is needed to determine if education during adulthood could lead to equivalent improvements in health status.[8]

Health Care Responses to the Literacy Issue

Social Policy Changes

With the growing understanding of the social determinants of health, health workers are lending increasing support to the need for societal change as a resolution to the health problems attributed to literacy problems. While medical solutions may be needed to treat certain impacts of low reading skills, a broader nonmedical approach is also required to prevent the recurrence of these events. A more just distribution of resources would improve living and working conditions for the poor, and would direct funding to literacy programs and programs that address the causes of limited literacy such as preschool programs for disadvantaged children. Rachlis and Kushner (1989) are two of the very few health critics to date to call for the redirection of some funding from medical services to literacy programs.

Increased Awareness of the Issue

Federal and provincial public health associations have paid considerable attention to raising awareness about the links between literacy and health. In the first phase of its Literacy and Health Project, the Ontario Public Health Association (OPHA) published two reports regarding the relationship between literacy and health (OPHA 1989 and Perrin 1989). The second phase of the Project was devoted to providing support for projects addressing the literacy and health issue, fostering working partnerships between literacy groups and health groups, and establishing a clearinghouse of literacy and health information at Alpha Ontario (Breen 1993).

The Canadian Public Health Association (CPHA) has built on this work by establishing a National Literacy and Health Program. Its goals are to raise awareness among health professionals about the links between literacy and health, to foster commitments to this issue by national health associations, and to establish links between literacy organizations and health organizations at the provincial level. The Program also promotes the use of plain language, provides information about the literacy and health issue to students in training in various health disciplines, and provides support to national health organizations as they work to establish literacy-sensitive strategies and policies within their organizations (CPHA National Literacy and Health Program Interim Report 1995). One excellent example of such

---

8. See Perrin (1989) for a full examination of these issues.

a strategy is the Canadian Association of Optometrists' *Sharing the Vision* campaign in which optometrists were matched with literacy learners for free vision care and eyewear for anyone enrolled in literacy programs. During 1995, the campaign was hoping to arrange eye care for 18,000 learners (Canadian Association of Optometrists 1995)!

The Alberta Public Health Association is also in the process of establishing a project aimed at increasing awareness of the impact of literacy on health and at supporting actions on these issues within health organizations.

The thrust of each of these programs has been to make health professionals aware of the prevalence of the problem, and to support changes that would lead to better quality care for all their clients/patients.

Collaboration between Health and Literacy Workers

One important response to this issue has been increased collaboration between literacy workers and health care workers. The benefits of such collaborations are many. Health workers can provide health information and resources to literacy workers and their students, and they can also help students negotiate their rights to better health care. In turn, literacy workers can provide health workers with information about the health issues their students face, and information about how the students currently understand their health problems. Together, literacy workers, health workers and learners can successfully collaborate to develop relevant health programs and program materials (Breen 1993).

Many models of this kind are being tried across the country (Breen 1993). A number of literacy, health and community workers joined together in Edmonton, Alberta, to jointly produce readable sexuality materials. An easy-to-read journal about pregnancy was developed in Montreal with an advisory group made up of low-income women, health professionals, a community organization in a low-income neighbourhood and two literacy groups. A literacy organization on Manitoulin Island, Ontario worked with a local band office to develop a readable survey about local health needs. In Arviat, Northwest Territories, because the literacy class was very interested in health topics, the teacher set up a program using their interest in health to teach literacy, and using their interest in literacy to teach about health (Norton 1992). And currently, a literacy group in Edmonton is designing a program called *Participatory Education for Literacy and Health Promotion* that integrates literacy with health promotion. The program is designed to help women with low literacy skills and/or low income access health information and resources through better literacy skills.

Experience of programs of this kind has shown that such collaborations are efficient and effective, and have the added benefit of building community cohesion.

Increased Access to Health Information

To work towards truly equitable access to information, organizations must examine their reliance on print and devise some alternatives. For example, some organizations have replaced and/or supplemented their pamphlets and brochures with posters, videos and audio tapes (Planned Parenthood Peterborough 1990). Others have used television and other mass media campaigns. Some are exploring the use of pictographs and illustrations to accompany print materials (Michielutte et al. 1992; Program for Appropriate Technology in Health 1989). Others are using one-on-one, personal instruction using no, or very little, print material. Some are asking people to identify a surrogate reader within their family or community to help them understand printed instructions.

Over the last 10 years, clear language has also steadily gained in popularity, particularly among health care and legal practitioners who are concerned with equitable access to information. Health workers have come to realize that not only should public documents and programs be inclusive in terms of gender, income, age, sexual orientation, disabilities, language, race, religion and culture; they should also be inclusive in terms of reading skills (Breen 1994). To support this, some organizations have developed equal access policies that include clear language as one important component.

While easy-to-read health documents are better than those that are hard to read, they are far from a complete solution as they are only useful for *some* lower-skilled readers. For those who cannot read or seldom read, and those who cannot read in the languages in which we write and those who don't learn well from print materials, and those who prefer to get information from other sources such as friends and family, easy-to-read materials are of very little benefit. Easy-to-read materials must not be seen a substitute for personal contact.

Some research has also gone into designing instruments to diagnose patients with low reading skills in clinical settings (TOFHLA [Williams et al. 1995]; REALM [Davis et al. 1993]). These instruments are intended to enable the health practitioner to identify lower-skilled readers and then to make easier-to-read health information available to them. Sometimes these patients are directed to local literacy programs, however, as noted above, upgrading classes are only of interest to a minority of lower-skilled readers, and learning to read is a slow process for most. Many more health care workers have recognized that since the number of people with lower reading skills is so great, rather than try to diagnose lower-skilled readers, it may be more cost effective to either rely less on print, or to use readable materials that could be used with both skilled and unskilled readers alike.[9] This shift of responsibility from expecting the patient to "catch up" to expecting the medical profession to change its practices is both significant and unprecedented.

SUCCESS STORIES

Beat the Street: Frontier College

Literacy programming for homeless people is a growing interest of community workers. Both St. Christopher House (Farmer 1995) and Frontier College (1992) offer flexible drop-in programs combining one-to-one literacy tutoring with some group classes. Literacy is not seen as an end in itself in either program. Instead, literacy is seen as a way to provide the severely disenfranchised with a means to control their lives better, a means to provide them with another form of social support, and a way to respond to the individual interests of the participants.

Overview

Beat the Street is a literacy tutoring program for homeless youth in downtown Toronto, Ontario run by Frontier College. Underlying this program is a belief in the right to literacy for all, and a belief that education can give people the tools to take control of their lives and to work towards their goals.

Purpose

Beat the Street was founded by two men who had lived on the street and who had learned to read through literacy programs at Frontier College. Since many street youth are school dropouts with limited reading skills, the founders believed that these young people need a chance to learn to read and write as a way to help them get off the street, reintegrate into society and further their education, where appropriate.

At *Beat the Street*, literacy teaching is done through one-to-one volunteer tutoring and support with a strong commitment to a learner-centred approach in which students know best what they want to learn and how. *Beat the Street* also believes that students should define their goals for success. They believe that learning must be built upon a person's strengths and

---

9. Eaton and Holloway (1980) have shown that skilled readers are not offended by easy-to-read materials provided they are not condescending. People prefer easy materials over difficult materials, *especially* when they or members of their family are in crisis.

successes and that everyone can learn—no matter how they have been labelled.

Key Players

In 1994, Toronto had about 10,000 homeless youth: 7,000 males and 3,000 females (Turner 1994). These young people either live on the street or make a living on the street, and many have problems with drugs and/or alcohol and prostitution. Many come from disrupted homes where they have been abused physically and sexually, and many are from foster homes. Most are school dropouts, and most, but not all, are from Toronto.

Tutors at *Beat the Street* are volunteers; some have lived on the street, and some have previously been students at *Beat the Street*. The program tries to match students with tutors who have similar interests.

Results

Beat the Street does not have formal classrooms; it operates from a store-front drop-in. In addition to tutoring in reading and writing and computer literacy, *Beat the Street* also offers counselling and moral support, and helps students with day-to-day issues such as finding a place to live. The program runs a drama group, an arts group and a women's group, and publishes student writing and student artwork. Programming is in English.

Many of the young people in the program have addictions and other high-risk behaviours. To address this issue, *Beat the Street* is also involved in a computer project to reach street youth with information regarding their health.

Replicability

Between 1987 and 1990, Frontier College set up similar programs in Winnipeg, Manitoba, and Regina, Saskatchewan, for Native youth. The program in Winnipeg has been successful and continues to operate, now under the direction of the Native community. The Regina project however, has closed. Frontier College is currently working on training other Ontario agencies that work with homeless youth regarding how they might include a literacy component in their programs.

Funding

Funding for *Beat the Street* comes from the Ontario Training and Adjustment Board, the Toronto Board of Education, Compugen Systems Ltd., the Metcalfe Foundation and individual donors.

Evaluation

Although programs for homeless people are difficult to evaluate because of the transient nature of homeless people's lives, Frontier College does conduct an annual evaluation of *Beat the Street*. In 1995, 300 to 400 young people were actively enrolled on an ongoing basis for literacy training. Most were white men, aged 16 to 24, but more women have become involved recently. Although the number of homeless youth attending the program represents only a fraction of the total number of homeless youth living in downtown Toronto, the evaluation did find very positive results for those who took part:

- 70 percent of the participants achieved or partly achieved the objectives they had set for themselves;
- 20 percent of the participants left the program to begin other educational or employment training; and
- 10 percent left for employment.

In addition, over 1,000 young people come to *Beat the Street* each year for help on a one-time basis. They do not come for literacy training, but instead for help with problems such as filling out forms, locating a service, cashing a welfare cheque or dealing with legal issues.

Both the students, the workers and the evaluators consider *Beat the Street* a success. Although *Beat the Street* only serves a small number of the homeless youth in downtown Toronto, for them the program is very important. For street youth whose lives are often chaotic, small victories like showing up regularly for tutoring can be read as an enormous vote of confidence in the program.[10]

BEST – Basic Education for Skills Training: The Ontario Federation of Labour

Please see the section "Literacy Programming" for a discussion of workplace literacy programming.

Overview

The *BEST* program is an Ontario-wide labour education project of the Ontario Federation of Labour (OFL) and its affiliated unions (Ontario Federation of Labour 1995).

Purpose

BEST was started in 1988 as part of the OFL's commitment to worker education and lifelong learning. The OFL sees *BEST* as a part of the "broader

---

10. An evaluation report is available through Frontier College: (416) 923-3591.

struggle of the labour movement that puts literacy into perspective—as a tool—as a means to an end, not the end in itself" (Turk and Unda 1991, 271). Therefore the intent of *BEST* is twofold: to help workers improve their self-identified individual reading, writing, math and communication skills, *and* to help them be more able collectively to shape their worlds. For these reasons, the curriculum is not preset, nor it is job specific; it is determined by what the workers at each workplace want to learn.

Key Players

In *BEST* programs, union and management work together to provide the programs. The learners are workers who have chosen to join the *BEST* program. The instructors are trained coworkers from the same union and workplace. They take part in an intensive training provided by *BEST*, and they are supported by one of six regional coordinators and the *BEST* project training officer.

Most *BEST* programs are held at the workplace in small groups of six to twelve people. The courses are free; they run for 36 weeks and classes are usually two hours long, twice a week. Employers usually provide the physical facilities and supports, such as photocopying; they also usually provide release time for the workers. In a typical two-hour session, one hour is on the employer's time and one hour is on the workers'. Additional resources are provided by the *BEST* program.

Results

BEST appears to be a resounding success. New programs are continually starting up around the province and dropout rates are low. At present, about 75 *BEST* programs are in operation in a wide variety of locations across Ontario: hospitals, hotels, diverse manufacturing sectors, municipal government offices, nursing homes and universities. *BEST* programs operate in both French and English.

Replicability

The Saskatchewan Federation of Labour runs a successful program modelled after *BEST*. The Canadian Labour Congress developed a similar project in New Brunswick that ran for three years, but it was forced to close because of inadequate funding.

Similar programs are run by the Labour Council of Metro Toronto and by the Hamilton and District Labour Council.

Funding

Funding comes from the Ontario Training and Adjustment Board with funds from the National Literacy Secretariat for special projects.

Evaluation

BEST is evaluated regularly at the class, program and project levels. The results show that the unions, workers and employers all consider *BEST* to be highly successful. Workers who go through the program become more capable and more confident—both within their jobs and their lives in general. They report changes such as being more involved with their union and/or their children's school. Employers also report very favourable outcomes: their workers have increased opportunities for job advancement, increased confidence, and are more able to handle advanced technologies (Unda 1995).

Learners assess their own progress throughout the courses but no external testing is used. Individuals develop portfolios documenting their goals and achievements, and these may be used to access further training. Individual results are confidential. An evaluation from the standpoint of the instructors will be published later in 1996.[11]

Intergenerational Literacy Program: Invergarry Learning Centre

In order to encourage linguistic development in young children, many family/intergenerational literacy programs have been established across the country. These programs usually focus on disadvantaged parents. Based on research findings that suggest that parents' literacy is a major predictor of both children's school achievement and health (Puchner 1993), the goals of these programs are usually (a) to increase the literacy levels of parents, and (b) to help the children's linguistic development, in particular by encouraging parents to read to their children.

The primary focus for intergenerational programs varies: some programs focus on the parents, others on the children, while others focus on the parents' relationship to their children. These programs are also run in a number of ways. Some are part of literacy programs and some are part of playschool programs. For example, some programs match seniors with small children, providing the children with opportunities both to improve their language and literacy skills and, depending on their age, to learn local history from the seniors. These programs also give the seniors opportunities to improve their reading skills as well as contact with more people in their

---

11. For more information, contact the Ontario Federation of Labour at (416) 441-2731.

communities. Other programs offer the parents literacy and/or language instruction as well as a variety of programs including pre-employment training, parenting classes and health classes. Programs of this kind usually offer a preschool program for the children to encourage their linguistic development and to better prepare them for school. Other programs have made reading to children a major focus of their public work, sometimes recruiting celebrities to read to children in public and organizing reading circles in neighbourhoods (O'Leary 1991). In all of these intergenerational programs, the focus is the important role of adults/parents in encouraging children to read.

Overview

The *Invergarry Learning Centre Intergenerational Literacy Program* in Surrey, British Columbia, was designed to improve the literacy skills of both the children and adults who attended the Invergarry Learning Centre.

Purpose

Unlike many programs where the adults and children are separated during most of the program, the goal of the *Invergarry Learning Centre Intergenerational Literacy Program* was to provide opportunities for children and adults to learn together. The premise was that parents could be provided with an opportunity to spend time with the children in the preschool setting, followed by time to reflect on what had happened and, in doing so, to learn more about child care and child development. A second goal of this reflective time was to improve literacy skills in the context of early childhood education, since the facilitator was both an early childhood education worker and an experienced literacy teacher. (Adults also attended other literacy classes during the day.) During the reflective time, while the adults were discussing children and child care, early childhood educators worked with the preschool children providing them with activities to foster their linguistic development.

Because the *Invergarry Intergenerational Literacy Program* was based on the concept of building on the participants' strengths in order ultimately to strengthen families and communities, the program relied on input from learners about their needs, and encouraged them to help plan curricula to reflect these needs. The program was continually adapted to reflect the needs and interests of the learners.

Key Players

Children were in the preschool program run at the Centre by the Surrey YMCA. Adults were part of the literacy program run by the Invergarry

Learning Centre. Staff consisted of experienced early childhood educators and experienced literacy workers.

Results

Between 20 and 25 children (fewer in the winter) attended for two and a half hours in the mornings, two to five days a week. They were mostly three- and four-year-olds. About a third of the children had limited English, and seven had parents in the literacy program.

Over the year, only 10 adults took part, and most were learning a second/other language. The program organizers were disappointed that so few adults participated, in particular, that few of the parents of the children in the preschool were involved. However, some parents had no other contact with the Centre, and many said that they wanted to spend the limited time they had away from their children on their own upgrading.

Replicability

The design of the program was based on extensive research conducted during the year before the program began (Isserlis et al. 1994). The research had indicated significant interest in such a program; however, logistics and time limitations for the literacy workers are major considerations in mounting a similar program elsewhere. A program of this kind requires space and equipment for both the literacy and the preschool components. Any adult education program with on-site child care could potentially provide a program of this kind provided that its staff was sensitive to cross-cultural issues (especially those pertaining to parenting), and committed to this model and the considerable organization it requires.

Funding

Funding was provided by a National Literacy Secretariat demonstration grant, and the program is no longer running.

Evaluation

Adults in the program reported that it was useful and interesting to them in terms of their own literacy learning, and in terms of learning about children's linguistic development and child development. They enjoyed the time with the children and the reflection time afterwards. These opinions are also revealed in their writing, which is included in the project reports. The participants reported that they spoke more with their children, were more involved with their children's school work and their children's schools. These reports were strengthened by the staff's observations of the adults. The children's linguistic development also improved. Staff reported that some immigrant children benefitted by being helped to fit into the preschool program by an adult who spoke their language. Through this program, the preschool obtained new books about on various cultural groups, and developed a greater commitment to reading to children.

After completing the pilot project, the staff was quite satisfied with the design of this learner-centred intergenerational program in large part because the model allowed them to modify the program until it best met the needs of the participants. The problems with the program were low enrollment, scheduling difficulties and other logistical problems.[12]

Intergenerational programs are a relatively new form of literacy programming and many important political questions have emerged from the work to date. Of particular concern are questions regarding what form literacy support should take when working with families with varied cultural, social and political histories, and questions regarding the wide range of opinions by literacy workers regarding the purposes of literacy within families (Gadsden 1994). Intergenerational work appears to be full of potential; however, it must be done with caution and sensitivity given the political nature of the work.

Something Special for Seniors:
Medicine Hat College and One Voice

Seniors are much more likely to have reading problems; for people aged 55 to 69, only about one in three is a skilled reader (Statistics Canada 1990). This is partly attributable to limited education since they grew up in a time when financial support for education was limited. Many had their schooling interrupted by the Depression and the Second World War, and, before the 1950s, education was not nearly as important a prerequisite for finding employment. In addition, certain health problems that can interfere with reading ability are associated with aging—problems with sight, hearing, manual dexterity and mobility, as well as those associated with mental impairment after a stroke.

The health implications of limited reading abilities for seniors are predictable, including increased dependence and vulnerability, and a much higher risk of medication errors (Petch 1992).

Overview

Something Special for Seniors is an innovative and successful literacy program for seniors in Medicine Hat, Alberta.

---

12. See Isserlis et al. (1994) and McDonald et al. (1995) for further details.

Purpose

The purpose of the program is to help less literate older adults live more independently by improving their literacy and numeracy skills.

Key Players

Older adults are trained as volunteer tutors to work with other older adults. The program also has coordinators who oversee the program and are essential to its success. At the time of the evaluation (1993), the tutoring program had 43 participants and the reading program had 11.

Results

Something Special for Seniors has two parts. The one-to-one Tutoring Program is for people who want to work on improving their reading and/or numeracy skills. The Read-To/Read-With Program is for seniors who are essentially nonreaders and who enjoy being read to and then discussing the stories, articles, etc. with the volunteer reader. Some seniors go from this program into the tutoring program. The "curriculum" is entirely dependent on what the learners are interested in reading.

Replicability

Other literacy programs for seniors operate across the country, and there appears to be no reason why this model could not be duplicated elsewhere.

Funding

Original funding was for a three-year pilot project. Program and evaluation funds were provided by the National Literacy Secretariat and One Voice (the Canadian Seniors Network); Medicine Hat College was the sponsoring organization. Funding is now provided by a Community Adult Literacy Council grant through Medicine Hat College.

Evaluation

Something Special for Seniors appears to be a highly successful program from the points of view of both tutors and learners. According to several evaluations, there is no question that older adults can learn many things, including how to read. Participants reported that they learned literacy and numeracy skills that would help them cope better in their daily lives. They also reported outcomes beyond reading and writing, including personal growth and increased independence and self-esteem—skills that allow them to be more involved in their communities. They said they enjoyed learning, and that the program made them enjoy life more. The tutors also reported that the program had enhanced their own lives. The seniors who take part in the program are its strongest advocates. "The evaluation team cannot stress enough the success this program has been" (Lothian 1993, 135).

POLICY IMPLICATIONS

Policy recommendations to address the literacy problem in Canada involve three domains: health, education and social equity.

Health Care

As health care policy broadens its focus from medical to social issues, literacy has emerged as a key determinant of health.

Raising awareness – Health care workers at every level need a better understanding of the prevalence of literacy limitations and the impact of these limitations on health status. In its health promotion role, the federal government has an ideal opportunity to support efforts to this end.

Clear language health materials – Clear language materials as well as audio and video materials can play a useful role in making more health information more accessible to more people. Until the literacy levels in our society are widely improved, clear language materials on both health and social issues are needed. Efforts made by health care workers to this end deserve support.

Research – Considerable research is needed to further explore the relationship between low literacy skills and health, as well as to determine mechanisms to minimize the negative impacts. In particular, longitudinal studies are required documenting potential changes in health status following changes in literacy skills in both children and adults, as well as research into the efforts to alter health status by raising awareness of the issue and by using easy-to-read materials.

Education

Lifelong learning – Policies supporting a culture of lifelong learning are vital in a rapidly changing world. Education must be supported for both lower- and higher-skilled readers. Commitments must be made to providing better learning opportunities for children of poor families so they will grow up with stronger reading skills. Research may also illuminate ways to increase literacy outside of formal literacy programming.

Coordination – Literacy work in Canada is fragmented—locally, provincially and nationally. Additional support for the two national coalitions, and for provincial networks and computer conferencing networks would provide a more permanent infrastructure to support literacy work, and would lead to better communication between programs and more collaboration and cooperation.

Workplace literacy – Policy is needed regarding the role of business in literacy training. More research is required on how literacy skills are needed and used in workplaces.

Family/intergenerational literacy programs – Since literacy skills within the family of origin affect children's reading skills, literacy programs to address these issues deserve support and careful documentation to better understand the potential cultural conflicts involved.

Programming – Since income affects literacy levels, a wide range of literacy training options is required to respond to the needs and circumstances of learners, especially those from vulnerable groups such as the poor, inmates and the disabled.

Research – Support for much more research about literacy is required. Efforts to bring the results of literacy research to literacy workers would benefit both groups involved. Research is needed in several areas such as quality standards, use of volunteers and learner involvement in program management. The goals and interests of learners must be made central to these discussions. Program evaluation regarding learner-centred programs is urgently required. Research is also needed regarding the optimal use of communication technologies, preschool and school literacy, mother tongue literacy and learning disabilities.

Social Equity

With the growing understanding of literacy as a social determinant of health, coordinated societal change is needed to address the underlying factors that cause literacy problems. Social policies must view literacy as more than an educational issue, and "literacy policy should not be developed in isolation from other relevant policy areas" (NAPO 1992). Along with support for education, support for job creation and job training is essential.

CONCLUSION

Everyone deserves the right to learn to read, write and use numbers. Literacy problems are widespread in Canada, and the consequences of limited literacy and numeracy skills have an impact on personal, social and political power. Limited literacy and numeracy skills result in less access to information, less ability to be involved in one's community and a greater likelihood of health problems and poverty. Since workplaces now require more literate workers, lower literacy skills also lead to many fewer employment opportunities. Adequate funding and support for literacy work are vital.

However, literacy work on its own is a limited solution. Literacy levels are but one important indicator of the widespread inequality in our culture.

Literacy problems seldom occur in isolation from other social factors, and cannot be resolved independently from these factors. Therefore, as Fingeret (1984, 52) points out:

> Education will not create additional jobs, solve the problems of crime and malnutrition, or make the world safe from terrorism. Social structures and social forces beyond the reach of literacy educators are at work maintaining the structures of social inequality. Education can, however, provide tools and access to opportunities for working together with others to change those structures and, in the process, create rather than merely accept the future.

Mary J. Breen *is a writer with a special interest in literacy and its impact on health. She has written and edited numerous easy-to-read health materials including the book* Taking Care: A Handbook About Women's Health *(1991), and has given many workshops and presentations on the need for easy-to-read health materials. From 1991 to 1993 she was the coordinator of the Literacy and Health Project for the Ontario Public Health Association. She lives and works in Peterborough, Ontario.*

BIBLIOGRAPHY

ABC CANADA. 1991. *Workplace Literacy: An Introductory Guide for Employers.* Toronto: ABC Canada.

ALBERT, J. L. and D. D'AMICO-SAMUELS. 1991. *Adult Learners' Perceptions of Literacy Programs and the Impact of Participation on their Lives.* New York: Literacy Assistance Center, Inc.

ALDEN, H. 1982. *Illiteracy and Poverty in Canada: Toward a Critical Perspective.* Unpublished, M.A. thesis, University of Toronto.

ANDERSON, D. 1995. *Native Literacy in Ontario: Areas for Development.* Toronto: Ontario Training and Adjustment Board.

BELFIORE, M. E. 1995. *A Summary of Principles of Good Practice in Workplace Education Development.* Toronto: ABC Canada.

BOUCHER, A. 1993. *Spelling It Out and In French: Illiteracy and Literacy Training among Francophones in Canada.* Montréal: Institut canadien d'éducation des adultes.

BOYD, M. 1991. Gender, nativity and literacy: Proficiency and training issues. In *Adult Literacy in Canada: Results of a National Study.* Ottawa: Statistics Canada. pp. 86–94.

BREEN, M. J., and J. W. CATANO. 1987. Can she read it? Readability and literacy in health education. Parts 1 and 2. *Healthsharing Magazine* 8, no. 3: 28–33; 8, no. 4: 13.

BREEN, M. J. 1993. *Partners in Practice: The Literacy and Health Project Phase Two Summary Report.* Toronto: Ontario Public Health Association.

————. 1994. Literacy and privilege: Reading the writings of the women's health movement. *Canadian Woman Studies* 14: 3.

BURNABY, B. 1992. Adult literacy issues in Canada. *Annual Review of Applied Linguistics* 12: 156–171.

CALAMAI, P. 1987. *Broken Words: Why Five Million Canadians are Illiterate: The Southam Literacy Report.* Toronto: Southam News.

CANADA, DEPARTMENT OF THE SECRETARY OF STATE. 1988. *Discussion Paper on Literacy.* Ottawa.

CANADIAN ASSOCIATION OF OPTOMETRISTS. 1995. *Optometrists Launch New Sharing the Vision Program.* Ottawa.

CANADIAN CONGRESS FOR LEARNING OPPORTUNITIES FOR WOMEN (CCLOW). 1996. *Isolating the Barriers and Strategies for Prevention.* Toronto.

CANADIAN COUNCIL ON SOCIAL DEVELOPMENT. 1996. *New Study Documents Impact of Child Poverty.* Ottawa.

DARVILLE, R. 1992. *Adult Literacy Work in Canada.* Toronto: Canadian Association for Adult Education.

DAVIES, R. 1995. *Men for Change.* Halifax: Private correspondence.

DAVIS, T. et al. 1993. Rapid estimate of adult literacy in medicine: A shortened screening instrument. *Family Medicine* 25(6): 391–395.

DESORMEAUX, M. 1994. *Where Are You Now?* Sudbury: Sudbury Literacy Network.

DOAK, C., L. G. DOAK, and J. ROOT. 1995. *Teaching Patients with Low Literacy Skills.* Philadelphia: J. B. Lippincott.

EATON, M., and R. HOLLOWAY. 1980. Patient comprehension of written drug information. *American Journal of Hospital Pharmacy* 372: 240–243.

EDWARDS, C. 1995. Due diligence: The challenge of language and literacy. *Accident Prevention* 42, no. 6 (Nov./Dec.): 18–21.

EVANS, R. G., and G. L. STODDART. 1994. Producing health, consuming health care. In *Why Are Some People Healthy and Others Not?: The Determinants of Health of Populations,* eds. R. G. EVANS, M. K. BARER, and T. R. MARMOR. New York: Aldine de Gruyter. pp. 27–64.

FARMER, K. 1995. *Literacy and Homelessness: Delivering Literacy in an Adult Drop-In.* Toronto: St. Christopher House.

FELLEGI, I. 1995. *Literacy, Economy and Society: Results of the First International Adult Literacy Survey.* Ottawa: Statistics Canada.

FINGERET, A. 1984. *Adult Literacy Education: Current and Future Directions.* Columbus (OH): ERIC Clearinghouse.

FRONTIER COLLEGE. 1989. *Learning in the Workplace.* Toronto.

_____. 1992. *Beat the Street.* Toronto.

FYLES, N. 1995. *alsoWorks: A Worker-Managed Business, Ten Years of Learning.* Ottawa: a.l.s.o.— Alternative Learning Styles and Outlooks.

G. ALLEN ROEHER INSTITUTE. 1990. *Literacy and Labels: A Look at Literacy Policy and People with a Mental Handicap.* Downsview (ON).

_____. 1991. *The Right to Read and Write: A Straightforward Guide to Literacy and People with a Mental Handicap in Canada.* Downsview (ON).

GABER-KATZ, E., and G. M. WATSON. 1991. *The Land that We Dream of...: A Participatory Study of Community-Based Literacy.* Toronto: OISE Press.

GADSDEN, V. L. 1994. *Understanding Family Literacy: Conceputal Issues Facing the Field.* Philadelphia: University of Pennsylvania, NCAL Technical Report TR94–02.

GEORGE BROWN COLLEGE. 1994. *Some Innovative Applications of Computer Telecommunications on AlphaCom.* Toronto: George Brown College, Concepts and Learning Centre.

HARDING, M. 1987. *The Relationship Between Economic Status and Health Status and Opportunities: A Synthesis.* Toronto: The Ontario Social Assistance Review Committee.

HIRSCH, D. 1991. Literacy and international competitiveness: The relevance of Canada's survey. *Adult Literacy in Canada: Results of a National Study.* Ottawa: Statistics Canada.

HORSMAN, J. 1990. *Something in My Mind besides the Everyday.* Toronto: Women's Press.

INDUSTRIAL ACCIDENT PREVENTION ASSOCIATION. 1989. *Workplace Literacy and Health and Safety.* Toronto.

INTERNATIONAL COUNCIL FOR ADULT EDUCATION. 1995. *Women, Literacy and Development: Challenges for the 21st Century.* Proceedings of the Fifth World Assembly. Toronto: ICAE. p. 3.

ISSERLIS, J. et al. 1994. *Community Literacy: An Intergenerational Perspective.* Vancouver: Invergarry Learning Centre.

JACKSON, R. H. et al. 1991. Patient reading ability: An overlooked problem in health care. *Southern Medical Journal* 84(10): 1172–1175.

JONES, S. 1991. Literacy programming and the survey of literacy skills used in daily activities. In *Adult Literacy in Canada: Results of a National Study.* Ottawa: Statistics Canada. pp. 95–101.

_____. 1993. *Reading, But Not Reading Well—Reading Skills at Level 3.* Ottawa: National Literacy Secretariat.

JURMO, P. 1996. *Comments on the January 29, 1996 Preliminary Draft Report of the Task Force on Education and Workforce Quality.* East Brunswick (NJ): Learning Partnerships.

LAPIERRE, G., and L. MALLET. 1987. Readability of materials. *CPJ/RPC* (Dec.): 718–728.

LEVINE, K. 1986. *The Social Context of Literacy.* London: Routledge and Kegan Paul.

LEWIN, T. 1996. Behind prison walls: Poor reading skills also pose a barrier. *New York Times,* Mar. 17.

LITERARY COORDINATORS OF ALBERTA. 1996. *Overview of STAPLE.* Calgary: Alberta Vocational College.

LLOYD, B. A. et al. 1994. *The Power of Woman-Positive Literacy Work.* Toronto: Canadian Congress for Learning Opportunities for Women (CCLOW).

LOTHIAN, T. 1993. *Evaluation of Something Special for Seniors.* Ottawa: Centre for the Study of Adult Literacy, Carleton University; Report 4.

MARMOT, M. G. 1994. Social differentials in health. *Daedalus* 123, no. 4 (fall): 197–216.

McDONALD, A., J. ISSERLIS, C. L. WEINSTEIN. 1995. *Intergenerational Literacy: Two Disciplines, One Goal.* Vancouver: Kwantlen University College & Community Language Access Society.

MEAGHAN, D., and F. CASAS. 1994. The myth of illiteracy: How not to debate educational reforms. *The College Quarterly* 2 (winter 1994–1995): 2.

MICHIELUTTE, R. et al. 1992. The use of illustrations and narrative text style to improve readability of a health education brochure. *J. Cancer Education* 7(3): 251–260.

MOVEMENT FOR CANADIAN LITERACY. 1994. *Brief to the Standing Committee on Human Resources Development.* Ottawa.

NATIONAL ANTI-POVERTY ORGANIZATION (NAPO). 1992. *Literacy and Poverty: A View from the Inside.* Ottawa.

NATIONAL ASSOCIATIONS ACTIVE IN CRIMINAL JUSTICE. 1995. *Between the Lines/Entre les lignes.* Ottawa: Literacy and Crime Prevention Project.

NATIONAL INSTITUTE FOR LITERACY. 1995. Adult learners talk about goal 6. *NIFL Newsletter* 3:2 (May-June): 3.

NATIONAL LITERACY SECRETARIAT. 1995. *Policy Conversation on New Technologies and Literacy: A Report.* Ottawa.

NEWMAN, A., W. LEWIS, and C. BEVERSTOCK. 1993. *Prison Literacy: Implications for Program and Assessment Policy.* Philadelphia: National Center on Adult Literacy.

NORTON, M. 1992. Linking literacy and health: A popular education approach. In *Voices from the Literacy Field,* eds. J. A. DRAPER and M. C. TAYLOR. Toronto: Culture Concepts. pp. 319–332.

ODELL, T. 1992. *Sentenced to Learn: Issues in Offender Education in Ontario.* Unpublished.

O'LEARY, J. D. 1991. *Creating a Love of Reading.* Ottawa: National Literacy Secretariat.

ONTARIO ASSOCIATION FOR CHILDREN AND ADULTS WITH LEARNING DISABILITIES. 1986. *Critical Issues Register,* ed. E. INGLIS. Toronto.

ONTARIO FEDERATION OF LABOUR. 1995. *What is BEST?* Toronto.

ONTARIO MINISTRY OF SKILLS DEVELOPMENT. 1988. *Literacy: The Basics of Growth.* Toronto.

ONTARIO PUBLIC HEALTH ASSOCIATION AND FRONTIER COLLEGE. 1989. *The Literacy and Health Project: Making the World Healthier and Safer for People Who Can't Read; Phase One.* Toronto: Ontario Public Health Association.

ONTARIO TRAINING AND ADJUSTMENT BOARD. 1994. *Framework and Quality Standards for Adult Literacy Education in Ontario.* Toronto.

PATH: PROGRAM FOR APPROPRIATE TECHNOLOGY IN HEALTH. 1989. *Developing Health and Family Planning Print Materials for Low-Literate Audiences: A Guide.* Washington (DC).

PAUL, C. 1991. *The Easier to Read: Easier to be Healthy Report.* Toronto: Lawrence Heights Community Health Centre.

PERRIN, B. 1989. *The Literacy and Health Project: Making the World Healthier and Safer for People Who Can't Read; Phase One Research Report.* Toronto: Ontario Public Health Association.

PETCH, E. 1992. *Wise Use of Medications: A Health Promotion Approach to Community Programming for Safe Medication Use with and for Seniors.* Toronto: South Riverdale Community Health Centre.

PLANNED PARENTHOOD PETERBOROUGH. 1990. *The Facts of Life Line.* Peterborough, Ont.

POWERS, R. D. 1988. Emergency department patient literacy and the readability of patient-directed materials. *Annals of Emergency Medicine* 17: 2, Feb.

PRITCHARD, R. R., and H. YEE. 1989. Johnny came back to school but still can't read. *Education Canada* 29: 1.

PUCHNER, L. D. 1993. *Early Childhood, Family, and Health Issues in Literacy: International Perspectives.* Philadelphia (PA): NCAL, International Paper IP93–2.

RADWANSKI, G. 1987. *Ontario Study of the Relevance of Education and the Issue of Dropouts.* Toronto: Ministry of Education.

RACHLIS, M., and C. KUSHNER. 1989. *Second Opinion: What's Wrong with Canada's Health Care System and How To Fix It.* Toronto: Collins.

STATISTICS CANADA. 1990. *Survey of Literacy Skills Used in Daily Activities.* Ottawa.

_____. 1992. *Reading Skills of Adults in Canada.* Ottawa.

_____. 1995. *Highlight Summary.* Ottawa.

STICHT, T. G. 1992. How fast do adults acquire literacy skills? *Mosaic* 2 (July): 2.

THE LEARNING CENTRE. 1996. *Information Sheet.* Ottawa.

THOMAS, A. M. 1990. *The Reluctant Learner: A Research Report on Nonparticipation and Dropout in Literacy Programs in British Columbia.* Victoria (BC): Ministry of Advanced Education, Training and Technology, and Ottawa: National Literacy Secretariat.

TURK, J., and J. UNDA. 1991. So we can make our voices heard: The Ontario Federation of Labour's BEST Project on Worker Literacy. In *Basic Skills for the Workplace*, eds. M. C. TAYLOR, G. R. LEWE, and J. A. DRAPER. Toronto: Culture Concepts. pp. 267–280.

TURNER, J. 1994. Beating the mean streets. *The Toronto Star*, Oct. 6, col. 1.

TURNER, T. 1993. *Literacy and Machines: An Overview of the Use of Technology in Adult Literacy Programs.* Philadelphia: NCAL Technical Report TR93–03.

UNDA, J.C. 1995. *Pilot Evaluation Project Report.* Toronto: Ontario Federation of Labour.

VENEZKY, R. L., P. S. BRISTOW, and J. P. SABATINI. 1994. *Measuring Gain in Adult Literacy Programs.* Philadelphia: NCAL Technical Report TR93–12.

WAGNER, D.A. 1993. *Myths and Misconceptions in Adult Literacy: A Research and Development Perspective.* Philadelphia: NCAL Policy Brief 93–1.

WEISS, B. D. et al. 1992. Health status of illiterate adults: Relation between literacy and health status among persons with low literacy skills. *Journal of the American Board of Family Practitioners* 5: 257–264.

WILLIAMS, M. V. et al. 1995. Inadequate functional health literacy among patients at two public hospitals. *Journal of the American Medical Association* 274(21): 1677–1682.

WINKLEBY, M. et al. 1992. Socioeconomic status and health: How education, income, and occupation contribute to risk factors for cardiovascular disease. *American Journal of Public Health* 82(6): 816–820.

WOODS, G. 1987. *The Cost of Illiteracy to Canadian Business.* Toronto: Canadian Business Task Force on Literacy.

YWCA OF MONTREAL. 1996. *Paroles de femmes/Words for Women: The YWCA of Montreal's Woman-Centred Literacy Centre.* Montreal.

Seniors

Maintaining and Enhancing Independence and Well-Being in Old Age

NEENA L. CHAPPELL, PH.D.

Director, Centre On Aging
Professor, Department of Sociology
University of Victoria

SUMMARY

This background paper discusses strategies for enhancing and maintaining independence and autonomy during old age. Severe mental declines resulting in cognitive impairment and dementia are not characteristic of the vast majority of seniors. Our physical health, however, does decline slowly and gradually throughout our lives and this decline becomes particularly evident during old age. Furthermore, chronic conditions—not acute infectious conditions—are characteristic of old age; chronic conditions are not dealt with well within our "medicalized" health care system. The nonmedical determinants of health are therefore particularly relevant when discussing old age.

This paper begins with a discussion of a broad definition of health that encompasses but goes well beyond a medical definition in terms of the absence of disease. It goes on to review the current situation of seniors and their preferences with regard to care. The nonmedical determinants of health are then discussed, including lifestyles and individual behaviours that can affect health. Selected health issues and behaviours—social ties, physical activity, nutrition, self-esteem, and a variety of negative personal health behaviours such as smoking or excessive intake of alcohol—are reviewed for their direct effects on health. This paper notes that seniors are knowledgeable about and adhere to a variety of well-established or traditional views on health promotion, such as refraining from smoking, from drinking alcohol and from skipping breakfast. However, the adoption of more recent perspectives on health promotion, such as having mammograms and minimizing the use of prescription medications, is more evident in younger populations. This suggests that seniors should be a target group for the dissemination of information in these new areas of health promotion.

The indirect and direct effects of social structures on health are then discussed. The influence of social structures on personal choice is perhaps most evident when looking at people who are born into poverty. Social structures, however, also have an independent effect on health, over and above their indirect effects through personal choices: two examples of this effect are unemployment and socioeconomic status. The social gradient, which demonstrates that people's relative position within society is related to health, is interpreted in terms of status within the particular culture or subculture, and need not necessarily refer to economic status. Education is key to enabling individuals to contribute—and to feel they are contributing—to society. Consequently, this paper highlights education as a potential key to self-empowerment and ultimately to good individual health.

Community development is also reviewed as a promising strategy. Five examples of success stories of seniors living in communities are presented, including Discover Choices *in Manitoba and Saskatchewan, the* Support Services to Seniors Program *in Manitoba,* Tenderloin Seniors Organizing Project *from the United States,* On Lok *from the United States, and an* Arthritis Self-Management Program *in British Columbia. Each success story involves aspects of community development, and each works through grassroots empowerment. They demonstrate that a community development health promotion approach can work with seniors and can also be cost effective.*

The section on policy implications elaborates the idea that there will not be cost savings in formal health care expenditures unless medical services to seniors do not continue to escalate in the present medical care system. Even if individuals make healthier choices concerning their lifestyle, and even if societal structures change in a way that improves people's well-being and health, there will be no formal savings until medical costs for services to seniors stop increasing.

The rhetoric of health reform with its emphasis on less expensive and more appropriate health care focused on wellness and healthy lifestyles rather than high-tech medicine, provides a vision which can incorporate the types of citizen empowerment and community development seen in the success stories. However, the rhetoric is not leading to action, and there is reason to believe that the health care system that the rhetoric promises will never become a reality. The success stories underscore the urgency for implementing a reformed health care system; a shift towards a more appropriate health care system would provide the support and means for empowering citizens.

Education emerges as a key tool for grassroots empowerment, as individuals must have the capacity to seek and acquire information, and they must possess the analytic skills to ferret through that information in order to make informed choices. Governments, however, have a role ensuring that there is equal opportunity, standard setting, and monitoring. The promise of health promotion in community development lies in its mediating role between people and their environment, allowing people to synthesize personal choice and social responsibility in health. The conclusion offers several specific suggestions for future action.

TABLE OF CONTENTS

FIGURE

INTRODUCTION

This background paper begins with a brief discussion of a broad definition of health which acknowledges the salience of nonmedical factors influencing health, and the situation of seniors. A more detailed discussion follows on two primary nonmedical determinants of health—individual lifestyles and social structural factors. A health promotion/lifestyle/community development approach is then elaborated as a comprehensive strategy which has the ability to encompass the broad spectrum of nonmedical determinants of health at both the individual and collective levels. The success stories provide examples of specific facets as well as comprehensive community development strategies that have worked with seniors, and, in particular, with those seniors who are frail and disadvantaged. The last part of this paper discusses the social policy implications of the earlier discussions, noting that curtailing the medical and institutional focus within the current formal health care system will not work without simultaneously strengthening the formal community social system and guaranteeing the empowerment of citizens.

HEALTH AND WELLNESS

Health encompasses more than the absence of illness. The definition of health proposed by the World Health Organization (WHO) more than 40 years ago is now widely accepted: "Health is a state of complete physical, mental, and social well-being, and not merely the absence of disease or injury" (Kickbusch 1984). In this definition health is viewed as a resource for living that includes the ability to realize one's aspirations and satisfy needs to cope with the environment. Health, in other words, is not strictly medical; it includes social, psychological, emotional and environmental aspects (some would also include spiritual aspects). This conceptualization of health directs attention not only to individuals who are at risk of particular diseases or medical conditions, but also to the majority of people in the everyday lives of these individuals. The appeal of this conceptualization of health lies in its broad vision which encompasses all people, and reduces their chances of disease and disability. In short, the WHO definition directs attention to lifestyles, environment, human biology and health care organizations (Lalonde 1974).

The definition, however, has been criticized for being too broad. Because the WHO definition appears to embrace all of human activity, critics such as Evans and Stoddart (1990) have relabelled the concept as "well-being", and issued their own definition of health from the individual's perspective as the absence of illness, injury, distressing symptoms and impaired capacity. Disease is a medical construct different from illness; generally speaking, just as disease affects illness adversely, so does illness have adverse effects on well-being.

Medicine and the health care system are only two of the many factors that can affect health. But individual lifestyle factors and social environmental factors—two nonmedical factors—are equally, if not more, important. Both can be affected through social policy.

In the late '70s and '80s when attention was focused on this broader definition of health, an interest on specific individual risk factors and specific diseases evolved. This individualistic interpretation led to interventions which focused on personal lifestyles, such as providing individual counselling on activities such as smoking cessation, seat belt use and dietary modification; such counselling became part of the clinician's work with individual patients. This response meant that the health care system extended its outreach and screening programs through counselling and increasing the number of individuals put on drug therapy and regular monitoring. The emphasis on individual risk factors and particular diseases extended the current way of thinking about health. However, the nonmedical determinants of health became medicalized. The focus was on the individual, preferably in consultation with their physicians, but did nothing to question the broader structural arrangements within society which lead to various individual choices. The lifestyles approach to health care placed a greater onus on the individual, and became known as the "blaming the victim" perspective (Evans and Stoddart 1990). It did little to alter the health care system or the health of the population.

This paper discusses lifestyle variables and their importance for health and wellness in old age, while arguing that these variables are subject to individual 'choice' which is in turn influenced by cultural and social structural factors.

SENIORS

This paper is focused on ways to promote health and wellness for seniors. There is compelling evidence (Berger 1983) that the environments and lifestyles of individuals very early in life—indeed going back to the fetal stage—may affect health during old age. While this evidence is interesting and should be researched, it will not be addressed in this paper.

Illnesses in old age tend to be chronic rather than acute. The formal health care system stresses short-term, medical, acute care in hospitals. However, the medical profession and the existing system of acute care hospitals have not been particularly successful in helping people cope with the chronic conditions of old age (Chappell et al. 1986). The major advances that have been made in the medical profession are related to the treatment of diseases, but they are not primarily responsible for the increased longevity that most Canadians are experiencing. The most common chronic illnesses among Canadian seniors are arthritis and rheumatism, hypertension, heart trouble, and respiratory problems (Chappell et al. 1986). The greatest need among seniors is for services to help them cope with chronic conditions and functional disabilities. Long-term care is often more appropriate than short-term acute care. With aging, there is a progressive decline of body functions that calls for care and support, but does not necessarily require medical attention. It has long been said in gerontology—the study of aging—that care is more important than cure.

Furthermore, elderly people prefer to stay in their own homes rather than in institutions (Chappell 1993a), a notion referred to as aging in place. Seniors want their homes to be adaptable to their changing needs, and they prefer housing and services as an integrated package. A wealth of geron-tological research over the last two decades (Kane and Kane 1985; Antonucci 1990; Chappell and Blandford 1991) has demonstrated that the vast majority of care provided to elders—at least three-quarters of it—comes from their informal networks, such as family and friends. Informal caregiving predominates over paid care, irrespective of whether a country provides comprehensive health care (Kane 1990). Family and friends are the first resort for seniors.

Moreover, while health does decline with aging, this is more the case with physical rather than mental health. Physical health, such as eyesight, begins to decline in early adult years and continues throughout the aging process. For most individuals, this is a gradual process that is adapted on a day-to-day basis, and changes are not particularly noticed when the age of 60 or 65 is reached. Most individuals adjust well and continue to function. Figures show that over 80 percent of Canadian seniors suffer from some chronic conditions, but that fewer (50 percent) suffer from functional disability. Figures for severe functional disabilities drop even further from approximately 50 percent to 17 percent (Chappell et al. 1986). In other words, most individuals continue to function and cope. The picture is even brighter when looking at mental health. While there are associated changes with certain aspects of memory and thinking, major declines in mental functioning, as in cognitive impairment and dementia, strike only a small proportion of individuals aged 65 and over (approximately 8 percent, according to the Canadian Health and Aging Survey, 1994, a national study to establish the prevalence of dementia in Canada).

There are both gender and ethnocultural differences in health and in the use of health services (Markides 1990; Verbrugge 1988). Women suffer more from symptomatology and use services more. Men suffer more from fatal illnesses and use services less. Similarly, differences are evident between ethnic and subcultural groups. Blacks are more likely to die earlier than Whites, but those who survive to old age tend to outlive Caucasians; Alzheimer's disease is very rare among Canadian Aboriginal peoples (Driedger and Chappell 1987). There has been much debate and research to ascertain the extent to which these differences are biological or due to differences in lifestyles, stress, etc. To date, the answer remains elusive. For both physical and mental health, the adage 'use it or lose it' seems to generally apply. Furthermore, as will be argued later in this paper, not all declines are necessarily inevitable. Contrary to the belief of many, health in old age can be maintained and, in many instances, enhanced (Spirduso 1995).

NONMEDICAL DETERMINANTS OF HEALTH

Lifestyles

Individual behaviours—even those defying medical categorization—can affect health. This section discusses several nonmedical factors and their importance to health, particularly in later life. The significance of larger structural factors affecting individual choice and consequently health are also discussed.

The term *personal health practices* denotes activities in which people engage, either consciously or unconsciously, that have implications for their health. These practices can include both potentially positive health practices (such as exercise and good nutrition) and potentially negative practices (such as cigarette and alcohol consumption), environmental protection and home safety practices (such as having a smoke detector), and health care practices (such as blood pressure checks and self-examination) (Penning and Chappell 1993).

There is both theoretical and empirical support for the notion that *social ties* positively influence health in old age. There is also evidence that social support protects individuals from the negative effects of highly stressful situations such as those encountered in serious illness, and these ties also promote the health of individuals when they are not undergoing stress (Berkman 1984). Strong social ties have been related to lower mortality, as well as enhanced physical and psychological well-being (House et al. 1988). Lubben and associates (1989) have shown that the relationship between social networks and hospitalization is as strong as the relationship between smoking and mortality that led to the Surgeon General's warning on cigarette packages many years ago.

Much research has been conducted on the effect of social support in old age. A review of this literature shows that there is a great diversity of:
- measures used for the various dimensions of the concept of social support;
- types of seniors sampled; and
- measures of health, including a number tracking psychological and physical health.

This research has been summarized and analysed in Chappell (1992) and will not be repeated here. Suffice it to say that social support is a necessary part of most seniors' lives. Social interaction provides support that contributes to enhancing health. The positive effects of this type of interaction are more apparent for women than men (Antonucci 1990), and vary from one subculture to another (Driedger and Chappell 1987).

Physical activity is important in maintaining good health in old age, but this concept is a relatively new one that few seniors recognize. Individuals who are seniors today grew up viewing old age as a time of passivity and rest—a reward for a life of hard labour (the rocking chair image). Only recently have both the physical and psychological health benefits of continued physical activity throughout old age begun to be documented. In a recent publication, Spiraduso (1995) brings together much of this research, demonstrating that it is never too late to make physical activity a regular part of life. Even for seniors with serious health problems, physical activity (tailored to take into account their ailments and to ensure appropriateness) can enhance health. Indeed, there are inspiring examples of very old seniors with many debilitating health conditions who have experienced miraculous effects from engaging in physical activity.

Canada's latest National Health Promotion Survey (Stephens and Graham 1993) shows that a greater proportion of Canadian adults aged 50 and over engage in frequent vigorous exercise than Canadians in younger age groups. However, the proportion of Canadians that never exercise is also greater among older adults. Among both old people (aged 70 and over) and young people (aged 15 to 29), more men than women report that they engage in frequent exercise. Women are more likely to report that they never exercise. Within middle-aged groups, the tendency is for women to be more active than men. The adage 'use it or lose it' applies in old age as well as in youth. Figure 1 illustrates the benefits of physical activity through-out life.

Much has been said and written about *nutrition*, and does not have to be repeated. However, the Canadian Health Promotion Survey (Stephens and Graham 1993) reveals that the proportion reporting not having had breakfast does decrease with age (from about 40 percent at ages 15 to 29 to 9 percent for ages 70 and over) for both men and women. It is also important to note that, among seniors, eating is frequently related to a social activity. Those living alone, particularly the recently bereaved, will frequently not take the time to prepare nutritious meals for themselves (the tea-and-toast syndrome among seniors). Physical health problems also interfere when it becomes difficult to peel, chop and cook certain types of foods. For these reasons, meal programs (both individual and group) have been established in many communities. People who are seniors today grew up before the era of fast foods, the widespread use of chemicals as preservatives, etc. They were raised in the tradition of three square meals a day, which emphasized the importance of fresh fruit and vegetables. Today's seniors have also lived with a greater gender division of labour, especially around food preparation. Many elderly men today are not adept at meal preparation. If they become widowed (which is usually not the case as men tend to die before their

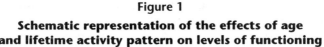

Figure 1

Schematic representation of the effects of age and lifetime activity pattern on levels of functioning

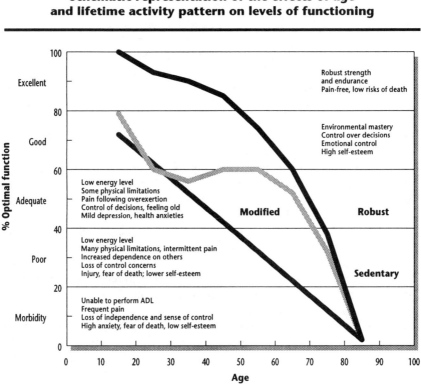

Source: Adapted from Fries (1988).

wives), they are particularly at risk of social isolation, depression and malnutrition, among other things. However, there is evidence that most widowed men remarry quickly (Bengtson et al. 1990). Nutrition could well become a greater concern as today's younger generations grow old.

An individual concept which needs to be highlighted at this point (a more in-depth discussion follows later) is *self-esteem*, which is tied to a sense of mastery, control and autonomy. There is substantial evidence that a sense of control is related to various health behaviours. For example, the health locus of control literature (Wallston et al. 1978; Lau 1982) demonstrates a relationship between locus of control and knowledge of disease, ability to stop smoking, ability to lose weight, compliance with medical regimens, effective use of birth control, having preventive inoculations, wearing seat belts, and having regular checkups. A sense of control can affect behaviours and attitudes that are self-maintaining. It is related to:

- Practicing preventive health measures, such as dieting, exercise and alcohol moderation;

- Making an effort to avoid harm from smoking by quitting, trying to quit or simply not smoking;
- Being more sanguine about early medical treatment for cancer;
- Achieving higher self-ratings of general health status;
- Reporting fewer episodes of chronic and acute illness; and
- Taking on a more vigorous management style with respect to illness, such as staying in bed less, and ensuring less dependence on physicians.

Self-esteem is considered particularly important for positive adjustment in old age and has been correlated with both objective and subjective measures of well-being including health. Those who have more self-esteem are more likely to engage in positive health behaviours and to resist pressures to engage in unhealthy behaviours (Tones 1986).

In terms of potentially *negative personal health behaviours*, the proportion of former smokers increases with age among men, but the proportion of current smokers decreases with age. Seniors are also less likely than younger adults to drink alcohol, and women are less likely to drink alcohol than men. Older adults use more medication than younger adults. Unhealthy behaviours such as smoking and drinking are the traditional risk factors which medical experts are now considering. Knowledge is key for choosing healthy behaviours at any age. How knowledge is acquired through education (including self-education) will be elaborated later.

When examining the lifestyle choices of seniors, it is important to recognize the differences in cohorts. Those who are elderly today are different from those who will be elderly tomorrow. This is reflected in health promotion survey findings (Penning and Chappell 1993); older adults are less likely than younger adults to report having made changes specifically to improve their health, such as changes in exercise or in diet, and they are also less likely to report planning to make a change in the upcoming year in order to improve their health. Older adults are also less knowledgeable about health matters such as the causes of heart disease, appropriate ways to lose weight, or methods for preventing the transmission of STDs. They are less likely to recognize the need for changes in personal lifestyles, environmental practices and government action on health issues. Older adults, that is, are less likely to reflect the "new" thinking on individual responsibility for health, and the "new" concerns such as environmental pollution.

However, the behaviours which reflect an adherence to well-established or traditional views of health promotion are more likely to be found among older adults. These behaviours include, among others: abstaining from smoking and drinking alcohol; ensuring that breakfast is not skipped; getting regular exercise; and having blood pressure checkups regularly. In contrast, younger individuals are more likely to practise home and environmental safety, to have mammograms and to avoid prescription drugs such as sleeping pills and tranquillizers. These behaviours are more consistent with recent views of health promotion. The differences, to a certain extent, also reflect age or life course differences. Older people are more likely to have worse health in terms of increasing chronic illness and increasing activity limitations. They may therefore be increasingly aware of the importance of health issues and the importance of positive personal health behaviours.

Dean (1991), an international scholar in self-care practices among elders, has argued that active health promotion and protection have not become a conscious part of daily life for most seniors. However, the most recent Canadian data in this area suggest that this is true only in terms of the more recent perspectives on health promotion that have received widespread acceptance over the last few years. In more traditional areas, elders appear active, engaging in a variety of activities to protect and improve their health. Research suggests seniors require information on the latest evidence in health promotion. As one of the success stories below demonstrates, seniors are receptive to such information. Before discussing success stories, it is necessary to address the issues around social structures. The following discussion argues that individuals do not have as much choice over their behaviour as they may think.

The Social Structure

The importance of the social structure lies in its double impact. It has independent effects on health, and it affects the personal choices that individuals make about their health. This section first addresses how the environment influences individual choice, and then how social structure is also an important direct contributor to health.

Social environment affects individual choices in a host of ways. Perhaps it is best illustrated by taking poverty as an example. Poor people frequently choose to eat food that is less healthy. Closer examination reveals that they have fewer choices. Fast foods, cigarettes and alcohol are all relatively accessible in an affluent society such as Canada's, but for the poor to choose what is accessible means having to forego other things. As stated in a document produced by the government of Ontario, *Nurturing Health* (1991), it is not money per se, but the conditions, opportunities and amenities that money makes available that are important to health. Income, by and large, determines the city neighbourhoods in which individuals live, the friends they make, the teachers their children have, etc. The cultural environment of the neighbourhood, and therefore the types of pressures that are put on individuals by their peers, are all highly correlated with economic status. Whether children choose to go on to university is heavily influenced by the neighbourhoods in which they grow up, the expectations of their parents, and peer pressure (Marmot et al. 1987). The point is simple: social structures have a major influence on individual choices, and they have long-term effects on individuals when they are older. The effects of social structures can be seen in today's seniors.

To be old and poor means fewer choices are available in terms of being able to afford fresh fruits and vegetables in the winter, a car for transportation (or taxis when mobility problems prohibit the use of buses), the necessary assistive devices not covered by health plans, or a trip out of town. Poverty is one of the greatest correlates of ill health for both men and women of all ages (Antonovsky 1967).

Despite considerable gain in average income status for Canadian seniors over the last two decades, many remain poor in the '90s (19 percent are below Statistics Canada's Low Income Cutoff). The situation is especially serious for women who live alone (45 percent fall below the low income cutoff) (Moore and Rosenberg 1995). There are also notable differences depending on an individual's ethnicity—for example, there is devastating poverty, as well as high morbidity and mortality rates among Canada's Aboriginal peoples (D'Arcy 1989; Strain and Chappell 1989).

Another example of the way in which social environment influences individual choice is the tendency of the current cohort of seniors to regard eating as a social activity. The choice not to eat, or not to eat healthy foods, when alone stems from a lifetime of experiences which taught today's seniors that eating is a social activity. Another example: a woman who has been battered and abused by her husband for 60 years is unlikely to have the confidence and self-esteem to choose to join the seniors' walk or seniors' lawn bowling in order to ensure that she has adequate social support and exercise. A woman whose husband refuses to give her enough grocery money to buy a good supply of fresh vegetables does not have the choice of healthy eating (Pittaway and Gallagher 1995). The point to stress through these examples is that personal health behaviours should not be used to blame individuals when they do not make the "right" health choices.

Social structure, however, also has an independent effect on health, over and above its indirect effect through personal choices. Unemployment is related to the structure of the economy in society, and is largely beyond the control of the individual (if individuals had control, most would prefer to be employed). Unemployment is related to higher mortality rates, higher levels of both poor mental health (including, for example, psychological distress, anxiety and depressive symptoms), and worse physical health (including more disability days, activity limitation, other health problems, hospitalizations, visits and telephone calls to physicians) (D'Arcy 1986). These health effects are evident not only among the unemployed and those in unstable economic positions, but also among their families and the community in general (Wescott et al. 1985).

During the '90s there has been much interest in the effects of socioeconomic status or structural position within the society on health. As noted above, the relationship between income and health has long been established in research circles. Prosperity is related to health in terms of the changes that it brings, such as being able to afford proper nutrition and living in healthy environments. For a long time, this strong and consistent relationship between poverty and ill health was interpreted to mean that there are basic necessities in life that everyone needs in order to live a healthy life. In other words, the situation of those who lack sufficient monetary resources in order to acquire a basic standard of living should be of primary concern.

However, more recent research has documented the effects of what is known as a social class gradient. That means, simply, that people with less socioeconomic resources have poorer health than those who have more resources. Those on the second highest rung of society are in better health than those on the third highest rung, but less than those on the highest rung. This has made a profound difference in interpreting the importance of economics because it means that it is not simply those with the bare necessities who need help. As Wilkinson (1994) has noted, mortality rates in the industrialized world are no longer related to per capita economic growth. Rather, they are related to the scale of income inequality in each society. The longest life expectancies are found, not in the wealthiest countries, but in those with the least gaps between incomes and the smallest proportion of the population in *relative* poverty. Standard reference is now made to the differences in health between Britain and Japan, or some other industrialized country and Japan, and their differential income distributions. For example, the income distribution in Japan has narrowed significantly since 1970 and, over the same period, life expectancy has increased by 6.9 years—now the highest in the world. In Britain, on the other hand, the income distribution has widened in this same time period, and British people have gained only 3.9 years in life expectancy, falling from tenth among all OECD countries to seventeenth in the two-decade period (Wilkinson 1994).

The importance of the findings regarding the social gradient is that they indicate that people's relative position within society is related to their health. But it is probably not income per se that is the primary factor affecting health; rather, in capitalist societies, income is a major determinant of social status or influence where an individual contributes in substantial ways. It is important to note in this regard that prior to 1989, Eastern Europe's smaller income differentials were not beneficial to health, and therefore income was not necessarily an indicator of social position (Wnuk-Lipinski and Illsley 1990). Whether standing in party status would be the main factor is unknown. Furthermore, the studies noted earlier demonstrating that unemployment is related to poor health have also found that areas of a country with higher overall unemployment rates show a weaker relationship between mortality and unemployment. That is, if an individual is unemployed and living in an area in which unemployment is the norm, then unemployment is unrelated to health differentials.

The importance of these findings is that they point to an underlying factor that is still not well understood. It would appear that, beyond destitute poverty itself, there are other complicated factors at work. An individual's control or influence over his own actions, and perhaps his feelings of contributing to the larger society, are of particular importance (Syme 1994). Or as Wilkinson (1994) asks: Is the individual's desire for more income a desire to improve his relative standing in the society? In other words, it is not a desire for a higher level of material consumption that causes an individual to desire a greater income. "Relative position" in a society is affected by how that society structures the opportunities available to its citizens, and whether the society offers a variety of different positions to its citizens. However, all individuals have a number of reference groups in their lives; an individual does not always have to be at the "top" level of society—he could hold a position of value and importance within his local community and, provided that the local community is the individual's reference group, this position would have a positive influence on his health.

Education is key to enabling individuals to contribute and feel they are contributing to society. Marmot (1994) suggests that education may be the tool that provides people with more life management skills which in turn lead to improved socioeconomic circumstances and health status. Education is highly correlated with income, a major indicator of socioeconomic status. Education is also related independently to health status, with the more educated less likely to be functionally limited. Indeed, research demonstrates that a lack of education is a significant predictor of having dementia in old age.[1] While initially this finding was not taken seriously, it is now receiving serious attention. Learning and memory depend on connections between nerve cells in various parts of the brain, and dementia involves the loss of these connections. Education enriches these interconnections, creating reserve capacity, which can then compensate for losses that occur with aging (Hertzman 1994). This general role of education (the importance of which will emerge again below when talking about the community development strategy) may be the key to both individual choice of healthy behaviours, and to ensuring a structure of society within which individuals can contribute—and have the capacity to contribute—in mutually beneficial ways. The current trend for provincial ministries of Education to emphasize trades training may ultimately lead to poorer health of the nation.[2]

How does the social environment affect individuals mentally/psychologically/emotionally and physically? It would appear that social

---

1. See, for example, Katzman (1993), and for Canadian research, D'Arcy's work on the CSHA.
2. See Nelson Mandela's recent autobiography in which he argues strongly that the apartheid system of education which saw Black people relegated to trade skills was a powerful contributor to creating the most hostile, embittered, and resistant generation of Black people ever. Mandela argues that this system of education was a powerful force leading to the overthrow of apartheid.

environment affects people first psychologically and then physiologically. There is evidence that the nervous and immune systems communicate with each other such that social environment can influence biological responses through its input to the nervous system (Evans and Stoddart 1990). Biological responses, however, include more than responses in the immune system. Apparently, hormonal systems also respond to stress. Currently much research is being conducted into linkages between social environment, emotional and physiological response, and physiology. What is clear is that there are connections which have not yet been acknowledged. Furthermore, the relationship seems to include a host response of the organism; that is, individuals who have little or no income are not susceptible simply to a particular disease, but to a host of illnesses. If a cure were found today for cancer, another illness would replace it, and the same relationship between social gradient and illness that is found today would prevail.

The effects of social structure are complex, especially when examined in light of a particular specification such as gender. Unemployment, for example, could be expected to affect men differently from women because, until recently, men were expected to be employed, whereas it was not expected of women; gender differences in food preparation have already been noted; monetary achievement has been more expected of men than women, and so on. Women have been the nurturers, and among today's seniors, women are more likely to have more close friends than men, to be the kin keepers and network builders within the family, to respond to stressful situations differently, and to reach out to others. However, because of these differences, women have also been excluded from many employment opportunities. As a result, many elderly, single women today live in poverty (Moore and Rosenberg 1995).

Having established that social structure has its own independent effect on health, and that both individual choice and social environment are important for the health of individuals throughout their lifetime, including old age, it is possible to discuss strategies for ensuring healthier actions, including changes in social structure as well as in individual behaviours.

COMMUNITY DEVELOPMENT: A STRATEGY WITH A PROMISE

Health promotion, healthy lifestyles, healthy cities, healthy communities, healthy public policy, community development—all words commonly used in Canada in the '90s. The appeal of these terms and approaches lies in their calls for collective action in the community, the workplace, the institution or wherever, in order to change and better the social environment while, at the same time, empowering the individuals involved so they attain a higher level of self-esteem. Such empowerment enables individuals to truly lead to healthier individuals and healthier communities. By definition, community development must include the people whose lives it is going to affect. As the World Health Organization (1984) has pointed out, health promotion represents a mediating strategy between people and their environments, synthesizing personal choice and social responsibility in health. It involves promoting positive health behaviour and appropriate coping strategies, but it also involves the development of an environment conducive to health. As Brown (1991) argues, a comprehensive health promotion strategy must both help individuals adopt health promoting behaviours, and adopt strategies targeted to the larger environment.

There is much talk these days about the implications of a health promotion perspective, a lifestyles perspective, healthy cities, and community development. The term "community development" as used in this discussion incorporates several elements, including both individual and collective action, and having health on the agenda of political decision makers. Central to this approach is a clear distinction between an enabling and a hierarchical concept of power—that is, having "power to" do something, as opposed to having "power over" something/someone (Kickbusch 1989). An emphasis on actual support systems and empowerment of individuals is also central to the approach. Green and Kreuter (1990) define health promotion as a combination of educational and environmental supports for action, and conditions of living conducive to health. They note that the purpose of health promotion is to enable people to gain greater control over the determinants of their own health.

Health promotion, like community development, requires action at the community level. Local and national governments have an important role to play in terms of funding, generating data, providing leadership, and formulating policies. Generally speaking, the greater number of individuals and groups that support the action, the more likely it is that the effort will succeed. In this context, empowerment can be defined as people having power to take action to control and enhance their own lives; the process for achieving this empowerment is to enable people to become empowered. Such an approach is strongly tied to the tradition of community development (Grace 1991). A community does not have to be geographically close; it can be small or large, and can include any combination of individuals. The approach does not refer to a homogeneous whole; instead, it refers to enabling those individuals that are currently disenfranchised to become full participants in the process, which necessarily entails conflict and confrontation as well as consensus and cooperation. Effective community-level action requires a fundamental shift in the distribution of power, and it is well known that groups and individuals who currently hold power are usually reluctant to give it up without a fight (Farrant 1991).

Several authors have itemized lists of the ingredients necessary for successful community development or health promotion. Typical of these lists is the one put forward by Lackey et al. (1987), in which they argue that the characteristics essential for an ideal community include:

- local groups with well-developed problem-solving skills and the spirit of self-reliance;
- a broad distribution of power in decision making, commitment to the community as a place to live, and broad participation in community affairs;
- leaders with a community-wide vision and residents with a strong sense of community loyalty;
- effective collaboration in defining community needs and the ability to achieve a working consensus on goals and priorities;
- citizens with a broad repertoire of problem-solving abilities who know how to acquire resources when faced with adversity;
- commitment to the community, and a government that provides enabling support for the people; and
- a formal or informal mechanism for exchange among conflicting groups.

They note further that there must be some form of community-wide, or at least neighbourhood-wide, organization where citizens volunteer their time over and above the formal structure of official government. There must be opportunities for all peoples and all groups, including the elderly, youth, minorities, and people living with disabilities, and they must have opportunities to not only participate in leadership activities, but also to develop leadership skills. Part of the promise of this approach is its inclusiveness and its flexibility to take subcultural uniqueness into account.

Another advantage of this approach is that it must, if implemented appropriately, respond to the needs of the community. This ensures that differing needs, including multicultural needs, are considered. A community development program in an Aboriginal community would necessarily be very different from one in a Chinese community.

A community development approach is necessarily multifaceted. Many health promotion programs have focused narrowly on self-care behaviours; indeed most are directed at instruction which improves individual health maintenance behaviour. At the end of the '80s, DeFriese et al. (1989) estimated that, in the U.S., approximately 60 percent of all health service organizations operated one or more self-care educational programs, but the vast majority (94 percent) offered instruction aimed at improving individuals' health maintenance behaviours. In contrast, less than half addressed advocacy or self-empowerment.

Particular facets or programs which are considered part of the health promotion and community development strategy include social support programs, self-help programs, and educational or informational programs. However, only when all or many of these strategies are adopted for the purpose of individual empowerment and change in social structure can it be said that a community development approach or a comprehensive health promotion strategy has been achieved. Part of the confusion in the literature comes from the fact that there may be, for example, one eight-week self-care or social support group launched in an entire community, without any other facets of health promotion put in place. It would be difficult to argue, in this instance, that a health promotion strategy had been tested.

Nevertheless, some of the examples provided in the success stories demonstrate that some of these more limited programs with a narrower focus can be successful with seniors. In the examples provided, the narrower programs include a grassroots involvement strategy which appears to contribute to their success. Examples of comprehensive strategies of community development with seniors are also provided.

SUCCESS STORIES

Discover Choices: **Manitoba and Saskatchewan**

Actions on Nonmedical Determinants of Health

Discover Choices was a community-based health promotion program for disadvantaged older adults which began in September 1988 and ran for a two-year period throughout Manitoba and Saskatchewan. The overall goal was to encourage disadvantaged older adults to make informed choices about their health by increasing their knowledge of the lifestyle, social, and environmental factors that affect health and quality of life. The primary target group of the program was persons aged 55 through 74 living in Manitoba and Saskatchewan, whose personal annual incomes were $10,000 or less (or whose family incomes were $18,000 or less), whose formal education was Grade 12 or less and who were not working full time. Of particular interest in this story is the short-term media project which successfully provided information to disadvantaged seniors, resulting in changed behaviours towards personal health.

The objectives of *Discover Choices* were:

1. To reach a higher proportion of seniors by means of television and other communications in order to:
   a) increase their knowledge about ways to maintain health and to cope with common problems;
   b) increase their knowledge of the resources available to assist them to achieve their goals;
   c) increase the number who perceive themselves as able and entitled to work with others for their mutual benefit and to work for changes which will increase opportunities and reduce barriers to their personal and shared goals;
   d) increase recognition of their interdependence and the knowledge of skills and resources available to promote the benefits of inter-dependence.

2. To increase the number of disadvantaged older adults who use community services programs.
3. To increase the amount of contact with family and peers to communicate among each other, provide mutual assistance and engage in satisfying activities.

The program for the short-term objectives included three major media components: television, print, and support and promotional materials. The television component consisted of a special TV series focusing on aging. The print component consisted of 24 educational articles dealing with a variety of health-related topics, as well as suggestions for ways in which seniors can maintain quality of life. These were assembled in a kit, along with a guide to resources listing the program services and resources available for older adults within the two provinces. A newsletter was distributed and articles printed in community newspapers, newsletters etc. A variety of promotional and support materials were designed and distributed to create awareness of the program (such as letterheads, pins, buttons, key chains, bags and bookmarks).

Reasons for the Initiative

The reason for the initiative was a recognition that there were many disadvantaged older adults (as defined above) throughout Manitoba and Saskatchewan. The intent was to assist in empowering these individuals. The Prairie Regional Office of the Health Promotion Directorate of Health and Welfare Canada was aware that little health promotion had been done with older people. There had been a prevailing belief that elders were too old to change. However, officers at the regional and federal levels felt that this would be a new approach with seniors, and at the time seniors were a priority of Health and Welfare Canada.

Actors

The actors were the Health Promotion Directorate, Prairie Regional Office of Health and Welfare Canada and the Federal Branch, and a project advisory committee consisting of provincial representatives, seniors and academics from both provinces. Little resistance was encountered for the media component discussed here.

Analysis of the Results

Process evaluations were conducted during the campaign, with participants giving strong, positive feedback. In addition, an outcome evaluation was conducted assessing data collected prior to the implementation of the

program, taken approximately six months following the initial implementation (shortly following completion of the television series), and data
taken one year after implementation. The goal of the short-term evaluation
was to assess the impact of the media. It was designed to be part of the
project right from the beginning.

The outcome evaluation of the short-term objectives for the primary
target group (persons aged 55 through 74 living in Manitoba and
Saskatchewan, whose personal annual incomes were $10,000 or less, or
whose family incomes were $18,000 or less, whose formal education was
Grade 12 or less and who were not working full time) revealed statistically
significant changes from time$_1$ (t_1: prior to the implementation of the
program) to time$_2$ (t_2: six months later) on several indicators including:
health-related knowledge; ability to cope with commonly encountered
problems; knowledge of the resources available within the community; and
use of community services and resources. Evidence indicated a change in
respondents' perceptions regarding their ability to assert control over their
own lives and choices. In virtually all cases the direction of change was
consistent with the goals and objectives of the *Discover Choices* program.
Similar changes were not evident for the secondary target groups (advantaged
seniors, i.e., those who were not disadvantaged, as well as the families of all
seniors). Furthermore, the short-term changes for the primary target group
were largely sustained after one year. The lack of change evident in the
secondary target groups lends more credence to the view that it was *Discover
Choices* per se which affected the primary target groups (disadvantaged
seniors) rather than other general changes which may have been taking
place in the provinces at the time of the program. Any general societal
changes which were occurring did not affect the secondary groups, and so
it can be assumed that they also did not affect the primary target group.

The outcomes study demonstrates that self-empowerment for seniors
can take place in a relatively short period time, in this instance over six
months; years do not go by before the effects of such programs are seen. It
also suggests that media coverage is effective. Part of the success of this
program can be attributed to the fact that it was not "just" a television show
or "just" a newspaper column, but took a comprehensive approach: a variety
of different media were selected to disseminate the messages, local grassroots
individuals were involved in the whole campaign (writing articles, designing
buttons, etc.), and local media such as community newspapers were a major
vehicle for disseminating the information. In other words, the media
campaign included a community development component in providing
information to its target audience.

Replicability of the Initiative

The *Discover Choices* program ended on schedule, and a movie (*Coming of Age*) was made and shown on Global television. One-page write-ups of the movie were widely distributed throughout Canada, and the videos were used in many foreign countries. There were, however, administrative changes in Ottawa; administration for seniors programs was centralized and run out of Health Promotion, and monies for seniors programs became more difficult to obtain. But *Discover Choices* has produced some spin-off effects: for example, TV programs targeted specifically to older adults are now more accepted (note the current program *50 Up*); more health-promoting groups aimed at seniors that now exist use a multimedia approach, such as mall walking programs. The short-term media target of *Discover Choices* was successfully reached, and added to the knowledge that such strategies can work with seniors. It should be stressed that the community development aspect of the campaign was largely responsible for its success.

Funding

Funding was provided by the federal government through the Health Promotion Directorate; it was time limited, terminating when the project was completed. Many people objected to the amount of money spent on the outcomes evaluation, arguing that these funds could have instead been channelled directly to program delivery. However, the percentage of funds spent on the evaluation was not inordinately high, and the researchers put in time and effort above and beyond the call of duty in order to meet deadlines and ensure scientific rigour. The importance of including rigorous evaluation research is not accepted in all circles. There is still a common perception that the money should go into the actual program or service. These individuals do not ask whether the funds are being misdirected by spending on this service in the first instance.

Evaluation

The evaluation was conducted by researchers at the Centre on Aging, University of Manitoba at a cost of $235,000. The program cost over $1 million over four years (the dollars for both the evaluation and the program included other aspects not discussed here). The evaluation was rigorous and included personal interviews with the primary target group (the disadvantaged elderly) who were selected from random listings of persons aged 55 through 74 from both the Manitoba Health Services Commission and Saskatchewan Health (from their medical records). People in long-term institutional care were excluded. Telephone screenings were conducted to determine membership within the primary target group. There were 720 disadvantaged seniors who participated in the first interview. A randomly selected sample of just under 400 of those interviewed at t_1 were subsequently reinterviewed for the short-term follow-up. The secondary target group (individuals aged 75 and over; those aged 55 to 74 with higher education income etc.; family and friends of the primary target groups; and the general public aged 18–54) were mailed questionnaires at t_1 and one year later. These respondents were selected from random listings of all persons aged 75 and over, or 18 through 54 residing within the two provinces. These lists were also obtained from the health records. Those aged 55 through 74 who did not meet the criteria for the disadvantaged category were also included in this group. There were 2,522 sampled in this secondary group. All who responded at t_1 were sent follow-up questionnaires at the one-year follow-up; 1,082 responded.

Each of the objectives was put into operation using established scales or, where scales did not already exist, by devising, testing, and revising new scales. Scenarios were also used in which seniors were asked to advise the person within a fictitious situation. The outcome evaluation called for quantitative data analyses following from large random samples so results could be generalized. Criteria for success therefore called upon conservative statistical tests of significance which demonstrated sizeable change from t_1 to t_2.

A publicly available report (Penning et al. 1991) resulted from the evaluation study. It argues that evaluations of health promotion programs generally should be broad and extensive in scope to do justice to the program and adequately measure the impact of such programs. Narrowly defined impacts will almost surely lead to a demonstration of no impact.

Support Services to Seniors Program

Actions on Nonmedical Determinants of Health

The *Support Services to Seniors Program* (SSS) program is a province-wide community-based program administered by Manitoba Health. It was initially introduced in 1984/85 to: 1) ensure consistency and continuity in support services that would enhance and expand rather than replace existing family and community supports; and 2) provide the supports necessary to allow seniors, particularly those who are frail or at risk, to maintain independent living in the community thereby deferring or precluding the need for home care services or institutionalization. The philosophy behind the program is that of prevention and maintenance. The program draws heavily on existing organizations within the community and on a strong volunteer component. The goal is to enhance quality of life through the maintenance of independence and autonomy, and to postpone—if not prevent—the use of other more costly services within the system.

Support services include meals, transportation, escorts, handymen, telephone reassurance, and home maintenance as well as others in the basic living category. Care services such as nursing services are excluded. The program provides provincial funding to communities to assist them in developing service delivery projects. It provides for staff support and coordinating services, as well as for direct service subsidies through operating grants for things such as: community resource co-coordinators, tenant resource co-coordinators, and volunteer co-coordinators; meal preparation; transportation; and socialization. Funding goes to an incorporated nonprofit community agency which has demonstrated that it has community support through sponsoring groups and volunteer commitment.

Reasons for the Initiative

The SSS program started with a pilot project at a single apartment complex in which a tenant resource co-coordinator was hired to coordinate formal and informal services to meet the needs of the tenants in the complex, many of whom had become quite frail. The usefulness and success of this position was evaluated (Blandford et al. 1989), deemed successful, and by the end of the first fiscal year four more SSS projects had been funded. Over the next few years additional projects were funded on a fairly regular basis. In 1991, in a climate of fiscal constraint and faced with growing budget requests from the SSS program, the government froze allocations at the level of the previous year and ordered a review. Funds to the program had increased by 100 percent in the first year, 400 percent in the second year, and over 100 percent for several years thereafter. Even though these funds represented small actual amounts, especially compared with the dollar increases going into acute care hospitals, the rate of growth was seen as problematic. Cabinet agreed to reopen the allocation process only if proof was found that the projects were effective and produced demonstrable cost savings to other programs.

Actors

The primary actors include a small number of provincial employees who allocate funding and assist projects, as well as the many community groups and volunteers who support the local projects. Many people who participate in the program are also volunteers within the project. Municipal governments and provincial MPs also support (in principle) the project.

Analysis of the Results

The evaluation demonstrated a wide regional variation in the nature and distribution of both meals-only and multiservice projects; while one region in particular had many multiservice projects, each region demonstrated a need for these types of projects to be implemented. Although increased funding has been associated with the program, more projects have been mounted with cost per project decreasing over time. Interviews with key informants revealed positive attitudes towards the program and its operation. Most understood the program and felt that it was very appropriate in meeting the needs of its clients. Both program staff and those representing the community gave overall high ratings in assessing the benefit to clients in terms of physical health, mental health and well-being, overall functioning, ability to maintain independence within their current residences, and relationships with family members and friends who provide assistance. Both types of informants identified the socialization component of the program and the importance of accessing a balanced meal as particularly beneficial to clients. Both groups identified the individuals most likely to be program clients as seniors who live alone or in seniors apartments, or who are frail and in poor health, but not totally dependent in terms of functional capacity. Concern was expressed that the program was not adequately funded.

The client interviews revealed that the clients who use the SSS program are more likely to be women belonging to the older elderly population who live alone, have lower incomes than most seniors, do not own their own homes, are widowed and have more chronic conditions, more functional disability, more days spent in hospital, and poorer perceived health than that of the general community sample. In other words, the clients most likely to use the program are at risk or disadvantaged according to several indicators; if an index of risk were constructed for all the clients, they are all at risk according to the typical definitions of what constitutes people "at risk". They were at risk when compared with seniors living in the community, and were considered prime candidates for using home care or nursing homes.

Just under one-third of the clients actually volunteered their time to the projects. The clients themselves considered the SSS program very important for their physical health, their psychological well-being, and their ability to live independently. Approximately one-third assess their quality of life as better after having received SSS services. In terms of cost, one region of the province is well served by the SSS program and consequently seniors in that region receive less home care services. Regions that receive fewer SSS services utilize more home care services, usually higher amounts than the percentage of seniors in the population. A specific example is the region of Westman, where approximately 14 percent of the population aged 65 and over reside in Westman, yet 23 percent of all SSS projects are located there, including 41 percent of all multiservice projects. However, while over 10 percent of all persons aged 65 and over receive home care services in Manitoba, only 6 percent of those in the Westman region do so. The second most well-served region in terms of the SSS program is Central Region (having 17 percent of all multiservice projects for 9 percent of the elderly population). Only 7 percent of the seniors in this region receive home care. Regions which are less well served in terms of SSS, especially in terms of multiservice projects include Norman/Thompson and Winnipeg and to a lesser extent Eastman, the Interlake and Parklands. Home care utilization in these regions ranges from 11 percent to 14 percent.

Crude cost figures reveal the potential for cost savings. The average annual cost per person for nursing home care at the time of the study was about $22,000. The average annual cost per person for home care was about $1,670 per person or $2,100 if administrative costs are included. In comparison, the average annual cost per person of the SSS program was approximately $184 for multiservice projects, of which $163 is the cost to government. The cost of meals-only projects is considerably lower. The average annual cost of a meal program to government is $4.70 (1990 figures).

Cost savings to home care can, therefore, be computed since regions with well-developed Support Services reveal half as many seniors in home care as do regions where Support Services are not well developed (roughly 6 percent vs. 12 percent). It costs approximately $27,944,700 (12 percent of persons age 65+ or 13,307 × cost per person of $2,100) to maintain seniors on the home care program outside of the Westman and Central regions. By expanding Support Services in all regions where multiservice projects are not well developed, the savings could equal 1/2 of the cost of 12 percent ($13,972,350) minus the cost of expanding support services to those regions to the level currently served well by Support Services (at 12 percent of seniors costing $2,448,488 in total or $2,169,041 to government) minus the multiservice clients currently being served outside of Westman and Central ($2,448,488 − $1,214,400). This represents the additional cost of expanding the program, i.e., $1,234,088 (in total) or $954,641 (to government) in 1990 dollars and a savings of $12,738,262 (in total) or $13,017,709 (to government) in home care costs if Support Services are expanded outside of the Westman and Central regions. These savings of course assume ceteris paribus, i.e., that other factors do not operate to expand home care utilization (such as increased early discharges from acute care hospitals).

The cost efficiency of the existing program can also be computed by examining costs saved by clients who would otherwise enter a personal care home. Using the predictors of nursing home care established by Shapiro and Tate (1988), the percent of Support Services clients who are at high risk of being in a nursing home if Support Services did not exist can be estimated. Taking only those considered at high risk of institutionalization, it is estimated that those who are aged 85 or over, have been admitted to a hospital in the last year, and have problems with basic activities of daily living; or are aged 85 and over, have no spouse, and have problems with basic activities of daily living; or were admitted to hospital in the last year, have problems with basic activities of daily living and have fair or poor perceived health, provides a total of 28 percent of the current clientele of Support Services who would likely be institutionalized. It would cost the province a total of $66,528,000 annually to maintain 28 percent of multiservice clientele in nursing homes.

Similarly, the number of seniors more likely to use home care services can also be calculated by drawing on Shapiro's work in Manitoba. These calculations include the 28 percent at "high risk" of personal care home placement, and provide an alternative cost of maintaining these individuals if SSS were not available. A figure of 41.6 percent is obtained when calculating the number of SSS clients most likely to use home care services who fall into the following categories: seniors aged 75 and over, have problems with activities of daily living, and have no spouse; seniors aged 75 and over, have problems with activities of daily living, have no spouse and have poor or fair perceived health; and seniors who have problems with activities of daily living, have no spouse and have fair to poor health. To maintain multiservice individuals only on home care would cost the province $7,503,310 annually in direct home care services, or $9,435,300 taking administrative costs into account.

The question arises as to whether it would be most cost efficient to maintain only those clients who would be in a nursing home or on home care in the SSS program without providing services to the remainder. It could be argued that in the long run such a strategy would lead to more expensive services. Whether or not the SSS program can keep people out of nursing homes or out of acute care hospitals for that matter is not simply a question for the SSS program. It is also a question for the more expensive institutional sector within the health care system, because the old saying "a built bed is a filled bed" has proven to be true. In other words, if governments insist on building beds in both the acute care and long-term care sectors, these beds will be filled. A cost-effective strategy calls for reallocation of monies to the community sector from the institutional sector. In other words, the SSS program cannot be blamed for dollars spent within the institutional sector which are out of its control.

Success of this program is due both to a small number of key individuals in the Ministry of Health who believed in and supported the program, as well as to the commitment to and contributions of the various community players involved in each project. the program suffers, however, from continual questioning from Treasury Board which accepts the necessity of expensive medical and hospital care without demanding rigorous outcome evaluations—despite the high price of those services—but demands outcome evaluations of low-cost SSS programs.

Replicability of the Initiative

This initiative has continued and is being expanded within the province of Manitoba. The initiative could clearly be replicated in other jurisdictions and in other provinces. There are many individuals available in Manitoba who could assist. The strength of the SSS program is that it draws on grassroots local initiatives from the community itself and is very low cost. Provided the principles of community development are followed so that the community itself decides on its needs, there is no reason why it cannot proceed elsewhere.

Funding

When the evaluation was undertaken, SSS was costing under $2 million per year. The report (Centre on Aging and WESTARC Group Inc. 1991) that was written from this study eventually went to government, and an academic publication is currently under submission (Chappell et al. delayed because government sat on the report for a long time). Despite a positive evaluation, the budget remained frozen. The report was shelved at a time when budgetary constraints were imposed on all government programs despite the fact that health reform proponents were arguing for more community care and less medical and institutional care, and for regionalization, two principles supported by the SSS program. However, there was no political will to proceed.

In May 1992, Manitoba Health produced a blueprint for health reform entitled *Quality Health for Manitobans: The Action Plan* (Manitoba Health 1992), which highlighted the SSS program as a "success story" and identified its place in the continuum of health services as the first line of defence to maintain seniors in the community. Identification of avoiding potential costs subsequently led to the funding of 24 new projects within the SSS program in underserved areas of the province for the fiscal year 93/94. A subsequent three-year new initiative has provided funds for up to 58 new or expanded projects by the end of 95/96 with a second evaluation to be done immediately.

Evaluation

Two external university-affiliated research groups were asked to conduct the evaluation (Centre on Aging, University of Manitoba and WESTARC Group, associated with Brandon University, also in Manitoba). There were many broad objectives, not atypical of government requests, which the researchers asked to be tailored to identify the key issues. The following were identified as the key questions to be answered in the evaluation:

- Is the program addressing the needs of those seniors for whom it was intended?

- To what extent will fees act as a deterrent to those needing service?
- What is the impact of the program on the demand for continuing care (home care) and institutional services?
- What is the cost-effectiveness of the SSS program?

In order to meet these objectives a number of strategies for data collection together with a multisample design were used. The strategies included: a file review; mailed questionnaires to project staff contacts; interviews with key informants; and interviews with clients.

The file review provided information on the program, the projects (N=141), and the sponsors. They included, for example: the nature and extent of services provided; staffing levels; volunteer involvement and cost; sources of funding; community service context; service delivery; and changes over time. Interviews with key informants included 33 persons representing the Interagency Committee for Support Service to Seniors, Housing Authorities and Project Councils, Regional Program Specialists, Regional Directors, and representatives of local community interests including business, church and voluntary organizations. These individuals were asked questions regarding the appropriateness of the program's objectives, the adequacy of the geographic distribution of projects, professional assessments regarding the impact of the program on elderly clients and their support networks, the effectiveness of the program for older persons with varying levels of health and functioning and living within various types of settings, the impact of user fees, and the complementarity/conflict with other community-based services. In other words, they were asked questions of an evaluative nature.

Interviews with the client group consisted of a sample of users of the various projects. The goals were to gather relevant information for producing a client profile, and to examine the perceived effectiveness of the services, the impact of fees on accessibility, the impact of the program on involvement with the informal social network, and quality of life. The sample of clients was drawn from a stratified (by project type and length of funding) random sample of 12 projects: six projects offering meals only and six multiservice projects, half of each funded prior to fiscal 1987 and half funded after that time. Projects randomly selected for inclusion in the study were asked to provide client lists. Ten clients were randomly selected from each of the meals-only projects, and 40 clients from each of the multiservice projects. A total of 279 clients were ultimately interviewed.

Finally, descriptive information concerning the specific projects which went beyond that available in the files was obtained using a mailed questionnaire sent to a staff contact person, one for each project. There were 113 questionnaires returned (80 percent). The main findings are listed in the earlier section on analysis of the results. Generally speaking, the criteria for success were indicators of the objectives that demonstrated overwhelming support for the program. The report contains the actual figures so the reader can judge for himself whether he agrees with the authors' opinion. Ultimately, the government agreed and has extended this program.

Despite the fact that the research was done under very tight time constraints and with an inadequate budget, and despite the fact that it demonstrated positive results, no action flowed from it because there was a lack of political will. It was only when a political advantage was perceived that action took place. Such political maneuvering seems to always take place regardless of the rigour and timeliness of the research.

Tenderloin Seniors Organizing Project (TSOP)

Actions on Nonmedical Determinants of Health

The *Tenderloin Seniors Organizing Project* (TSOP) is an excellent example of grassroots community development. The 45-block Tenderloin area of San Francisco had long been recognized as a high-crime, red-light area, housing large numbers of sex offenders, prostitutes, substance abusers, and former mental patients. It was also one of the countries largest 'gray ghettoes', with some 8,000 elderly men and women in its single room occupancy (SRO) hotels. A multiplicity of health problems were common among these seniors, including alcoholism, depression, malnutrition and hypertension.

TSOP had two main goals: 1) to improve the physical, mental, and emotional health of elderly residents by increasing social support and providing relevant health education; and 2) to facilitate individual and community empowerment by helping residents to identify common problems or needs, and to collectively seek solutions to these problems.

Reasons for the Initiative

TSOP was established in 1979 to address the interrelated problems of social isolation, poor health and powerlessness common among the elderly residents of the Tenderloin district's low-income SRO hotels. TSOP actually started operating one year after the completion of an ambitious earlier program which used support groups as a means of combatting social isolation among the elderly hotel residents in this area of San Francisco. That project experienced only modest and short-term success, which has been attributed to failing to spend sufficient lead time in establishing trust and building a sense of community among the residents, and failing to develop a plan for continuing the project when funds ran out. The TSOP project was founded by a Berkeley University professor and her students. For eight years the project operated with more than 250 student volunteers who were spurred by a commitment to demonstrate that social support and education for critical consciousness could work in this setting.

Actors

The professor and her students were initially the key actors who spent time gaining an understanding of which local agencies were accepted by the elderly SRO residents. They identified a Catholic church in the area as the agency most accepted by Tenderloin seniors, and worked through that agency to offer their services (free blood pressure checkups) in one hotel. This entrée into the first hotel permitted informal interaction with residents, which in turn led to the development of trust. After over one year, hotel residents formed a seniors activity club which met weekly and was facilitated by student volunteers. Different activities were organized, and as trust and rapport increased the elders started to share their personal concerns. The volunteers encouraged leaders to emerge, and eventually residents of other hotels were included in the group discussions. It took some time before the residents began to take ownership of the process, and to see beyond the walls of their respective hotels. An interhotel coalition was eventually formed around issues of common concern, such as the high crime rate and low nutrition. The project has grown from a small university-sponsored project to a nonprofit community-based organization with a small paid staff (2.5 full-time employees), 15 student volunteers, 22 resident leaders, and an active board of directors. The greatest strength of this project appears to be the actors' understanding and ability to nurture the involvement of the residents, and to enable participants to experience their own successes and take control of their own lives.

Analysis of the Results

TSOP has experienced many successes. For example, the residents recruited local businesses, agencies, bars and restaurants to be places of refuge where residents could go in time of danger or medical emergency; each of these "safe houses" was identified by a decal. Within the first two weeks, TSOP had recruited 14 safe houses, and after one year it had recruited 48 safe houses. From the time the safe houses were established, crime in the area dropped by 18 percent in the first year (and eventually by 26 percent) and the police attribute the drop in large part to the program (Minkler 1996). The weekly group meetings have been a major success. Discussions on malnutrition in these meetings led to the development of a comprehensive nutrition project including hotel-based minimarkets and cooperative food buying clubs. Moreover, a health resource centre with health promotion material oriented towards low-income elders was established. It created social networks and support groups within the residential hotels where the elderly had been living frequently in isolated despair. It organized a tenants association that was successful in rolling back an illegal rent hike charged by a hotel owner. It improved local transportation services. During the project residents evolved from being targets of change to agents of change (Minkler et al. 1982–1983).

Minkler attributes much of the success of TSOP to the fact that social planning activities accommodated and blended well with the social action organizing focus, and that these activities remained TSOP's key philosophical and practice orientation. There have been difficulties with the high rates of alcoholism and mental health problems of some of the seniors involved in the project, so that it has been difficult to achieve group autonomy and continuity without outside backup. This has been identified as one of the greatest difficulties with TSOP. A further difficulty has been the dilemma of trying to meet the sometimes conflicting agendas of community residents on the one hand, and funding sources on the other. Volunteers and staff walk a fine line, trying not to take over control. Residents do on occasion discuss burnout with staff (Wechsler and Minkler 1986).

Replicability of the Initiative

Projects based on community development can be, and are being, replicated elsewhere. However, such projects are not so easily implemented, which is why the Tenderloin experience stands out as such a success. Minkler has listed seven prerequisites for true replication, including:

- Willingness on the part of the senior residence management to allow informal discussion groups one morning a week in the lobby/recreation area;
- A cadre of volunteers knowledgeable in group process and community organization methods, and able to make a commitment of several hours per week for at least several months;
- A commitment among all parties to the principle of starting where the people are;
- Sufficient resources to enable follow-through by residents, volunteers and staff on action plans developed by residents;
- Realistic plans for continuity over time;
- Ongoing leadership development and a commitment to increasing levels of resident control and group autonomy; and
- Respect for the social as well as the task-oriented needs of residents, and a commitment to meeting both sets of needs to the extent possible.

In Minkler's terms, the project started out empowering residents and later helped create the conditions for groups of residents to empower themselves. It can be replicated, but with great difficulty. Because of the fame of this project and the many inquiries about replication, TSOP staff have written a replication manual for others to follow. Efforts to replicate TSOP include:

- A 1987 New York City project among chronically schizophrenic veterans. After several months, a support group led to a variety of positive outcomes, but it did not evolve into a community organizing group; and
- A Vancouver-based project. In 1990, the Vancouver Mile High Society received government funds to operate in SRO hotels, building supportive networks and trying to link isolated residents with the broader community. The project is now in its fifth year, and includes nine hotels.

Funding

TSOP was funded through a small university project and was heavily subsidized through the commitment of student and faculty volunteers. Ongoing funding was a problem. TSOP staff approached several funding sources for gifts and grants in the order of $100,000 per year. Ultimately, after 16 years, it could not secure ongoing funding and was closed in 1995. The original professor underscores the difficulty the funders had with "ongoing" projects.

Evaluation

There have been several evaluations of TSOP. Almost all have included evidence of effectiveness and have described the changes made as a result of the program as positive. These changes included mobilizing to reduce the crime rate, establishing a nutrition program, arranging for vacant lot clean-up, as well as a host of other actions which improved the quality of life of the members of the neighbourhood. For TSOP, the actions demonstrate the possibility of successful problem solving at the community level. A more quantitative evaluation was undertaken (Shaw 1995) in the mid-'90s to document the success of the program in more traditional terms. The evaluation was hampered by the fact that TSOP closed when the evaluation was only halfway completed. The evaluation included a comparison of buildings in the Tenderloin district in which TSOP was active and those where it was not. It demonstrated that residents in TSOP buildings felt safer at night, had more social contacts, changed more of the buildings rules, brought about more improvements in the general conditions of their buildings, had superior knowledge of where to find a safe haven in the streets, and had higher morale and higher quality of life scores. One of the major difficulties with this evaluation is that many of the individuals Tenderloin is believed to have helped moved out of this very disadvantaged area as a result of being empowered, and were not tracked. The Shaw evaluation is the only one that was conducted by an outsider. The evaluator concludes that TSOP can only be deemed successful from a programmatic point of view. It succeeded in helping many people, a striking success when considering that many of the participants have been described as people without hope. In the view of the evaluator, TSOP is easily replicable. TSOP's major weakness was its inability to obtain ongoing funding which was the direct result of organizational weaknesses such as a lack of realistic short- and long-term plans, a lack of goals and objectives, a lack of engaging in monitoring activities, and a lack of an effective fundraising strategy.

For all of the evaluations, success was defined by a broad spectrum of indicators of quality of life and empowerment, including changing rules, the participation of seniors in events, and enabling seniors to become more active and less isolated.

On Lok: "Peaceful, happy abode"

Actions on Nonmedical Determinants of Health

On Lok provides comprehensive, inclusive, long-term care for elderly residents of the Chinatown/North Beach/Polk Gulch neighbourhoods in San Francisco. Its goal is to enable frailer seniors to stay in their communities, preferably in their own homes, as long as is medically, socially and economically feasible. The program is flexible, allowing direct service providers full control over all health and health-related services. The program has three objectives:

- To rehabilitate participants as much as possible through a variety of therapeutic services;
- To maintain the health and independence of participants by providing comprehensive medical, social and nutrition services; and
- To sustain the highest possible quality of life while controlling health care costs through the flexible use of resources.

Only frail seniors who meet functional eligibility requirements for institutional care are admitted to the *On Lok* program. No other community-based program in the U.S. offers all supportive and medical, both acute and chronic, services through the same program reimbursed by both Medicare and Medicaid capitated payments (Miller 1991).

Reasons for the Initiative

During the late '60s, a group of concerned citizens recognized that 18,000 residents in the area who had limited incomes and little or no command of English had needs that were not being met. Many of the seniors experienced physical impairment and confusion, and lived in hotel rooms above night clubs and behind stores. *On Lok* seniors health services began in 1971 with the U.S.' first adult day health program in a renovated Broadway night club, providing a hot meal and a place to see friends (Yee

1980). In 1975, the day health centre expanded to two facilities and added in-home care, home-delivered meals, and housing assistance. In 1980, hospital and skilled nursing facilities were added. Other additions included the *On Lok* house, comprised of 54 apartments for the frail elderly, a third day care centre and a respite unit. In 1983, *On Lok* became the first organization in the country to assume full financial risk for the care of the frail elderly population it was serving.

Actors

Key actors in this story are the individual citizens of the area who saw the need and organized creatively to meet that need, as well as the *On Lok* staff who followed the original philosophy and created an innovative program to meet the needs of this frail senior population. One feature of the program to emphasize is that as *On Lok* evolved, it provided all services which its participants required—anything from friendly visiting to intensive care and surgery. This also included delivering a prescription to someone's home, repairing a broken window, or calling a participant on the telephone for reassurance.

Analysis of the Results

Since the program began, there have been a fairly steady stream of evaluations which praise its success. The specific results are noted in the section on evaluation. There seems to be no room to doubt *On Lok*'s success at maintaining a group of frail, marginalized old people in the community, while enhancing their independence.

Replicability of the Initiative

On Lok has been such a success that there has been great interest in replicating it elsewhere. In 1985, the Robert Wood Johnson Foundation awarded a grant to *On Lok* to study the feasibility of extending their model of risk-based long-term care services to the frail elderly to other parts of the country. The *Program of All-Inclusive Care for the Elderly* (PACE) enabled legislation under which Medicare and Medicaid waivers were granted to 10 community-based public or nonprofit organizations in order to replicate *On Lok*. In 1987, *On Lok* embarked on the implementation phase of the replications. Proposed sites had to operate an adult day health centre for 12–24 months before becoming eligible for waivers and capitated financing. In this time, they had to demonstrate adequate development of the consolidated service model and enrollment of approximately 100 participants. The replication is complex with a framework for site development which consists of three transitional stages and nine development areas each in logical progression.

Each stage must be successfully completed before proceeding to the next (Der-McLeod and Hansen 1992; Miller 1991).

As of mid-1994, there were nine replications operating under dual capitation payments and a tenth site that proved not to be viable. The beginnings of an evaluation are documented in Branch et al. (1995), who discuss slow enrollment rates which may imply target clients who were less enthusiastic than the designers of this site. Branch et al. report evidence of "niche marketing" or "skimming". Consequently, they question the long-term viability of PACE. Despite these difficulties, implementation does seem to be sensitive to variations in local state conditions, as well as variations in the projects themselves, including differences in personnel, organization and finances. All projects were able to obtain a sponsor, and some financial and administrative support from their sponsor. All of the replication sites are in larger areas than is *On Lok*, proving that the *On Lok* model is viable in areas as big as 14,000 square miles. None of the replication sites have yet developed the housing component, which could prove critical to their success. The most important barriers appear to be the required attendance at the day centre, financial limitations and loss of freedom of choice.

Funding

Funding evolved over time. At the beginning, the day centre was funded by the Administration on Aging as a research and demonstration project. Two years later, it became a pilot project under Medicaid by contractual agreement with the California Department of Health Services. This lead to the inclusion of day health services as a permanent benefit under Medical, California's Medicaid. In 1975, when the day health centre expanded to two facilities and added in-home care, home-delivered meals, and housing assistance, it was through an Administration on Aging model project grant. In 1978, it became a legislative Medicaid program and received federal funding from the office of Human Development Services to develop a program of complete medical care and social support for nursing home–eligible elderly. In 1979, Health Care Financing Administration authorized the reimbursement of *On Lok* with Medicare section 222 waivers for the Community Care Organizations for Dependent Adults. In 1980, the hospital and skilled nursing facilities came under this same package. In 1983, *On Lok* became the first organization in the U.S. to assume full financial risk for the care of a frail elderly population, with program funding changing from cost-based reimbursement to six-monthly premiums covering all services. *On Lok* diversified its funding sources to include Medicare, Medicaid, and private funds. In 1986, landmark legislation approved *On Lok* to continue operating under its special Medicare and Medicaid provisions, conditional upon maintaining the programs cost and quality. It became the first community-based long-term care program to move beyond demonstration status. *On*

Lok is ongoing, but as noted above it is not clear whether the replication projects will continue.

Evaluation

On Lok has been the subject of several process and outcome evaluations, many of which are published. While some evaluations have focused on evaluating the health of participants, most have been interested in cost savings when compared to traditional institutional care. For example, Yordi and Waldman (1985) compared service utilization and cost impacts of traditional long-term care with *On Lok's* consolidated model. Using a longitudinal design with a matched comparison group, the study found that *On Lok* participants had fewer days in hospital and nursing home care, and received a broader range of less costly community-based services compared with those receiving traditional institutional care. Nursing homes and acute hospital costs were much higher for the comparison group while the reverse was true for community-based service costs. When all costs were combined, the cost for the *On Lok* group was still less.

Lurie et al. (1976) report evaluating *On Lok* services by using intake medical status evaluations at baseline, after six months, and evaluating the participants' status as perceived by family and friends. Medical status improved the most as a result of the program, but so did functional capacity (40 percent of the participants were functionally poor at intake and this figure declined to 20 percent after program participation). The program had a homogenizing influence on cognitive skills, reducing people at both extremes. *On Lok's* cost was less than traditional care in an institution and was less expensive than skilled care, but found to be more costly than intermediate care.

The criteria of success vary depending on the evaluation being conducted. In Lurie et al.'s study (1976), more traditional health measures such as medical status and functional capacity were examined. *On Lok* evaluations have not included broader health promotion measures, such as client participation, individual empowerment, or resultant changes in community institutions.

Arthritis Self-Management Program: B.C. Project

Actions on Nonmedical Determinants of Health

The *Arthritis Branch Community Support Program* (ABC) is a health promotion project involving three projects (the arthritis self-management program, support groups, and telephone contact) aimed at improving the quality of life and independence for an aging population experiencing chronic health problems. Arthritis, while not fatal, is the most prevalent chronic condition among people aged 65 years and over. Over half of all seniors in Canada suffer from arthritis (Zimmer and Chappell 1994). The project uses self-help and mutual aid health promotion mechanisms to foster enhanced coping abilities and increased access to services for people in rural and remote areas of B.C. Implementation relies heavily on planning and decision making by grassroots volunteers. The arthritis self-management program, which is of particular interest to this paper, was implemented using media promotion, liaising with Stanford University experts in order to implement the strategy, cotraining and popular support. It is presented here as an example of a strategy targeted to a broader audience than the frail and disadvantaged seniors who were the concern of the preceding stories.

The arthritis self-management program was developed, piloted, implemented and evaluated by the Stanford Arthritis Center, School of Medicine, Stanford, California in order to teach people to become "health self-managers". The course is designed to strengthen and enhance self-advocacy—the belief and sense that someone has about his personal capabilities and accomplishing everyday life activities. The course is based on two assumptions: that people can learn the general principles of managing health conditions, and that knowledgeable persons practising self-care will experience improved physical function, less pain and reduced health care costs. The course teaches skill development and is lead by two trained instructors. The course is comprised of six two-hour sessions spread over a two- or three-month period, offered in a community setting. It costs approximately $10 per participant. The program was initially implemented in B.C., Alberta and the Yukon on a demonstration basis to determine feasibility and viability of the program for the Canadian population.

Reasons for the Initiative

The project was initiated by individuals involved with arthritis societies in Canada, who were aware of the success of the program in the U.S., and were interested in bringing the benefits to the Canadian population.

Actors

Several actors are involved: staff of the arthritis societies, a provincial coordinator, trainers, lay leaders and participants. Using the existing service infrastructure is considered extremely important. Branch volunteers who already had a relationship with the arthritis society were the first to contact target populations and recruit course leaders. Branch offices were contacted and invited to become course leaders themselves, or to ask branch managers if they were interested. Course leaders were required to take a three-day training workshop.

Analysis of the Results

According to the outcome evaluation, the objectives of the program were met and the program was deemed successful. The evaluation demonstrated that all changes in the target population after participation in the course followed the direction predicted by the program: fewer visits were made for doctor-suggested routine checkups, fewer patient-initiated visits to the physician were made concerning a specific problem, and significant increases in levels of relaxation were noted. Significant differences in pain and disability levels were experienced, but the direction of change was toward improvement; however, because there were very low levels of pain and disability at the beginning of the projects, there was little room to determine whether or not the program effected improvements in these areas.

After 20 months, the project was fully implemented in 22 communities in three provinces; there were eight trainers and 218 leaders. The projects demonstrated that individuals with chronic arthritis are interested in the program, and they are utilizing and able to follow the protocols and procedures to deliver the program in their own communities. The group recommended that a longer lead time be given to recruit volunteers, particularly the lay leaders, and that a clear understanding of what is involved must be conveyed to the volunteers from the beginning (McGowan 1994).

Replicability of the Initiative

The project was itself a replication of a U.S. program; the Canadian replication was deemed successful. After completion of the project, provincial offices in B.C., Alberta and the Yukon established it as a permanent program, and the National Arthritis Society of Canada adopted the program for national implementation.

Funding

The program (including the self-management course, the support groups, and the telephone contact) was funded by the Seniors Independence Program (SIP) of Health Canada for $200,000 in 1988. From 1992–1994, SIP contributed an additional $500,000. Monies for the national permanent program have been obtained from corporate sponsors, and amount to approximately $30,000 per province.

Evaluation

The arthritis self-management program, as noted earlier, was originally implemented in the U.S. A series of research studies in the U.S. demonstrated that:

- Lay leaders are able to offer the program and obtain results similar to those led by health professionals (Lorig et al. 1986);
- The program leads to improved behaviour and increased levels of self-advocacy and improved health status (Lorig et al. 1985; Lorig and Holman 1993);
- Self-advocacy is the key mechanism in the program responsible for bringing about improvements in health (Leneker et al. 1984);
- The improvements are maintained without reinforcement for at least four years (Lorig and Holman 1989; Holman et al. 1989); and
- These programs can bring about important cost savings (Holman et al. 1989).

In addition, the pre- and posttest evaluation conducted by McGowan (1994) in B.C. suggests that this program works in Canada. The evaluation results helped lead to the establishment of a permanent national program.

All of the success stories described here have been subjected to scientific evaluation. The methodologies have varied, as have the number of evaluations each project has undergone. Similarly, the outcome measures (the criteria by which success was measured) vary considerably from more traditional health measures such as medical status and functional disability, through to broad community development or health promotion measures of individual empowerment and institutional change. In all instances, there is evidence that these examples are successful and, taken together, demonstrate that community development with seniors can be effective. The fact that these examples are all community-based does not necessarily mean that institutionally-based programs cannot succeed. However, community-based programs that have been subjected to rigorous evaluation are, while not plentiful, nevertheless more numerous than those that are institutionally based.

Furthermore, the stories selected for this paper were purposely chosen from the community level on account of two factors: that health reform promotes—at least in rhetoric—community rather than institutional care, and that seniors themselves prefer to remain in the community for as long as possible. It is important to note that while there are many examples of community-based programs for seniors, the vast majority of them have not been evaluated with any sort of rigour. Moreover, community programs for seniors have only started to be developed recently, so in many cases there has not been enough time to judge their long-term effects. The examples provided here not only support the notion that community programming with seniors can be effective, but also that it has longer-lasting effects.

POLICY IMPLICATIONS

This paper has not focused on the health care system. Instead, it has emphasized nonmedical factors that affect health. However, the health care system is relevant if many of the factors discussed here are to bear fruit. As others have argued, the overall decline in mortality evidenced in the industrialized world in this century cannot be attributable to advances in medicine.[3] Both the introduction of specific medical measures and the expansion of medical services tended to occur after the major advances in the health of the population were made, advances that can be attributed both to public health measures, and to an increased standard of living. Furthermore, the increasing numbers of elders (those aged 65 and over) are not causing the general increase per se in health care costs, despite the alarmist language used by many. Rather, there has been an increased medical servicing of seniors within our society without clear evidence that this increased servicing by clinicians is leading to better quality of life. In fact, there is reason to believe (Markides 1990; Verbrugge 1984) that the years being added to life are primarily years of illness and disability. That is not to say that increased servicing is not always appropriate; however, the measure of the adequacy of the intervention should be the quality of life of the individual. The critical question here is whether the health care system is, in Evans' terms (1989), simply assisting people to take longer to die or whether there is real benefit to these interventions.

There is general consensus that the greatest improvements in human health in the near future will come from healthier lifestyles and changed environments rather than from biomedicine. This includes smoking cessation, dietary improvement, exercise and stress management (Taylor and Voivodas 1987). The point to emphasize is that, even if individual choices concerning lifestyle and the societal structure in which people live are changed in ways that improve people's well-being and health, but the medical care system continues to escalate its medical servicing, there will be no cost savings in formal health care expenditures.

It could be argued that current health reform, with its emphasis on less expensive and more appropriate health care focused on wellness and healthy lifestyles rather than high-tech medicine, is the answer which will incorporate the types of citizen empowerment and community development evident in the success stories described above. After all, the new rhetoric promotes a paradigm that suggests governments should not necessarily relieve families of their traditional caring tasks, that most of the time people can take care of their own needs. This new vision is a rediscovery of community care and informal caregiving. The new rhetoric includes the catchwords of the nineties such as empowerment, citizen or consumer participation, and partnership. At present there is acknowledgment that there are many legitimate players in the health care provider arena, including informal caregivers, social care services, community care services, the volunteer sector and the private

---

3. See, for example, McKinlay and McKinlay (1977) and Barer et al. (1986).

sector—in Europe this is referred to as the mixed economy of welfare (Chappell 1993b).

This is a significant shift. Under the old paradigm, public policy operated largely in ignorance of family care despite the fact that informal caregiving has always contributed the vast majority of care to seniors. The family is not only recognized now, but has become a major cornerstone in the rhetoric of health care reform. And the *rhetoric* of health reform is indeed consistent with the philosophical perspective on the nonmedical determinants of health put forward in this paper and exemplified within the success stories. Unfortunately the rhetoric is far from reality.

In addition, even the rhetoric in many instances lacks an in-depth and realistic understanding of the message. This oversimplification is unlikely to lead to the reform necessary for the creation of the type of health care system promoted by the rhetoric. For example, the new rhetoric argues that Canadians want medical and institutional care to be more efficient, and they want to expand community care and home care so that caregiving is brought closer to home. It rests on the assumption that family care—which is provided primarily by women—is available, and that when such care is not available, the care will be provided by paid professionals. These policies reinforce traditional family values, structures and authorities. To say it another way, the policies do not question why it is women who are primarily the people who provide care, and they do not ask whether this is a just or equitable situation. As Neysmith (1991) and McDaniel and Gee (1993) point out, Canadian policies assume that the family is the correct place for care, and that within the family women are the most appropriate members to provide this care. If, however, women are to be truly free to choose their roles, there must be alternatives to only women providing health care and support. If alternatives are available— whether they involve men or formal agencies being available to provide care— women would be free to choose their participation.

This is not to argue that the values of belonging and sharing and loving are any less important today than they have ever been. But the forms in which we find those values expressed and lived do change. For example, some people spend more time caring for elderly parents today than raising children (Bengtson et al. 1990). There are more single-parent households and one-parent families in absolute numbers and proportionally than in the '50s and '60s, and lesbian relationships appear to be more numerous than they have ever been (or at least more visible). In other words, new forms are emerging for people to live together and to share their lives together. Policies which support only the traditional family structure of husband, wife and children will penalize all the other forms which are becoming more prominent in today's society (Chappell 1993a).

An examination of the gender split in the formally paid workers in the health professions reveals that women are also the primary caregivers in this area. Women far outnumber men in professions such as nursing, social work, homemaking and working in social agencies; in other words, women tend to occupy the roles that have a nurturing component. The occupations dominated by women are not at the apex of power among health professions; physicians wield that power and they still tend to be males. While today a far greater number of women become physicians, and the power structure within that profession is being realigned, women physicians still hold the most powerless positions (Riska 1993), and tend to be at the bottom of the hierarchy within the medical profession. This fact has been demonstrated in England, the U.S. and Norway (Elston 1993; Lorber 1993; Riska and Wegar 1993). While female physicians no longer face the formal discrimination which denied them access to medical schools or residences in the past, they do not occupy the top positions. They are rarely the heads of large prestigious services or of large teaching hospitals or medical centres. They experience a 'glass ceiling' in their upward mobility, being kept down by subtle and informal processes, but no longer by explicit legal barriers. All of the studies cited found that female physicians tend to be in general practice, family practice, and primary care without the same types of occupational autonomy and powers enjoyed by male physicians.

The rhetoric for more appropriate social and community care is particularly relevant for women because it calls for more informal caregiving (done largely by women especially wives and daughters) and more formal health care workers (expansion in any sector other than physicians means expansion in the female-dominant jobs). At present, these positions in the community (outside of the institutions, particularly hospitals) are less expensive than institutional care partly because they are staffed largely by women who do not have much formal educational training, who are not unionized, and who frequently do not work on a full-time basis and therefore do not receive benefits. If community care is expanded on the backs of these women without changing the circumstances in which they work, it will be at the expense of greater burden on both the shoulders of informal caregivers and community care workers.

Health reform rhetoric, in addition, does not clearly distinguish between community care and family care, yet this distinction is critical and especially relevant for women. More of a focus on community care may or may not mean more family or informal care. In some situations, it is preferable for both family members and the person who is ill or disabled to remain apart. All the recent attention on child sexual and physical abuse, spouse abuse, and elder abuse should highlight the dangers of simply encouraging families to stay together no matter what. Said differently, if informal care is given unwillingly, it loses its emotional warmth and affection. Few would argue in this instance that it is superior to formal care. Is there enough knowledge available to prevent people from encouraging families in situations which may be abusive, or may lead to abuse if the situation continues?

While the rhetoric argues for more community care and politicians everywhere are now recognizing informal caregivers, it is not clear what this means. It could be interpreted as a plea for family and friends to do more. However, as noted earlier, informal caregivers have always been the mainstay of care for seniors throughout history, providing between 75 percent and 80 percent of all personal care irrespective of whether the country in question has a comprehensive universal health care system or not (Chappell 1993b). Indeed, the issues involved in the relationships between the two are not even being raised. Part of the issue for home care is that it provides assistance with activities of daily living which represent an area of overlap with the informal care system and with self-care. This is where friends and family provide assistance when an individual cannot cope entirely on his own. In Canada, home care and other community services are not considered part of universal health care. The discussion over the legitimacy of home care is still apparent (see below on current actions). Research, however, has shown again and again that seniors and their families are likely to use home care services only very judiciously, and that the provision of home care services to these individuals and families does not lead to a "dumping of care" onto the formal system; rather, it helps informal caregivers maintain their assistance and prevent burnout.[4]

The relevance of these assumptions becomes obvious in light of what has actually been happening in health care reform in the recent past. Consistent with the rhetoric urging a shift from medical and institutional care, there is evidence throughout Canada (and throughout the industrialized world) of earlier discharges from hospital, closure of hospital beds, moratoria on additional long-term care beds, lower enrollment into medical schools, etc. There is also a shift from inpatient to outpatient services being offered through acute care hospitals. For example, in Toronto nearly 80 percent of surgeries are now performed on a day surgery basis (Deber and Williams 1995). A corresponding extension of community care services is not evident, however. Instead, Manitoba's world-renowned health care system is being cut back, Nova Scotia was just starting to provide home care when the cutbacks came, and in B.C., homemaking-only services have been cut from community services. The rhetoric is being used to put caps on the monies going to medicine and hospitals (without seeing major decreases in these areas), but a strengthening of the community care system is not apparent.

However, the transformation occurring in medicine and in acute care hospitals means that individuals who are sicker and who require short-term intensive servicing are being returned to the community, which puts additional pressure on the community care system. Yet the resources (whether in terms of dollars to hire additional staff or to provide training for current staff who were never hired to provide the types of intensive servicing they

---

4. See Chappell (1992) for a review.

are now being asked to provide) are not forthcoming. Furthermore, the types of cuts occurring in community home care systems take *social services* out of the system, leaving behind a medically oriented support system for the medical care being received in physician offices and in hospitals. The latest B.C. cut which resulted in the "homemaking-only"service being taken off B.C.'s community home support service list is a prime example. Social care is being deemed ineligible, rather than medical support. (This trend also occurred in the U.S. a few years earlier with the introduction of DRGs.) The community care system is not being supported, but is being forced to become more medicalized.

A very important question at the present time is whether or not community care is going to be extended, or whether the new rhetoric is simply being used to shift a greater burden onto families and onto women. In order to have a more appropriate and cost-effective health care system, resources and decision-making powers must be shifted away from the medical pharmaceutical complex and the acute care institutional complex as it exists today. It is essential that both resources and decision-making powers are enhanced at the grassroots level both within community care settings and among citizens.

The success stories presented in this paper demonstrate that in fact there are strategies which can be used to enhance the health and quality of life of seniors, indeed of very frail and disenfranchised seniors. Walker (1995) argues that the frail and vulnerable can be assured of influence and power over service provision only if their advocates are guaranteed a voice in the organization and management of services. This user-centred or empowerment approach aims to involve users in the development, management and operation of services, as well as in the assessment of need. Seniors with mental incapacities must be represented by independent advocates. Usually little attention is paid to who participates in "public consultation", and who becomes politicized. To assume that local interest groups represent the general public is rarely accurate. Consumer groups who speak up are frequently are dominated by the elderly who are in relatively good health and who want good aging-in-place services, as well as seniors living with disabilities, who exempt themselves from the process. The belief that there is one consumer voice or one view which represents *the* seniors community is misleading. The rhetoric does not even admit to a diversity of views.

The narrower strategies presented in this paper worked, and it should be recognized that they involved the grassroots within local communities, which was no doubt a major reason for their success. The broader, more comprehensive strategies also worked. In all instances, women, men, the physically frail, and subcultural minorities were involved.

The perspective and the success stories outlined here suggest that the rhetoric of health reform should indeed be implemented. Within the shift towards a more appropriate health care system, there must be support and resources for truly empowering citizens. The educational process emerges as key to this strategy. Education in any of its guises is critical (whether it's self-education, didactic, interactional, for credit, not for credit, etc.). Rather, individuals must have the capacity to search out and attain information. They must possess the thinking and analytic skills to ferret through that information so they can decide for themselves the choices they wish to make. But governments also have a role in ensuring equitable opportunity, standard setting, and monitoring. Governments, however, must play their roles without their agents usurping power and decision making from the citizens. The promise of health promotion and community development lies in its mediating role between people and their environment, allowing people to synthesize personal choice and social responsibility in health. While much can go awry in implementing policy, good policy is nevertheless a necessary, if insufficient, condition for improving health.

SPECIFIC SUGGESTIONS

From the discussions in this paper, it is obvious that significant changes must be made in the current health care system in order to both free up resources for an expanded community care system, and also to ensure that the appropriate roles are assumed for medicine and the other specializations within a comprehensive health care system. Many suggestions can be made, including:

- Creating an expert panel/council that has the credibility and acceptance to pass judgement on a variety of medical interventions. This panel should include researchers (epidemiologists, health sociologists, as well as clinical researchers), and should work by forming subcommittees or working groups whose members vary depending on the type of intervention being considered. The task of the panel would be to validate medical intervention for reimbursement within the health care system only for those services that have proven beneficial. Those which cause no harm but have not been proven beneficial should not be included. This panel should make evidence-based decisions instead of decisions that bow to political or interest group pressures;
- Removing obvious conflicts of interest within the current medical care system. For example, either physicians should be forbidden from having business/monetary interests in medical laboratories and drug companies, or they should be forbidden by law to have a clinical practice that has anything to do with their monetary interests;
- Scrapping the fee-for-service system for physicians. The scare tactics used recently suggesting that physicians in Canada will all move to the U.S. are unwarranted. Many physicians and many big businesses in the U.S. are now arguing for a system more similar to Canada's because businesses say that their obligations to contribute to employer-employee

health plans are making them uncompetitive, and physicians are finding the overhead costs of having to employ specialized personnel who understand the frequently inconsistent and conflicting rules from the various insurance companies time consuming and frustrating;

- Ensuring governments decide that physicians must practice in areas where their services are needed, particularly since the public purse provides the vast majority of medical education;

- Ensuring that physicians learn only medicine rather than being trained from a broader perspective. A host of other specialties including alternative medicines should be viewed as legitimate players within the system. The current practice of many insurance schemes, where a policy-holder is reimbursed for visiting a nonphysician health care worker only when referred by a physician (for example, a physiotherapist or a social worker), should be terminated. Such practice promotes use of the most expensive service within the system, namely physicians; and

- Enacting policies such as reference-based pricing currently being implemented within Pharmacare in B.C. throughout the country in order to stop unjustified increases in the cost of medications. Under such a policy, expert panels decide whether a reference drug exists for a classification of drugs which is just as effective and with no more side-effects than more expensive drugs. Pharmacare reimburses to the cost of this drug, unless a more expensive drug is medically indicated. It is incumbent on medical schools and medical associations to ensure continuing education of physicians in this country and, in particular, to take a strong position against the "detail" men who are the salesmen for the pharmaceutical firms. Medical education should also ensure a greater appreciation for research and aggregate findings on the clinician's part, and a more circumspect and realistic view of their individual clinical experience with patients.

These are only a few examples of a host of specific actions that could be taken. Outside of the Medicare arena, there are many recommendations that warrant action. These include:

- Governments must ensure that the social care component of their home care/home support programs is not curtailed, leaving only medical support within the community;

- Funding must be available for grassroots developments such as the *Support Services to Seniors Program* in Manitoba. While these programs should be accountable, they should be no more accountable than physicians or hospitals;

- Health implications in other jurisdictions must be examined explicitly, in a manner similar to environmental impact studies;

- Resources should be provided to communities for grassroots devel-opment, but these projects must be reviewed. Those that are successful should be continued, and those that are not should be cut. The variety of health councils and health boards that are being formed through the process of regionalization in order to broaden the base of decision-making power for the allocation of health dollars must not be controlled by the old vested interests of physicians and hospitals;

- Appropriate training and career paths for nonphysician health workers must be examined; and
- A major commitment with resources must be made to build a proper community support system.

Neena L. Chappell *is a professor of sociology and the first director of the Centre on Aging at the University of Victoria (1991–). She was also the founding director of research of the Centre on Aging at the University of Manitoba. She has written more than 150 academic articles and reports, authored books and spoken extensively on health, health care policy, and formal and informal caregiving relevant to seniors. She is an editorial board member of the* Journal of Aging and Ethnicity, *the* Canadian Journal of Sociology, *the* Journal of Aging Studies, *the* Journal of Applied of Gerontology, *the* Journal of Gerontology, Sociological Inquiry, Social Sciences, *and* The Gerontologist.

BIBLIOGRAPHY

ANTONOVSKY, A. 1967. Social class, life expectancy and overall mortality. *Milbank Memorial Fund Quarterly* 41: 31.

ANTONUCCI, T. C. 1990. Social supports and social relationships. In *Handbook of Aging and the Social Sciences*, eds. R. H. BINSTOCK and L. K. GEORGE. New York (NY): Academic Press.

BARER, M. L., R. G. EVANS, C. HERTZMAN, and J. LOMAS. 1986. *Toward Effective Aging: Rhetoric and Evidence*. Paper presented at the 3rd Canadian Conference on Health Economics, Winnipeg, Manitoba.

BENGTSON, V., C. ROSENTHAL, and L. BURTON. 1990. Families and aging: Diversity and heterogeneity. In *Handbook of Aging and the Social Sciences*, eds. R. H. BINSTOCK and L. K. GEORGE. San Diego (CA): Academic Press.

BERGER, K. S. 1983. *The Developing Person Through the Life Span*. New York (NY): Worth Publishers, Inc.

BERKMAN, L. F. 1984. Assessing the physical health effects of social networks and social support. *Annual Review of Public Health* 5: 413–432.

BLANDFORD, A. A., N. L. CHAPPELL, and S. MARSHALL. 1989. Tenant resource coordinators, an experiment in supportive housing. *The Gerontologist* 29(6): 826–829.

BRANCH, L. G., R. F. COULAM, and Y. A. ZIMMERMAN. 1995. The PACE evaluation: Initial findings. *The Gerontologist* 35(3): 349–359.

BROWN, E. R. 1991. Community action for health promotion: A strategy to empower individuals and communities. *International Journal of Health Services* 21(3): 441–456.

CANADIAN STUDY OF HEALTH AND AGING, MULTIPLE AUTHORED. 1994. The Canadian Study of Health and Aging: Study methods and prevalence of dementia. *Canadian Medical Association Journal* 150(6): 899.

CENTRE ON AGING, UNIVERSITY OF MANITOBA AND WESTARC GROUP INC. 1991. *Review of the Support Services to Seniors Program, Manitoba Health*. Final Report.

CHAPPELL, N. L. 1992. *Social Support and Aging*. Toronto: Butterworths.

_____. 1993a. Implications of shifting health care policy for caregiving in Canada. *Journal of Aging and Social Policy* 5(1 and 2): 39–55.

_____. 1993b. The future of health care in Canada. *Journal of Social Policy* 22(4): 487.

CHAPPELL, N. L., and A. A. BLANDFORD. 1991. Informal and formal care: Exploring the complementarity. *Ageing and Society* 11: 299.

CHAPPELL, N. L., L. A. STRAIN, and A. A. BLANDFORD. 1986. *Aging and Health Care, A Social Perspective*. Toronto (ON): Holt, Rinehart and Winston.

D'ARCY, C. 1986. Unemployment and health: Data and implications. *Canadian Journal of Public Health* 77 (Suppl.1).

_____. 1989. Reducing inequalities in health: A review of literature. In *Knowledge Development for Health Promotion: A Call for Action*. Health Services and Promotion Branch Working Paper HSPB 89–2, 11–21. Ottawa: Minister of Supply and Services Canada.

DEAN, K. 1991. Relationships between knowledge and belief variables and health maintenance behaviours in a Danish population over 45 years of age. *Journal of Health and Aging* 3(3): 386–406.

DEBER, R. B., and A. P. WILLIAMS. 1995. Policy, payment, and participation: Long-term care reform in Ontario. *Canadian Journal on Aging* 14(2): 294–318.

DEFRIESE, G. H., A. WOOMERT, and P. A. GUILD. 1989. From activated patient to pacified activist: A study of the self-care movement in the United States. *Social Sciences and Medicine* 29: 195–204.

DER-MCLEOD, D., and J. HANSEN. 1992. On Lok: The family continuum. *Generations* 17(3): 71–72.

DRIEDGER, L., and N. L. CHAPPELL. 1987. *Aging and Ethnicity: Toward an Interface*. Toronto (ON): Butterworths.

ELSTON, M. A. 1993. Women doctors in a changing profession: The case of Britain. In *Gender, Work and Medicine—Women and the Medical Division of Labour*, eds. E. RISKA and K. WEGAR. London: SAGE Publications Ltd.

EVANS, R. G. 1989. Reading the menu with better glasses: Aging and health policy research. In *Aging and Health: Linking Research and Public Policy*, ed. S. J. LEWIS. Chelsea (MI): Lewis Publishers, Inc. pp. 146–167.

EVANS, R. G., and G. L. STODDART. 1990. Producing health, consuming health care. *Social Science and Medicine* 31: 1347–1363.

FARRANT, W. 1991. Addressing the contradictions: Health promotion and community health action in the United Kingdom. *International Journal of Health Services* 21(3): 423–439.

GRACE, V. 1991. The marketing of empowerment and the construction of the health consumer: A critique of health promotion. *International Journal of Health Services* 21(2): 329–343.

GREEN, L. W., and M. W. KREUTER. 1990. Health promotion as a public health strategy for the 1990s. *Annual Review of Public Health* 11: 319–34.

HERTZMAN, C. 1994. The lifelong impact of childhood experiences: A population health perspective. *Daedalus, Journal of the American Academy of Arts and Sciences* 123(4):167–180.

HOLMAN, H., P. MAZONSON, and K. LORIG. 1989. Health education for self-management has significant early and sustained benefits in chronic arthritis. *Trans Association of American Physicians* 102: 204–208.

HOUSE, J., K. R. LANDIS, and D. UMBERSON. 1988. Social relationships and health. *Science*, 241(July 29): 540–545.

KANE, R.L. 1990. Introduction. In *Improving the Health of Older People: A World View*, eds. R.L. KANE, J.G. EVANS, and D. MACFADYEN. New York (NY): Oxford University Press. pp. 341–345.

KANE, R. A. and R. L. KANE. 1985. The feasibility of universal long-term care benefits. *New England Journal of Medicine* 312:1357.

KATZMAN, R. 1993. Education and the prevalence of dementia and Alzheimer's disease. *Neurology* 43: 13–20.

KICKBUSCH, I. 1984. *Health Promotion: A Discussion Document on the Concept and Principles*. WHO discussion document. Health Promotion Programme, World Health Organization.

_____. 1989. Healthy cities: A working project and a growing movement. *Health Promotion* 4(2): 77–82.

LACKEY, A. S., R. BURKE, and M. PETERSON. 1987. Healthy communities: The goal of community development. *Journal of the Community Development Society* 18(2): 1–17.

LALONDE, M. 1974. *A New Perspective on the Health of Canadians*. Health and Welfare Canada.

LAU, R. R. 1982. Origins of health locus of control beliefs. *Journal of Personality and Social Psychology* 42: 322–334.

LENEKER, S. L., K. LORIG, and D. GALLAGHER. 1984. Reasons for the lack of associations between changes in health behaviour and improved health status: An explanatory study. *Patient Education and Counselling* 6: 69–72.

LORBER, J. 1993. Why women physicians will never be true equals in the American medical profession. In *Gender, Work and Medicine: Women and the Medical Division of Labour*, eds. E. RISKA and K. WEGAR. Newbury Park (CA): Sage Publications. pp. 27–61.

LORIG, K., P. FEIGENBAUM, C. REGAN, E. UNG, and H. R. HOLMAN. 1986. A comparison of lay-taught and professional-taught arthritis self-management courses. *The Journal of Rheumatology* 13(4): 763–767.

LORIG, K., and H. HOLMAN. 1989. Long-term outcomes of an arthritis self-management study: Effects of reinforcement efforts. *Social Science and Medicine* 29: 221–224.

_____. 1993. Arthritis self-management studies: A twelve-year review. *Health Education Quarterly* 20: 17–28.

LORIG, K., D. LUBECK, R. G. KRAINES, M. SELEZNICK, and H. R. HOLMAN. 1985. Outcomes of self-help education for patients with arthritis. *Arthritis and rheumatism* 28(6): 680–685.

LUBBEN, J. E., P. G. WEILER, and I. CHI. 1989. Health practices of the elderly poor. *American Journal of Public Health* 79: 731–34.

LURIE, A., R. KALISH, D. WEXLER, and R. ZAWADSKI. 1976. *Highlights from the Evaluation Report of On Lok Senior Health Services: Evaluation of a Success.* On Lok Senior Health Services, San Francisco (CA).

MANITOBA HEALTH. 1992. *Quality Health for Manitobans—The Action Plan; A Strategy to Assure the Future of Manitoba's Health Services System.* Winnipeg (MB): Manitoba Health.

MARKIDES, K.S. 1990. Trends in the health of the elderly in western societies. Paper presented at the annual meeting of the International Sociological Association, World Congress, Madrid, Spain.

MARMOT, M.G. 1994. Social differentials in health within and between populations. *Daedalus, Journal of the American Academy of Arts and Sciences* 123(4): 197–216.

MARMOT, M. G., M. KOGEVINAS, and M. A. ELSTON. 1987. Social economic status and disease. *Annual Review of Public Health* 8: 111.

McDANIEL, S. A., and R. M. GEE. 1993. Social policies regarding caregiving to elders: Canadian contradictions. *Journal of Aging and Social Policy* 5(1 and 2): 57–72.

McGOWAN, P. 1994. *Arthritis Self-Management Program National Implementation: Evaluation of Impact on Participants' Health Status.* The Arthritis Society National Office.

McKINLAY, J. B., and S. M. McKINLAY. 1977. The questionable contribution of medical measures to the decline of mortality in the United States in the twentieth century. *Health and Society* (summer): 405–428.

MILLER, J. 1991. *Community-Based Long-Term Care: Innovative Models.* Newbury Park: Sage Publications.

MINKLER, M. 1996. Empowerment of the elderly in San Francisco's Tenderloin district. In *Society and Health: Case Studies*, eds. AMICK and RUDD. Mass: Harvard University Press.

MINKLER, M., S. FRANTZ, and R. WECHSLER. 1982–1983. Social support and social action organizing in a "gray ghetto": The Tenderloin experience. *International Journal of Community Health and Education* 3(1): 3–15.

MOORE, E. G., and M. ROSENBERG. 1995. *Population Health among Canada's Elderly: Sociodemographic and Geographic Perspectives.* NHRDP.

NEYSMITH, S. M. 1991. Closing the gap between health policy and the home care need of tomorrow's elderly. *Canadian Journal of Community Mental Health* 8(2): 141–150.

ONTARIO PREMIER'S COUNCIL ON HEALTH STRATEGY. 1991. *Nurturing Health: A Framework on the Determinants of Health.* Healthy Public Policy Committee.

PENNING, M. J., and N. L. CHAPPELL. 1993. Age-related differences. *Canada's Health Promotion Survey 1990: Technical Report.* Minister of Supply and Services, Health and Welfare Canada.

PENNING, M. J., A. A. BLANDFORD, and N. L. CHAPPELL. 1991. *Outcome Evaluation of the "Discover Choices" Community Program, Final Report.* Centre on Aging, University of Manitoba.

PITTAWAY, E. D., and E. GALLAGHER. 1995. *Services for Abused Older Canadians.* Victoria: Ministry of Health and Ministry Responsible for Seniors.

RISKA, E. 1993. The medical profession in the Nordic countries. In *The Changing Character of the Medical Profession: An International Perspective*, eds. F. HAFFERTY and J. McKINLAY. Oxford University Press.

RISKA, E., and K. WEGAR. 1993. Women physicians: A new force in medicine? In *Gender, Work and Medicine: Women and the Medical Division of Labour*, eds. E. RISKA and K. WEGAR. Newbury Park (CA): Sage Publications. pp. 27–61.

SHAPIRO, S., and R. TATE. 1988. Who is really at risk for institutionalization? *The Gerontologist* 28: 237–245.

SHAW, W. F. 1995. *Tenderloin Senior Organizing Project Evaluation*. Shaw International Associates.

SPIRDUSO, W. W. 1995. *Physical Dimensions of Aging*. Champaign (IL): Human Kinetics.

STEPHENS, T., and D. F. GRAHAM. 1993. *Canada's Health Promotion Survey 1990: Technical Report*. Ottawa: Ministry of Supply and Services Canada.

STRAIN, L. A., and N. L. CHAPPELL. 1989. Social networks of urban native elders: A comparison with non-natives. *Canadian Ethnic Studies* 21: 104–117.

SYME, S.L. 1994. The social environment and health. *Daedalus, Journal of the American Academy of Arts and Sciences* 123(4): 79–86.

TAYLOR, H., and G. VOIVODAS. 1987. *The Bristol-Myers report: Medicine in the next century*. Louis Harris for the Bristol-Myers Company.

TONES, B. K. 1986. Health education and the ideology of health promotion: A review of alternative approaches. *Health Education Research* 1(1): 3–1.

VERBRUGGE, L. M. 1984. Longer life but worsening health? Trends in the health and mortality of middle-aged and older persons. *Milbank Memorial Fund Quarterly* 62: 475–519.

_____. 1988. Unveiling higher morbidity for men: The story. In *Social Structures and Human Lives*. M. W. RILEY (Ed.). Newbury Park (CA): Sage Publications.

WALKER, A. 1995. The future of long-term care in Canada—A British perspective. *Canadian Journal on Aging* 14(2): 437–446.

WALLSTON, K. A., B. S. WALLSTON, and R. DEVELLIS. 1978. Development of the multidimensional health locus of control (MHLC) scales. *Health Education Monographs* 6: 160–170.

WECHSLER, R., and M. MINKLER. 1986. A community-oriented approach to health promotion: The Tenderloin senior outreach project. In *Wellness and Health Promotion for the Elderly*. ed. K. DYCHTWALD. Rockville (MD): Aspen Publishers. pp. 301–312.

WESCOTT, G., P. SVENSSON, and H. F. K. ZOLLNER. 1985. *Health Policy Implications of Unemployment*. World Health Organization. Copenhagen: World Health Organization.

WILKINSON, R. G. 1994. The epidemiological transition: From material scarcity to social disadvantage? *Daedalus, Journal of the American Academy of Arts and Sciences* 123(4): 61–77.

WNUK-LIPINSKI, E., and R. ILLSLEY. 1990. Introduction. *Social Science and Medicine* 31: 833–836.

WORLD HEALTH ORGANIZATION. 1984. *Health Promotion: A discussion document on the concept and principles*. Working Group on Concept and Principles of Health Promotion.

YEE, D. 1980. On Lok senior health services: Community-based long term care. *Aging* (July–Aug. 319–320): 26–30.

YORDI, C. L., and J. WALDMAN. 1985. Consolidated model of long-term care: Service utilization and cost impacts. *The Gerontologist* 25(4): 389–397.

ZIMMER, Z. and N. L. CHAPPELL. 1994. Mobility restriction and the use of devices among seniors. *Journal of Aging and Health* 6(2): 185.

Promoting Active Living and Healthy Eating among Older Canadians

SANDRA O'BRIEN COUSINS, M.P.E., ED.D.

Faculty of Physical Education and Recreation
University of Alberta

SUMMARY

Understanding the broad social determinants of better eating and more active living are considered to be key pieces of the puzzle of healthy aging. Healthy eating and active living are essential partners in health promotion and disease prevention among older Canadians. Indeed, both are essential to survival and quality of life in old age; without adequate food and adequate mobility, older people succumb rapidly to chronic disease, a need for daily care, and early death. Food security and active living vary considerably according to the broad social determinants of health: economic disparity, education, self-worth, social support networks and physical environment. Canadians most likely to be lacking access to good food and adequate physical activity are elderly women who have low incomes and are socially or geographically isolated. Without financial resources and personal skills, without first-hand knowledge of the benefits, and without a supportive and accessible environment, healthy eating and active living are not available and realistic choices for many older Canadians.

The following table summarizes the five broad determinants of health, their scientific application, and their implications for policy.

Table 1
Broad health determinants

Broad health determinant	Scientific application	Policy implication
Income disparity	Create economic incentives and improve efficacy to take action.	Healthy choices need to be easy to make and affordable.
Education	Outcome expectations must be positive. Positive attitudes about the behaviour and knowledge about the benefits are needed through first-hand experience with the action.	Increase knowledge about the benefits. Improve skills through first-hand experience with health promotion professionals and consultants free to target populations.
Social network	Encouragement, companionship and social support facilitate health and healthy actions.	Access food and activity programs in social settings; promote networks of support in communities which bring older adults together for the purposes of promoting health.
Physical environment	Physical and structural supports facilitate action.	Food services, recreation facilities and supportive experts must be accessible and affordable to older adults. Winter transportation to group programs are needed.
Self-worth	Social norms and stereotypes are fostered when individuals are segregated or ghettoized. The meaning of retirement and old age needs re-creation.	Intergenerational systems of support can prevent isolation and promote self-worth. Children's daycare and elderly home care services can be met with intergenerational partnerships.

TABLE OF CONTENTS

FIGURE

LIST OF TABLES

INTRODUCTION

Background

For optimal growth and development in childhood, and for maintaining full function, avoiding disease and for high-quality living throughout life, the stimulation of enjoyable physical activities combined with a satisfying and nutritious diet are basic health requirements for both young and old. Contemporary evidence suggests that a high-variety, high-fibre, low-fat diet with a focus on fruits and vegetables is clearly a significant force in disease prevention. Moreover, nutritional benefits are likely to be most effective in populations such as the elderly, many of whom are currently impoverished.

Similarly, a variety of daily physical activity brings about physical fitness, or an improved ability to adapt to the diverse challenges of everyday living. As with nutrition studies, active living research confirms a strong link to numerous positive health and disease prevention outcomes. Additionally, the impact of exercise on health is most effective when the most sedentary people undertake some physical activity on a regular basis. Thus, both eating and moving adequately have the greatest effect on population health when the behaviour changes occur *with the least affluent members of a society*. The challenge facing policymakers is to ensure that health promotion initiatives have an impact on those who could benefit most—people with little or no education, and people who are marginalized.

Framework

The intent of this report is to focus on elderly Canadians and their active living and healthy eating behaviours in an effort to seek more effective and affordable ways to promote their health. The report is organized around five broad determinants of health: income disparity, education, social network, physical environment, and self-worth. The literature for active living and healthy eating is examined separately in order to tease out the unique relationships of these two components to the broad determinants of health.

Theoretical Support

Theoretical frameworks provide scientific foundations for understanding why economic disparity, education, self-worth, social networks and the physical environment are so important to health. For example, social cognitive theory conceptualizes that the situational environment, personal factors and human agency are reciprocal and interacting determinants of each other. The model described by Bandura (1989) is a triangle of "reciprocal determinism" (figure 1).

Figure 1
Triangle of "reciprocal determinism"

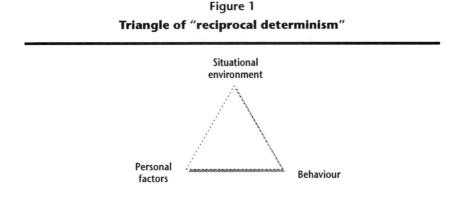

According to social cognitive theory, the environment provides the social and physical situation and events within which a person must function, and thus also provides incentives and barriers to individual behaviours. Certain life situations act as external forces that provide real structural barriers to making healthy choices. For example, when one partner of an elderly square dance couple falls ill, the other partner cannot do that activity anymore. Or, when an elderly man is suddenly widowed, he may not have adequate skills to make his own meals.

In addition to structural barriers, internalized beliefs can act as barriers. Ageist stereotypes, social norms and socialized beliefs can become disempowering forces that lead people to a sense of helplessness, worthlessness and loss of life control. Social cognitive theory predicts healthy human agency will only occur when people:

- Believe that their action will solve a problem or lead to a desired goal;
- Judge they are efficacious or capable of doing the behaviour;
- Expect positive outcomes for their effort;
- Believe that the environment will support their action.

For example, older people with limited income may be unmotivated to pursue healthy behaviours: they may believe that sedentary living is not a threat to their health (belief number 1—value or incentive), and they may judge that eating fresh fruits and vegetables is too expensive for them (belief number 2—efficacy).

Internalized patterns of eating and moving the body are also governed by the social, historical and contextual situation of older Canadians. Having enough to eat to be productive at physical work was a typical concern earlier in this century. Daily exercise was not an issue as many older Canadians engaged in hard physical labour on the job, whether at home or in an employment setting. Therefore, people with this productive work ethic enter retirement without any understanding or skills for healthy leisure-time pursuits. Moreover, eating is no longer as important since food energy is not needed for productivity. Recent research has shown that without feelings of self-worth, without purchasing ability or skills for leisure, without a supportive environment and access to food and activity resources, older Canadians lack motivation to promote their health and ask: "Why bother?" Lacking knowledge, skills, resources, and self-value in contemporary society, it is not surprising that many older Canadians feel that they have little control, and see no point in seeking healthier ways of living.

KEY CONCLUSIONS FROM THE LITERATURE ON ACTIVE LIVING

One hypothesis advanced to explain lack of participation in regular and vigorous exercise, especially among older women, is that "personal and societal barriers or obstacles in the lives of women make it difficult for them to exercise" (Yoshida, Allison, and Osborn 1988, 105). Dishman (1990) documents as many as 44 variables that are possible determinants of active living. Under "personal attributes," education, white-collar occupation, past exercise participation, and perceived good health are positively linked to current activity behaviour. Under "environmental factors," past family influences and school programs are predictive of physically active lifestyles in adulthood (Dishman 1990). In another study, Yoshida and colleagues (1988) report that cost and access to exercise programs, and lack of time due to family and work responsibilities are structural barriers to regular exercise.

Other research suggests that key influences of late life exercise are closely linked to five broad determinants of health: income disparity, education, social network, the physical environment and self-esteem, or self-worth, of older Canadians. The following section presents key conclusions from the scientific literature.

Income Disparity

Being employed, or having good income and higher socioeconomic status are general features of physically active adults (Clark 1995; Health and Welfare Canada 1988). In the 1991 Canada Census of Population and Housing, Norland (1994) reports that "few seniors had no income at all, because old age pension programs in Canada are almost universal" (43). Although 90 percent of all seniors have income of $5,000 to $49,999, 0.8 percent of seniors, or nearly 24,000 older people had no income, and average income for older men and women are highly disparate (see table 2 from Clark 1995). This income disparity focuses attention on the social and health disadvantages facing Canadian women who are significantly affected by "systemic, unearned male advantage" (Phillips 1995, 508).

Table 2
Older Canadian's average annual income by gender

Age	Male	Female	Income ratio
65–69	27,500	14,800	1.85
70–74	24,400	15,400	1.59
75–79	22,100	15,600	1.42
80–84	20,600	15,600	1.32
85+	18,700	15,300	1.22

Source: Clark 1995.

Despite indicators that low-income seniors are less likely to be physically active, there is some evidence to suggest that seniors with high incomes are not necessarily highly active individuals either. For example, Eggers (1988) found that among elderly women, employment status was actually an interference to their physical activity patterns. Other studies have found that health and cultural background are more important than economic status to older adult physical activity (O'Brien Cousins 1993). One interesting point is that major consensus statements about the determinants of physical activity do not even mention financial means as an important barrier to participation (Bouchard, Shephard, and Stephens 1993).

To some degree, older Canadians with low incomes are financially buffered with various forms of pensions and social security that guarantee at least a minimal monthly income. Also, older people with high incomes may purchase recreational services which undermine their physical activity (such as automated golf carts or power boats rather than pullcarts and canoes). Low-income seniors are likely to use walking as a key form of transportation, whereas wealthier seniors tend to use cars. Part of the challenge in studying the impact of financial status on physical activity patterns is the inclination of researchers to focus on the leisure-time activities of well and community-dwelling elderly, who are more likely to have adequate income. The elderly most needing study are least likely to volunteer.

Education

There is strong and consistent evidence that better-educated individuals are more likely to participate in health-promoting forms of physical activity and sport (Clark 1995; Health and Welfare Canada 1988; Yoshida et al. 1988). Rates of physical activity are low among adults with eight or fewer years of education even while accounting for differences in income, health, functional status, body mass and chronic disease (Clark 1995). With income and health already accounted for, it is not clear what features of being more educated relate to prospects for increased physical activity. Clark (1995) surmises that "perhaps due to stress from limited resources and poorer health, older persons with limited education appear to place somewhat less emphasis on physical activity" (479).

Increased opportunities for sport and recreation may occur with higher education, thereby increasing skills and knowledge about the beneficial side of being more active. Another possibility is that, with higher forms of education, people learn how to learn, raise their awareness and self-worth, and improve their literacy skills. Poorly educated adults may have literacy problems which make the reading and understanding of health promotion information too challenging. In addition, poorer education tends to lower prospects for social status and good employment income.

Education and the sport opportunities provided in schools, colleges and universities may play a central role in the formation of a lifelong personal efficacy for specific tasks (Clarke 1995). Older people must have a robust sense of personal efficacy to sustain the persevering effort needed to succeed in physical activity, exercise and sport settings. Self-referent perceptions of efficacy are at least partly responsible for the kinds of challenges that people choose to undertake, how much effort they will spend on that activity, and how long they will persevere in the face of obstacles (Bandura 1986, 1989). According to Bandura (1989), "when faced with difficulties, people who are beset by self-doubts about their capabilities slacken their efforts or abort their attempts prematurely and quickly settle for mediocre solutions, whereas those who have a strong belief in their capabilities exert greater effort to master the challenge" (1176).

Self-efficacy, the belief that one is able to perform a specific activity, is the most powerful correlate of adult walking (Hofstetter et al. 1991). Efficacy in physical activity settings is enhanced by experience and practice (McCauley, Courneya, and Lettunich 1991) and is generally stronger for males and younger adults (Duda and Tappe 1989).

Social Network and Support

Some literature suggests that having a smaller family size may facilitate leisure-time physical activity (Fishwick and Hayes 1989; Yoshida et al. 1988) while other research suggests that a bigger social network is better for older women's physical activity (Branigan and O'Brien Cousins 1995). Clearly, having social freedom to participate in physical activity is necessary and raises questions about gender issues related to social encouragement and support. Many older women are constrained from their own personal activities by an ill spouse or relative who requires ongoing home caregiving, or the presence of their company at home.

Of particular interest to this topic are the socializing forces or cues that are perceived by older people relative to late life physical activity—perceptions of endorsement versus disapproval, and advocacy versus discouragement for more vigourous forms of active living. In broad terms, these socializing forces reflect the processes of the family and community, as well as the larger views of society. Expectations about how others may view older adult physical activity are important. Social feedback from friends, family and significant others such as physicians can provide positive reinforcement or feelings of embarassment and foolishness (O'Brien Cousins 1995). For women, affiliative benefits have been emphasized as important personal incentives for physical activity involvement (Duda and Tappe 1989).

Historically, older people have learned to conserve their energy for work tasks, and until recently in this century, few people lived to the kind of old age that is common today. The concepts of "active living" and "leisure time" are foreign to many older adults whose living patterns were, by nature, already active and now, in retirement, they consider themselves to be taking a "well-deserved rest" (O'Brien Cousins and Burgess 1992). Role models of active older adults are visible in major Canadian health promotion programs such as *Vitality* and *ParticipACTION*, but most older people lack role models in their own communities and can easily explain older athletes seen in the media as exceptions, fanatics or movie stars.

Having strong social support to exercise in late life is regarded as an important environmental catalyst for older people, since many of them may well experience weakening cues such as:
- disapproval from their spouse (Perusse, LeBlanc, and Bouchard 1988;
- lack of companionship and negative peer interest (Hauge 1973);
- discouragement by the immediate family (McPherson 1982); and, perhaps most importantly,
- inadequate advocacy by physicians (Branigan 1995).

In its more conservative and fragile treatment of the aged body, the medical profession has played a key role in exacerbating negative attitudes toward old age. Rather than advocating modest physical activity as a remedy for aches and pains, general practitioners have had a propensity to advocate rest. Moreover, there is reluctance to make referrals and follow through with the aggressive care awarded to younger patients. Aging becomes "... likened to a worn-out and degenerating body-machine—an affliction for which there seemed to be few remedies" (Vertinsky 1995, 230).

Physical Environment

The present activities of older adults are thought to be a reflection of environmental and structural barriers. For example, about 70 percent of older Canadians claim to be walking and gardening, but less than 20 percent claim to be swimming or cycling (Stephens and Craig 1990). Of all age groups, older adults are more likely to exercise alone (about 60 percent), and at home (40 percent). The reasons for these findings are neither clear, nor likely simple, but a number of situational barriers may be operating.

For example, many older people do not own swimsuits or bicycles; for many, lycra swimsuits and 21-speed dirt bikes are too expensive and beyond their needs. Swimming requires convenient and affordable pool facilities with warm water, private changing facilities with hair dryers, easy steps in and out of the water, and preferably a serene atmosphere with little splashing. Older women feel vulnerable to stares from young people in the locker room and on the pool deck. Further they must be confident about moving in water. Wave pools, competitive swimmers, or boisterous children are not very compatible with the needs of older people pursuing aquatic activity (Etkin 1994). In Canada, few facilities offer the kind of environment conducive to attracting older people on an informal basis. However, aquafit programs for seniors can be highly popular among those older people who enjoy formal structure and group exercise.

Severe Canadian winters are just one of the reasons why so few older people use cycling as a means of transportation and recreation. Physical risk is a serious concern associated with cycling outdoors. Older people fear traffic and the speed needed on roadways, and are not very confident about their balance and reaction time. An additional deterrent is the awareness that sidewalks and roadways have ridges and potholes, and sometimes are icy or wet. To enhance safety, older people need to purchase a bicycle helmet, and then not feel foolish wearing it.

Physical activity becomes less structured and more informal with age (Stephens and Craig 1990). Ironically, people may become more and more independent from supervised exercise at the very life stage when they may feel at increased risk. However, casual participation does provide a degree of personal control over the pace (intensity level) of an activity, and likely reduces perception of risk by removing social pressures to "keep up" (O'Brien Cousins and Burgess 1992).

While many older adults enjoy regular walking regimes, women in particular, are reluctant to walk anywhere in the darkness of night. Mall walking is popular in northern cities where early darkness and long nights are a feature of Canadian winters. Well-lit pathways, even pavement, and sidewalks free of ice and snow are some of the prerequisites that need to be met to ensure that those who brave the outdoors are not at risk of falling or in fear of criminal activity.

Self-Worth and Empowerment

Social scientists have argued convincingly that older people have learned their social roles well. Aging individuals apparently live up to the self-fulfilling prophecy that as they get older they are "less" than they once were—less physically competent (Kuypers and Bengston 1973), less productive (Vertinsky 1995), and less healthy (Statistics Canada 1990). The image of aging held by most North Americans does tend to exaggerate the health, loneliness and financial problems of older persons.

Vertinsky (1995) notes a deepening of negative attitudes towards the physical capabilities of the elderly occurred at the end of the nineteenth century. Definitions of aging as a period of decline, weakness and obsolescence still persist today. Although the majority of older adults do not fit the prevalent stereotypes, in contemplating certain physical activities, they face the serious risk of being accused of not acting their age, or of entering "their second childhood" (Arluke and Levin 1984). The self-worth of older individuals certainly comes into question as they approach the retirement years.

Upon retirement, Canadian society officially requires older people to cease employment, whether they want to or not. Men who enjoy paid employment at age 65 are usually forced to retire anyway. Removing work activity makes them feel powerless and useless, and predictably, their self-worth is dashed. O'Brien Cousins and Janzen (in press) report from focus group interviews that the low self-esteem arising from mandatory retirement undermines older men's motivation for maintaining their health. Mandatory retirement is viewed by many older men as an indication that they are no longer useful to society. When society regards them as no longer useful, older men see no point in trying to promote themselves with better health behaviour.

Similar situations can also happen to older women, some of whom may have just restarted employment after decades of raising their families. In addition, women's retirement is often a long life stage—a life stage as long as 40 years. In Canada, women live on average seven more years than men, and those who reach their nineties find that they have long outlived their husbands, and some of their children too. These situations leave aged women passively existing with no particular roles, and no particular meaning for life. Vertinsky (1995, 223) examined the gendered nature of myths and stereotypes concerning aging and physical activity and explored those social and cultural factors that have historically persuaded aging women to practice "being" old and inactive before "becoming old." "Indeed, it is a paradox that one of the main reasons given in surveys of elderly women for not being more physically active is their declining health and the perception that they are 'too old', while at the same time scientific research increasingly demonstrates that one of the certain benefits of physical activity is health improvement" (Vertinsky 1994, 8).

The main stereotype of aging is one of inevitable decline and disease, a theme that has gone unchallenged by many health professionals even though the profound ability of regular exercise to correct most health problems in late life are well known to medical scientists.

KEY CONCLUSIONS FROM THE LITERATURE ON HEALTHY EATING

Nutritional well-being is an essential component of the health, independence, lifespan and quality of life of older individuals. Diet is related to overall survival in elderly people (Trichopoulou et al. 1995). Enhanced resistance to diseases such as cancer (Rasmussen 1994; Willett 1994), optimal functioning of the brain, and prevention of osteoporosis are all related to adequate diet (McIntosh, Shifflett, and Picou 1989).

Food insecurity is affected by availability, affordability, and accessibility of food (Burt 1993). Individuals who most need meal programs are older, less likely to be married, less well educated, more likely to be renters, and are more likely to be ill and isolated than other seniors (Burt 1993).

Although the majority of older Canadians are in good to excellent health, it is estimated that 85 percent of independently living seniors have one or more chronic conditions that could be improved with better nutrition (Posner, Jette, Smith, and Miller 1993). There is evidence that even the type and amount of dietary carbohydrate can significantly affect the health and lifespan of elderly people (McDonald 1995) and that only a minority of seniors may be meeting the guidelines for key nutrients (Alstad, Osterberg, Steen, and Birkhed 1994).

Canadians over age 65 are more likely than Canadians in any other age group to be eating three regular meals daily (Stephens and Craig 1990), but still, this applies to only 55 percent of older women and 58 percent of older men. About one-third of Canadians over 65 are following the Canada Food Guide—a statistic that tends to be associated with an active lifestyle.

When asked to compare their dietary patterns with those of seven years earlier (1981–1988), reduced consumption of red meat and total calories were most commonly reported among older adults. Women over age 65 reported reducing caloric intake by over 40 percent while men of the same age reduced their intake by 32 percent. Almost 70 percent of women over age 65 were limiting their dietary fat, as were 57 percent of men. Still, peak health risk for obesity peaks in both women and men between the ages of 45 and 64. At 65 years and over, 50 percent of all men and 41 percent of all women are still at risk of future health problems leading to premature death. Fewer seniors than middle-aged Canadians are at risk possibly due to increased activity levels at retirement and to the survival of leaner, healthier individuals.

Inactive Canadians are the least likely to improve their eating habits by reducing consumption of fat, sugar, salt and red meat. The disinclination of inactive Canadians to change their eating behaviours "is consistent with their lower adherence to Canada's Food Guide and their greater consumption of fat and fried foods" (Stephens and Craig 1990, 21).

Undernourishment in recently hospitalized elderly people was found to be a problem in 53 percent of males and 61 percent of females (Mowe,

Bohmer, and Kindt 1994). Lack of income, eating fewer than two meals per day, and eating too few fruits and vegetables were the strongest predictors of inadequate nutrient intake in a Boston study (Posner et al. 1993). Numerous studies indicate that intakes of calcium, protein, iron, vitamins A and C, riboflavin, zinc and thiamine are inadequate for a significant portion of the elderly population (McIntosh et al. 1989), although there is currently some debate about appropriate recommendations for older adults (Wood, Suter, and Russell 1995).

Income Disparity

Factors with the strongest causal impact on food security are income and other financial factors, health conditions, rural setting, and race/ethnicity (Burt 1993; Talbot 1985). Few Canadian seniors are destitute, but there are "pockets of older people, particularly of women and minority group members, whose sparse work histories have placed them in economic jeopardy" (Silverstone 1996, 27). According to *Profile of Canada's Seniors* (Norland 1994), older Canadians spend about 14 percent of their monthly income on food—the third biggest expense after shelter and personal taxes. Some rural families raise most of their own food so that low income has less effect on the their nutritional status.

The relationship of income to health behaviour is not always clear cut. While lower-income adults seem to adopt a more passive approach to their health (waiting for problems to arise), one study found a "general lack of difference existed among people of different SES with respect to food habits, sports and exercise, smoking and alcohol use" (Cockerham, Lueschen, Kunz, and Spaeth 1986). They concluded that a "culture-of-medicine" thesis may be more likely the case than attempting to explain these results from a "culture-of-poverty" perspective.

Among the one million Canadian seniors with disabilities, 47 percent of men and 45 percent of women say they have "excellent" eating habits; almost 50 percent of both groups report "fair to good" eating habits, and 3.7 percent of men and 4.7 percent of women with disabilities report "poor" eating habits (Lavigne and Morin 1991). According to Lavigne and Morin (1991), "eating less food and eating a greater variety of foods are the measures most frequently selected for improving eating habits" (36).

Lavigne and Morin (1991) report on the kinds of changes older Canadians think are important to improve their eating habits, according to income and health status (table 3). Overall, almost 70 percent of seniors gave no response or did not know. Over 12 percent felt they should eat less, and 11 percent wanted more variety. Indeed, beliefs about needed changes in food patterns were not very different among low- and higher-income elderly. The minority of older Canadians in poor health (146,875 people) feel that they need to eat more food, have more variety and eat more regularly, while those reporting excellent health (1,217,655 people) felt they should eat less but with improved variety.

Table 3

Measures to improve eating habits among disabled Canadian seniors

Variable	Eat More	Eat Less	More Variety	Regular Meals	Don't Know
65 + years	4.6%	12.3%	10.7%	3.8%	68.6%
< $10,000	5.4%	15.6%	15.1%	7.3%	56.6%
> $30,000	3.3%	18.2%	18.8%	11.2%	48.5%
Poor health	21.4%	10.9%	22.4%	18.8%	26.5%
Excellent	1.5%	17.4%	9.0%	3.6%	68.6%

Source: Lavigne and Morin 1991.

Education

Younger seniors generally have a better education than older Canadians. Close to one-third of seniors aged 65–69, compared to only 20 percent of 85+ seniors, had a postsecondary education (Norland 1994). Social and cultural contexts that vary by age and education "produce different expectations, perceptions, barriers and priorities regarding health and health behaviour" (Clark 1995, 473). Low levels of education and income tend to form a combination that undermines healthy eating among older people. Less educated people tend to also be compromised financially making the purchase of fresh and attractive food produce more difficult.

Significant relationships have been found between food consumption, food beliefs, and socioeconomic characteristics (Rothenberg, Bosaeus, and Steen 1980). Older individuals, especially those lacking education and good reading skills, could be targeted for free nutrition education programs (Brun and Clancy 1980). Furthermore, older people often need more information and support to take advantage of the many social services already available to them. Homebound people need special assistance to acquire and interpret the forms needed to receive benefits (National Senior Citizens Law Center 1992).

Social Network and Support

Attempting to change health habits is not merely an individual problem, but a group and societal problem. The general hypothesis is that one individual trying to change a health behaviour may be influenced (positively or negatively) by significant others during the course of the change process.

For example, elderly adults with more extensive friendship networks and companionship have better appetite, more protein intake and more calories in their diet (McIntosh, Shifflett, and Picou 1988).

Zimmerman and Connor (1989) studied 116 individual self-reports of health behaviours at baseline and 7 weeks later at the end of a health promotion program. Fifteen to twenty percent of participants strongly agreed that their family, friends and/or coworkers had encouraged them to maintain their health habit change. Behaviours most influenced by others were exercise and fat consumption. For exercise behaviour, encouragement was the only significant interpersonal influence variable. The researchers concluded that "long-term change requires more than education, persuasion, behaviour modification, or occasional follow-up; it requires an environment that is supportive of change, in fact is 'actively' supportive of change" (Zimmerman and Connor 1989, 58). The Zimmerman study highlights the need to study the nature of the support systems for individuals trying to improve their health behaviour.

Physical Environment

Access to food, and its preparation into high-variety meals, is more than a financial consideration; access very much depends on the nature of the physical environment, and the mobility of older individuals within it. Evidence of nutritional risk is found in the number of home-delivered meal services—services which are likely to see an increase in demand (Frongillo, Williamson, Roe, and Scholes 1987). By age 85, 37 percent of men and 50 percent of women have some degree of disability related to mobility, agility, hearing, seeing, and speaking (Norland 1994). Up to 30 percent of seniors rate their current health as only "fair" or "poor." The poor health of many older individuals is compromised further in terms of the difficulties they face in getting to and from the grocery stores, being able to shop "at one stop" (Kassner 1992), being able to make wise food choices from those that are affordable, being able to lift and carry food produce, and being able to prepare food safely.

Healthy eating is a challenge at times even when older adults are well cared for. Gilani (1995) and Molis (1993) have examined the importance of providing appetizing, varied meal selections in retirement communities. Large resident care communities require the preparation of large quantities of food while accommodating older people's varied cultural backgrounds, food preferences, age-related declines in taste and smell, and individual nutritional needs. In addition, elderly people who are members of a minority group may find that the only food available to them does not satisfy their taste for the ethnic cuisine they may be used to.

Gilani (1995) reports that the basic strategy is to treat residents with the flexibility and choice of a restaurant rather than same-for-everyone meals more typical of a health care setting. For example, the resident council does the planning for holiday menus, considers requests for new items, and proposes special events such as ethnic meals and nonalcoholic cocktail parties. A cooked to order menu, and "homestyle" approach to dining (table spread with food choices) is recommended by Molis (1993). Providing appealing meal selections, compatible individuals at the table, and a comfortable dining atmosphere can boost resident enjoyment, improve mood, and enhance quality of life (Lengyel 1995).

Healthy seniors who live independently may also encounter problems with food security. Little recognition has been given to the role of neighbourhood senior centres where a hot daily meal is often purchased (Ralston 1991). Harsh winter conditions or temporary bouts with illness may prevent independent seniors from travelling to stores or preparing nutritious meals for themselves. Temporary supports need to be examined to assist independently living older adults from entering a downward spiral simply because they are temporarily set back with health problems or seasonal barriers.

Self-Worth and Empowerment

Aging is often referred to as being about losses. Losing control over bodily functions, losing control over the environment, and losing control over mental capacities makes people uncomfortable and nervous. Fear can easily build up in older people, and this can lead to alienation and the shifting of responsibility from themselves to others (Etkin 1994). The way in which older people care for their teeth is a good example of how low self-worth and a sense of finitude can undermine health. Often major dental work goes undone because the expense is great, and older people may not think their teeth are worth the expense. An older person can spend many years not eating well, mainly because of the decision they made to stop fixing their teeth.

Older people may shun service programs aimed at healthier eating because they do not want to be perceived as a social burden; others may feel that admitting that they are needy of food and better nutrition hints at incompetence and will require them to give up their independent living. Becoming institutionalized is rated as the number one fear among older adults. Yet, a combination of self-care incorporating the basics of healthy eating and an active lifestyle are key elements working in favour of extending independent living.

THE HEALTHY EATING–HEALTHY ACTIVITY CONNECTION

Daily energy expenditure declines progressively throughout adult life in all societies. Under sedentary conditions, the main determinant of energy expenditure is fat-free mass or muscle (Evans and Meredith 1989). In elderly people, most of whom have lost a good deal of their muscle mass through sedentary living, energy intake is remarkably low and tends to be substantially below the recommended dietary allowance (Shephard 1990; Voorips et al. 1991). Nutrition surveys suggest that a typical daily intake for women is only 1400 kcal/day and for men 1850 kcal/day (Evans and Meredith 1989). Declining physical activity partly accounts for the low energy intake, such that in the "oldest old," where disability is prevalent, energy needs are so low as to make it impossible for individuals to obtain adequate nutrition. This leads experts to say: "An increase in activity leading to greater food intake could be the best strategy for reducing the risk of malnutrition in ambulatory elderly people" (Evans and Meredith 1989, 96).

In Canada, the health concern which links eating and activity is obesity; Canadians are significantly *under*active (in terms of expending physical energy), and significantly *over*nourished (in terms of fat intake and total calories). These phenomena should not be divorced from each other in social marketing approaches to disease prevention and health promotion. People seem to think they can eat their way to better health, when in fact their ability to eat is directly limited by their inclination (or disinclination) to move the body. A key conclusion from the literature is that healthy eating and active living are mutually interdependent, and that social marketing and community support of these behaviours should be concurrent.

Although Canadians are facing difficult economic times, food abundance is no longer the issue it was in historical times. Rather the contemporary focus is on "a rainbow of healthy choices" that emphasizes variety and moderation in eating patterns (Bell-Moore 1992).

SUCCESS STORY

A case study on a community-driven health promotion initiative among the elderly poor demonstrates the role of community organizing as a vehicle for enhancing individual and community-level empowerment (Minkler 1992). The 12-year-old *Tenderloin Senior Organizing Project* (TSOP) reflects the World Health Organization definition of health as a means of helping individuals and communities to take increasing control over the factors influencing their health. Through the Project, undernourishment, among other health and social problems, was one of the main community concerns addressed.

Actions on the Nonmedical Determinants of Health

Three theoretical models guided the project: social support theory, Friere's "education for critical consciousness" and community organization theory. The general strategy was to assist the older residents to look for the problem behind the problem.

Student volunteers from the School of Public Health of the University of California, Berkeley, began in a single hotel in the Tenderloin neighbourhood, offering blood pressure screenings and bringing coffee and refreshments as a means of encouraging resident interaction. With the help of these inducements, an informal discussion group was formed which met weekly and included a core of 12 residents and two outside facilitators. As levels of trust and rapport increased, members began to share personal concerns regarding such issues as fear of crime, loneliness, rent increases, and their own sense of powerlessness. The initiative created dissatisfaction with the status quo, and channelled frustration into action. Facilitators helped people identify specific "winnable" issues among the concerns raised.

Among the early issues confronted by several of the elderly hotel groups was the problem of undernourishment and particularly lack of access to fresh fruits and vegetables. Following much discussion of alternative approaches, the residents of three hotels contracted with a local food advisory service and began operating their own hotel-based "minimarkets" one morning per week. In a fourth hotel, residents began running their own hotel-based modest cooperative weekly breakfast program, thereby qualifying their hotel for participation in a food bank where large quantities of food could be purchased in bulk at reduced prices.

Reasons for the Initiative

The project was established in the late 1970s with the dual goals of: a) improving physical and mental health by reducing social isolation and providing relevant health education; and b) facilitating through dialogue and participation, a process through which residents were encouraged to work together in identifying common problems, and seeking solutions to these shared problems and concerns. The overall goal was to empower residents to take action customized to their needs.

Actors

The 45-block Tenderloin area in San Francisco, California, is one of the most notorious neighbourhoods in the U.S., housing some 8,000 elderly men and women, a similar number of Indo-Chinese refugees, and smaller numbers of ex-offenders, substance abusers, and former mental health patients. A multiplicity of health problems are common among the elderly residents, including undernourishment, alcoholism, depression and suicide. University students initiated the project.

Analysis of the Results

Over time, decreased reliance on the facilitators was observed. Resident participation broadened in discussion and decision making. Residents within each hotel came to know each other very well, and a common bond was formed among them. They developed strategies to involve the community-at-large in helping solve their problems. For example they started a Safehouse Project which recruited 49 businesses to act as places of refuge from crime. Coalition members convinced the mayor to increase the number of patrolling officers in the neighbourhood, and an 18 percent reduction in crime in the first 12 months was achieved.

TSOP was also engaged in significant leadership training, focusing on small group activities so that residents could improve interpersonal skills and find effective ways to work through bureaucracies to bring about change. They conducted media workshops and met with journalists and reporters who provided advice on how to maximize their efforts through the media.

Replicability of the Initiative

TSOP now works only in hotels whose residents have invited the organization to help them organize and work collectively for change. But the TSOP model lends itself to replication in communities where large numbers of socially isolated individuals live alone in densely populated areas. The TSOP model differs considerably from more traditional health and social service approaches in that the agenda in each discussion group is determined entirely by group members, and not by outside professionals. The TSOP model can be useful in a variety of settings, especially in economically depressed urban areas.

Funding

The project started with student volunteers, and over time was able to obtain a variety of supports, including funding, from the local community and businesses. Foundations provided the bulk of the financial support, but without tangible deliverables for some of the community solutions, new sources of revenue generation are an ongoing concern.

Evaluation

Evaluation of the project was difficult because of inherent distrust of outside researchers. Project staff were committed to avoiding any data-gathering activities that might confuse the residents as to the true mission of the organization. Success was seen in the empowerment of the residents to take action, and to tackle the "problems behind the problem".

POLICY IMPLICATIONS

Broad health determinants such as income disparity, education, social network, physical environment and self-worth are playing important roles in the eating and active living patterns among older Canadians. In reality, these five health determinants have complex interrelationships, but are dealt with more simply in this section to better represent our modest understanding.

Income Disparity

Some of Canada's richest and poorest citizens are seniors. Income disparity is reflected in the aging and health experiences of today's seniors, some of whom die at a young age, while others are robust, healthy and active into their eighties and nineties. In order for Canadians to age more successfully as a group, and being sensitive to the reality of limited funding for social programs, differential treatment targeted at the most vulnerable people is recommended. Burton (1994, 210) states: "paradoxically, equity requires unequal provision of services."

The most vulnerable groups among older Canadians are those over age 70, women, and people who are members of ethnic minorities and is already experiencing health limitations. These social groups are most likely to perceive barriers, lack incentives, and feel least able to engage in healthy eating and active living. These target groups are most likely to benefit from programs which enhance self-confidence, empowerment, and provide financial incentives to participants. Therefore, programs and services which require little knowledge and are enjoyable, culturally meaningful, easy to do and require personal participation are advocated. A local community empowerment approach is most likely to succeed in making these kind of social changes. For all of society, the general policy should be that the healthy choices are the easiest and most affordable choices.

Education

In addition to income, educational level provides another type of social status that alters possibilities for health-promoting behaviour. To compensate the most vulnerable social groups, adult education for late life seniors will be essential. Increasing knowledge, raising awareness, increasing literacy, elevating self-esteem, and building skills are all important elements dependent on education. Seniors need to feel more welcome and able to contribute in all educational settings including colleges and universities where tuition is often waived or nominal.

While most older Canadians will agree that "poor nutrition will affect your health" and "exercise is good for you," these rhetorical phrases are apparently quite meaningless unless seniors know in more detail, and preferably by direct experience, the enormity of the health benefits they can receive. Seniors cannot make informed choices about how to spend their time and resources if they are ignorant of the positive and negative outcomes of certain lifestyles. Moreover, they are less likely to change their behaviour if they do not actively participate in programs for learning new skills for healthy living.

Specific details about the range of health benefits are currently overshadowed by feelings that in old age, it is too late to be promoting health, that buying less expensive, but fattier and lower-fibre foods will not have serious impacts, and that physical activity is not all that necessary. Expected outcomes are unclear; people perceive that a great deal of effort and resources must go into these behaviours, and that health benefits are neither guaranteed nor even likely. The evidence is quite the contrary. Older people can generally expect a good nutritional health return, especially if they maintain a modest level of daily physical activity. Regular walks of about 30 minutes a day (or 10 minutes, three times a day), at a comfortable to brisk pace, combined with some gentle stretches and strengthening exercises, will virtually ensure that most older people will maintain the adequate fitness necessary to live a full and independent lifespan.

Older Canadians dread the prospect of losing their independence. Therefore Canadian seniors need to know that fit and nourished older adults are rarely institutionalized, and if they are, it is only for serious cognitive disorders. Older Canadians will always encounter bouts of illness, but fit and nourished seniors recover more rapidly and have a stronger immune system to ward off illness. Active older people have the benefit of noticing physical problems, and seeking professional help, before these problems become major health issues. Active older people have larger appetites and increase their food intake to levels closer to or exceeding the RDA.

Social Networks and Support

Canadians, while socially considerate of seniors, hold quite low opinions of the elderly. A small proportion of elderly people are ill and frail, but they are the most conspicuous elderly people to the public eye. Myths about aging and negative stereotypes form and are generalized to all older people. While having companionship, having friends, and having family members available are positive factors for health, social networks in themselves do not foster healthy behaviours.

The key to promoting healthy eating and more active lifestyles is to create a supportive and open-minded society in which institutions, communities, families, physicians and friends empower old and aged adults to take an active role in all aspects of life. The community development philosophy advocated by Labonte (1996) is one of local empowerment and citizen action. Encouraging older people to sit back and "take it easy" is an invitation to low-quality living and premature illness. Rather, the preferable social systems advocate older adult agency, self-determination, and taking a proactive stance to late life.

Social systems become most supportive when they view older people as simply older versions of their formerly competent selves. While social supports are effective at local community levels, television, print media, and other forms of entertainment need to attend to the reality of the age wave by presenting realistic images of contemporary aging, and reflecting the actual proportion of older Canadians in the presentations. Without this macro-level support, older Canadians are invisible and marginalized— where is the AGE channel?

Physical Environment

Both healthy eating and active living are more likely to be found in enjoyable social settings, and therefore a general principle to foster these behaviours is to advocate for mechanisms which bring older Canadians together in convivial settings, daily if possible, to enjoy other people, to enjoy some physical activity, and to enjoy a nourishing meal. The evidence suggests that developing transportation supports to bring isolated older people to social settings for health promotion activity would be worth the cost in care savings. The settings might be schools, churches, daycare centres, shopping malls, workplaces, and recreation centres.

Winter is a major barrier to getting out, walking, visiting friends, and replenishing food stocks. Innovative solutions can be found if communities are motivated and creative. In most neighbourhoods, drivers commute to and from work with empty cars. Older people could take advantage of these free shuttles if willing drivers would register their commute times and locations to needy older people. Empowering Canadian communities, both urban and rural, leads to solutions to the isolating effects of geography and climate.

Self-Worth and Empowerment

Canadian society expects little from its older citizens, who are rewarded with pensions for a lifetime of work. In expecting no further contribution from seniors, it could be argued that contemporary Canada ignores the vast wealth of skills and expertise of its oldest members. In expecting so little, perhaps Canada gets little in return. Many older people feel devalued and discon-nected from society because they are forced to retire when they are among the most productive employees available.

Stereotypes about older people are harmful because many seniors live out a self-fulfilling prophecy of being "less than" they are. Institutional settings provide little incentive for older people to maintain their skills, a level of productivity and social utility. Without self-worth, the aged enter a downward spiral in terms of health. Homes for the aged may need to take a stronger role in attempting rehabilitation and reversal of this downward spiral, thereby giving hope to all its residents, and making the last years the best years.

Evidence suggests that intergenerational programs are fruitful means of increasing communication, improving understanding and respect, and creating mutual helping relationships among people of all ages. Segregating seniors into residential communities of their own serves to isolate aging adults further from children, youth, young adults, and maturing families. Integration of multiage communities and intergenerational activities involving healthy physical activity and nutritious eating events can bring older people back into everyone's lives, thereby promoting a healthier situation for all of us.

Sandra O'Brien Cousins *is a professor in the Faculty of Physical Education and Recreation at the University of Alberta. She is a world authority on healthy aging through physical activity. Her research as a social scientist in gerontology and health promotion has captured international interest. She has a prolific research and publication record on motivation and late life exercise that is changing scientific understanding of the barriers to improving older adult health.*

Acknowledgements

A number of national agencies and researchers provided me with samples of their research findings and community "stories." Although most of their stories could not be used in this report, I would like to briefly recognize them here for their support.

The Bernard Betel Centre for Creative Living, North York
Art Burgess, Campus Fitness & Lifestyle, U. of Alberta
Sandra Crowell, Atlantic Health Promotion Research Centre
Ruth Chapple, Canadian Association for Community Care
Stan Dyer, U. of Agers, Edmonton
Norah Keating , Human Ecology, U. of Alberta
Christina Lengyel, Nutrition Studies, U. of Alberta
Marian MacKinnon, U. of P.E.I.
Lydia Makrides, Dalhousie Cardiac Rehabilitation Program
Ethyl Marliss, Alive and Well Program, U. of Alberta
Robert McCulloch, Vice-President's Office, U. of Regina
Arlis McQuarrie, Physical Therapy, U. of Saskatchewan
Anita Myers, Health Studies, U. of Western Ontario

Margaret J. Penning, Centre on Aging, U. of Manitoba
Jenny Shaw, West End Seniors Network, Vancouver
Roy Shephard, Professor Emeritus, U. of Toronto
Catrine Tudor-Locke, The Centre for Activity and Ageing, London
Lita Villalon, Université de Moncton, New Brunswick
Sally Willis, Vancouver General Hospital, U.B.C.

BIBLIOGRAPHY

ALSTAD, T., T. OSTERGERG, B. STEEN, and D. BIRKHED. 1994. Carbohydrate intake in elderly people: cohort and longitudinal comparisons from a population study. *American Journal of Clinical Nutrition* 59(Suppl.): 773S.

ARLUKE, A. and J. LEVIN. 1984. Another stereotype: Old age as a second childhood. *Aging* 346: 7–11.

BANDURA, A. 1986. *Social Foundations of Thought and Action.* Englewood Cliff (NJ): Prentice Hall.

_____. 1989. Human agency in social cognitive theory. *The American Psychologist* 44: 1175–1184.

BELL-MOORE, K. 1992. *A Rainbow of Healthy Choices.* Safeway Nutrition Awareness Program. Ottawa, ON: Minister of Supply and Services, Canada.

BOUCHARD, C., R. J. SHEPHARD, and T. STEPHENS (Eds.). 1994. *Physical Activity, Fitness and Health: International Proceedings and Consensus Statement.* Champaign (IL): Human Kinetics Publishers.

BOWNE, D. W., M. L. RUSSELL, J. L. MORGAN, S. A. OPTENBERG, and A. E. CLARKE. 1984. Reduced disability and health care costs in an industrial fitness program. *Journal of Occupational Medicine* 26: 809–816.

BRANIGAN, K. 1995. Physician advocacy of exercise for older adults. Master's thesis, Edmonton (AB): The University of Alberta. Faculty of Physical Education and Recreation.

BRANIGAN, K., and S. O'BRIEN COUSINS. 1995. Older women and beliefs about exercice risk: What has motherhood got to do with it? *Journal of Women and Aging* 7: 47–66.

BRUN, J. K. and K. L. CLANCY. 1980. Low-income and elderly populations. *Journal of Nutrition Education* 12: 128–130.

BURT, M. R. 1993. *Hunger among the Elderly:Local and National Comparisons: Final Report of a National Study on the Extent and Nature of Food Insecurity among American Seniors.* Washington (DC): Urban Institute.

BURTON, T. 1994. Issues in policy development for active living and sustainable living in Canada. In *Toward Active Living,* eds. H. A.QUINNEY, L. GAUVIN, and A. E. WALL. Champaign (IL): Human Kinetics. pp. 187–212.

CANADIAN FITNESS AND LIFESTYLE RESEARCH INSTITUTE. 1994. Activity reduces the cost of heart disease. *CAHPER Journal* 60: 41.

CARNET. 1994. *Healthy Choices for Healthy Aging.* Toronto: Canadian Aging Research Network.

CLARK, D. P. 1995. Racial and educational differences in physical activity among older adults. *The Gerontologist* 35: 472–480.

COCKERHAM, W. C., G. LUESCHEN, G. KUNZ, and J. SPAETH. 1994. Social stratification and self-management of health. *Journal of Health and Social Behaviour* 27: 1–14.

DAVIS, S. K., M. A. WINKLEBY, and J. W. FARQUHAR. 1995. Increasing disparity in knowledge of cardiovascular disease risk factors and risk reduction strategies by socioeconomic status: Implications for policymakers. *American Journal of Preventive Medicine* 11: 318–323.

DISHMAN, R.K. 1990. Determinants of participation in physical activity. In *Exercise, Fitness and Health: Consensus of Current Knowledge,* eds. C. BOUCHARD, R. J. SHEPHARD, T. STEPHENS, J. R. SUTTON, and B. D. McPHERSON. Champaign (IL): Human Kinetics Publishers. pp. 75–101.

DUDA, J. L. and M. K. TAPPE. 1989. Personal investment in exercise among middle-aged older adults. *Perceptual Motor Skills* 66: 543–549.

EGGERS, J. L. 1988. Well-elderly women's entrance and adherence to structured physical fitness programs. *Activities, Adaptation and Aging* 11: 21–30.

ETKIN, S. E. 1994. Reaching the hard to reach: Active living programs for low socioeconomic individuals. In *Toward Active Living,* eds. H. A.QUINNEY, L. GAUVIN, and A. E. WALL. Champaign (IL): Human Kinetics. pp. 263–268.

EVANS, W. J. 1992. Exercise, nutrition and aging. *Journal of Nutrition* 122: 796–801.

EVANS, W. J., and C. N. MEREDITH. 1989. Exercise and nutrition in the elderly. In *Nutrition, Aging and the Elderly*, eds. H. N. MUNRO and D. E. DANFORD. New York: Plenum. pp. 89–125.

FEINGOLD, R.S. 1994. Making connections: An agenda for the future. *Quest* 46: 356–367.

FIATARONE, M. A., E. F. O'NEILL, N. D. RYAN, K. M. CLEMENTS, G. R. SOLARES, M. E. NELSON, S. B. ROBERT, J. J. KEHAYIA, L. A. LIPSTIZ, and W. J. EVANS. 1994. Exercise training and nutritional supplementation for physical frailty in very elderly people. *New England Journal of Medicine* 330: 1769–1775.

FISHWICK, L. and D. HAYES. 1989. Sport for whom? Differential participation patterns of recreational athletes in leisure-time physical activities. *Sociology of Sport Journal* 6: 269–277.

FRONGILLO, E. A. JR., D. F. WILLIAMSON, D. A. ROE, and J. E. SCHOLES. 1987. Continuance of elderly on home-delivered meals programs. *American Journal of Public Health* 77: 1176–1179.

GILANI, S. 1995. Tempting the tastes of seniors. *Spectrum: National Association for Senior Living Industries* 9: 20–22.

HALL, N., P. DE BECK, D. JOHNSON, K. MACKINNON, et al. 1992. Randomized trial of a health promotion program for frail elders. *Canadian Journal on Aging* 11: 72–91.

HAUG, M. R., M. L. WYKLE and K. H. NAMAZI. 1989. Self-care among older adults. *Social Science and Medicine* 29: 171–183.

HAUGE, A. 1973. The influence of the family on female sports participation. *DGWS research reports: Women in sport*, ed. D.V. Harris, Washington (DC): AAHPER Press.

HEALTH AND WELFARE CANADA. 1988. *Health Promotion Survey: Technical Report*. Ottawa (ON): Minister of Supply and Services.

HOFSTETTER, C., M. HOVELL, C. MACERA, J. SALLIS, V. SPRY, E. BARRINGTON, L. CALLENDER, M. HACKLEY, and M. RAUH. 1991. Illness, injury and correlates of aerobic exercise and walking: A community study. *Research Quarterly for Exercise and Sport* 62: 1–9.

KASSNER, E. 1992. *Falling through the Safety Net: Missed Opportunities for America's Elderly Poor*. Washington (DC): American Association of Retired Persons, Public Policy Institute.

KRETCHMER, N. 1994. Nutrition is the keystone of prevention. *American Journal of Clinical Nutrition* 60: 1.

KUYPERS, J. A. and V. L. BENGSTON. 1973. Social breakdown and competence: A model of normal aging. *Human Development* 16: 181–201.

LABONTE, R. 1996. Community empowerment. Public lecture at the University of Alberta, Edmonton (AB), April 1.

LAVIGNE, M., and J. P. MORIN. 1991. *Leisure and Lifestyles of Persons with Disabilities in Canada*. Ottawa, (ON): Statistics Canada.

LEIGH, J. P., and J. F. FRIES. 1992–1993. Associations among healthy habits, age, gender, and education in a sample of retirees. *International Journal of Aging and Human Development* 36: 139–155.

LENGYEL, C. 1995. There's no place like home. Unpublished research report. Department of Sociology c/o Dr. H. C. Northcott, University of Alberta, Edmonton (AB). December 18.

MCCAULEY, E., K. S. COURNEYA, and J. LETTUNICH. 1991. Effects of acute and long-term exercise on self-efficacy responses in sedentary, middle-aged males and females. *The Gerontologist* 31: 534–542.

MCDONALD, R. B. 1995. Influence of dietary sucrose on biological aging. *American Journal of Clinical Nutrition* 62(Suppl.): 284S.

MCINTOSH, W. A., P. A. SHIFFLETT, and J. S. PICOU. 1989. Social support, stressful events, strain, dietary intake and the elderly. *Medical Care* 27: 140–153.

MCPHERSON, B. D. 1982. Leisure lifestyles and physical activity in the late years of the life cycle. *Recreation Research Review* 9: 5–14.

_____. 1994. Sociocultural perspectives on aging and physical activity. *Journal of Aging and Physical Activity* 2: 329–353.

MEREDITH, C. N., W. R. FRONTERA, K. P. O'REILLY, and W. J. EVANS. 1992. Body composition in elderly men: Effect of dietary modification during strength training. *Journal of the American Geriatrics Society* 40: 155–162.

MINKLER, M. 1992. Community organizing among the elderly poor in the United States: A case study. *International Journal of Health Services* 22: 303–316.

MOLIS, D. B. 1993. Classic cuisine: Innovations in food service. *Provider* 19: 18–22.

MOWE, M., T. BOHMER, and E. KINDT. 1994. Reduced nutritional status in an elderly population (over 70 years) is probable before disease and possibly contributes to the development of disease. *American Journal of Clinical Nutrition* 59: 317–324.

MULLINS, L. C., C. COOK, M. MUSHEL, G. MACHIN, and J. GEORGAS. 1993. A comparative examination of the characteristics of participants of a senior citizens nutrition and activities program. *Activities, Adaptation and Aging* 17: 15–37.

NATIONAL SENIOR CITIZEN'S LAW CENTER. 1992. *Access to Federal Public Benefits Programs by the Elderly.* Washington (DC): American Association of Retired Persons, Public Policy Institute.

NORLAND, J. A. 1994. *Profile of Canadian Seniors: Focus on Canada.* Scarborough (ON): Prentice-Hall Canada, Inc.

O'BRIEN COUSINS, S. 1993. The determinants of late life exercise among women over age 70. Doctoral dissertation, University of British Columbia, Vancouver.

_____. 1995. Social support for exercise among elderly women in Canada. *Health Promotion International* 10: 273–282.

O'BRIEN COUSINS, S. and W. JANZEN. In press. Lay beliefs of older adults regarding exercise. In *Exercise, Aging and Health.* Washington (DC): Taylor and Francis.

O'BRIEN COUSINS, S. and A. C. BURGESS. 1992. Perspectives on older adults in physical activity and sport. *Educational Gerontology* 18: 461–481.

O'BRIEN, S. J. and P. A. VERTINSKY. 1991. Unfit survivors: Exercise as a resource for aging women. *The Gerontologist* 31: 347–358.

PAVLOU, K. N., W. P. STEFFEE, R. H. LERMAN, and B. A. BURROWS. 1985. Effects of dieting and exercise on lean body mass, oxygen uptake, and strength. *Medicine and Science in Sports and Exercise* 17: 466–471.

PERUSSE, L., C. LeBLANC, and C. BOUCHARD. 1988. Familial resemblance in lifestyle components: Results from the Canada Fitness Survey. *Canadian Journal of Public Health* 79: 201–205.

PHILLIPS, S. 1995. The social context of women's health: Goals and objectives for medical education. *Canadian Medical Association Journal* 152: 507–511.

POSNER, B. M., A. M. JETTE, K. W. SMITH, and D. R. MILLER. 1993. Nutrition and health risks in the elderly: The nutrition screening initiative. *American Journal of Public Health* 83: 972–978.

RACETTE, S. B., D. A. SCHOELLER, R. F. KUSHNER, and K. M. NEIL. 1995. Exercise enhances dietary compliance during moderate energy restriction in obese women. *American Journal of Clinical Nutrition* 62: 345–349.

RALSTON, P. A. 1991. Determinants of senior centre attendance and participation. *Journal of Applied Gerontology* 10: 258–273.

RASMUSSEN, L. B., B. KIENS, B. K. PEDERSEN, and E. A. RICHTER. 1994. Effect of diet and plasma fatty acid composition on immune status in elderly men. *American Journal of Clinical Nutrition* 59: 522–527.

RODGERS, A. B., L. G. KESSLER, B. PORTNOY, A. L. POTOSKY, B. PATTERSON, J. TENNEY, F. E. THOMPSON, S. M. KREBS-SMITH, N. BREEN, O. MATHEWS, and L. L. KAHLE. 1994. "Eat for health": A supermarket intervention for nutrition and cancer risk reduction. *American Journal of Public Health* 84: 72–76.

ROSENBERG, I. H., and J. W. MILLER. 1992. Nutritional factors in physical and cognitive functions of elderly people. *American Journal of Clinical Nutrition* 55(6 suppl.): 1237S–1243S.

ROSENBLOOM, C. A., and F. J. WHITTINGHAM. 1992. The effects of bereavement on eating behaviors and nutrient intakes in elderly widowed persons. *Journal of Gerontology: Social Sciences* 18: S223–S229.

ROSS, R., H. PEDWELL, and J. RISSANEN. 1995. Effects of energy restriction and exercise on skeletal muscle and adipose tissue in women as measured by magnetic resonance imaging. *American Journal of Clinical Nutrition* 61: 1179–1185.

ROTHENBERG, E., I. BOSAEUS, and B. STEEN. 1994. Food habits, food beliefs, and socio-economic factors in an elderly population. *Scandinavian Journal of Nutrition* 38: 159–165.

SHEPHARD, R. J. 1990. Measuring physical activity in the elderly: Some implications for nutrition. *Canadian Journal on Aging* 9: 166–203.

_____. 1993. Exercise and aging: Extending independence in older adults. *Geriatrics* 48: 61–64.

SHERWOOD, S. 1973. Sociology of food and eating: Implications for action for the elderly. *The American Journal of Clinical Nutrition* 26: 1108–1110.

SHIFFLETT, P. A., and W. A. MCINTOSH. 1986–1987. Food habits and future time: An explorative study of age-appropriate food habits among the elderly. *International Journal of Aging and Human Development* 24: 1–17.

SILVERSTONE, B. 1996. Older people of tomorrow: A psychosocial profile. *The Gerontologist* 36: 27–32.

STATISTICS CANADA. 1990. *Women in Canada: A Statistical Report.* Ottawa (ON): Minister of Supply and Services

STEPHENS, T. and C. L. CRAIG. 1990. *The Well-Being of Canadians: Highlights of the 1988 Campbell's Survey.* Ottawa (ON): Canadian Fitness and Lifestyle Research Institute.

TALBOT, D. M. 1985. Assessing needs of the rural elderly. *Journal of Gerontological Nursing* 11: 39–43.

TORRES, C. C., A. A. MCINTOSH, and K. S. KUBENA. 1992. Social network and social background characteristics of elderly who live and eat alone. *Journal of Aging and Health* 4: 564–578.

TRICHOPOULOU, A., A. KOURIS-BLAZOS, M. L. WAHLQVIST, C. GNARDELLIS, P. LAGIOU, E. POLYCHRONOPOULOS, T. VASSILAKOU, L. LIPWORTH, and D. TRICHOPOULOS. 1995. Diet and overall survival in elderly people. *British Medical Journal* 311: 1457–1460.

VAN DER WIELEN, R. P. J., G. M. DE WILD, L. C. DE GROOT, W. H. L. HOEFNAGELS, and W. A. VAN STAVEREN. 1996. Dietary intakes of energy and water-soluble vitamins in different categories of aging. *Journal of Gerontology: Biological Sciences* 51A: B100–B107.

VERBRUGGE, L. M., and J. L. GRUBER-BALDINI. 1996. Age differences and age changes in activities: Baltimore Longitudinal Study of Aging. *Journal of Gerontology: Social Sciences* 51B: S30–S41.

VERTINSKY, P. A. 1994. *The Eternally Wounded Woman: Doctors, Women and Exercise in the Late Nineteenth Century.* Manchester: Manchester University Press.

_____. 1995. Stereotypes of aging women and exercise: A historical perspective. *Journal of Aging and Physical Activity* 3: 223–237.

VOORIPS, L. E., W. A. VAN STEVEREN, and J. G. HAUTVAST. 1991. Are physically active elderly women in a better nutritional condition than sedentary peers? *European Journal of Clinical Nutrition* 45: 545–552.

WILLETT, W. C. 1994. Micronutrients and cancer risk. *American Journal of Clinical Nutrition* 59(Suppl.): 116S–5S.

WOOD, R. J., P. M. SUTER, and R. M. RUSSELL. 1995. Mineral requirements of elderly people. *American Journal of Clinical Nutrition* 62: 493–505.

YOSHIDA, K. K., K. R. ALLISON, J. W. MARR, D. C. PATTISON, and J. N. MORRIS. 1988. Social factors influencing perceived barriers to physical activity among women. *Canadian Journal of Public Health* 79: 104–108.

ZIMMERMAN, R. S. and C. CONNOR. 1989. Health promotion in context: The effects of significant others on health behaviour change. Health Education Quarterly 16: 57–75.

Facilitating the Transition from Employment to Retirement

VICTOR W. MARSHALL, PH.D. AND
PHILIPPA J. CLARKE, M.SC.

*Department of Public Health Sciences and
Institute for Human Development, Life Course and Aging
University of Toronto*

SUMMARY

Any life transition can have positive or negative consequences for health, and retirement is no exception. Because work is so central to people's lives, and provides the major resources required to attain life goals, the transition from employment to retirement is particularly important for health. Most retired Canadians claim to enjoy the retirement years and most working Canadians say they prefer to retire before age 65. However, the relationship between employment and retirement is changing dramatically in Canada. In contrast to an earlier pattern of relatively stable career employment leading to retirement around age 65 (for men), increasing numbers of men and women are leaving their major employment situation earlier. Whether or not this is voluntary, many people then go on to hold "bridge" jobs. The process of retirement takes on new meaning and duration.

The extent to which retirement leads to worse health is likely exaggerated because some people retire because of declining health. Their postretirement health status may have nothing to do with the retirement transition. For most people, retirement is either a neutral or health-enhancing transition. In the case of typical retirement at the traditional age of 65, the few negative effects on health that have been found have been very modest in intensity. However, unscheduled, early and involuntary retirement can lead to worse health or adversely affect health indirectly by influencing other social determinants of health such as self-esteem, sense of control, and income. Women may be particularly vulnerable to unscheduled or involuntary loss of employment because of their economic dependence relative to men and because they typically have less control over the transition from employment to retirement.

As the nature of the transition from employment to retirement changes, that portion of a person's life between stable career employment and permanent retirement at pensionable age can be quite disruptive, involving difficult job searches, lower-level employment, lower wages and repeated job displacement. There is virtually no research about the health effects of life course instability from middle age to late life, but limited research on instability early in the working life shows a strong and significant relationship, with instability leading to increased mortality. The possibility that labour force instability later in life has adverse consequences merits further investigation.

Programs and policies to ease the transition from employment to retirement have not been well assessed, but some evaluation studies and more descriptive studies suggest the benefits of programs to employers, older workers, displaced workers and retirees. Retirement preparation programs can enhance the sense of control over the important life change of retirement. In several model programs, retirees participate in community service for nominal pay, and these can be used as adaptation programs following retirement at any age. Bridge jobs frequently provide employment in an industry or sector different from their career jobs. Training for bridge jobs needs to take into account the learning needs of older persons, and company managers can benefit from educational initiatives that counter myths and stereotypes about older people's strengths and capacities.

Women and those of lower socioeconomic status are particularly vulnerable to job displacement associated with the increased use of early retirement incentives. Preretirement programs should be conducted well in advance of age 65, should strive to enhance feelings of control, and should explicitly take into account the possibility of early retirement with or without subsequent bridge jobs until the age of the state pension.

Policy initiatives should support gradual and phased retirement; develop and support retiree service programs; support retirement education programs that recognize the diversity of the transitions from employment to retirement; develop and support programs explicitly directed to training and placing older workers and early retirees in bridge jobs; promote positive images and counter negative stereotypes of older workers through social marketing and educational programs; recognize the greater vulnerability of women and those of lower socioeconomic status to career disruption; and foster research on the health effects of a life of disrupted employment.

TABLE OF CONTENTS

LIST OF FIGURES

The most striking feature about today's generation of older workers is the extent to which they are withdrawing from the labour market. There has been a marked increased in both voluntary and involuntary early retirement, to the extent that most men and women retire before age 65, the traditional age of retirement. Increasingly in recent years, downsizing in organizations has resulted in many older workers leaving the workforce, with varying degrees of financial and counselling support. ... As more and more "baby boomers" enter their fifties, the transition from full-time employment to retirement will become an increasingly significant issue.

Advisory Group on Working Time and the
Distribution of Work 1994, 24.

INTRODUCTION: THE NEW TRANSITION FROM EMPLOYMENT TO RETIREMENT IN RELATION TO HEALTH

In our society, most adults are employed for a large part of their lives, and most eventually reach a point when they cease to be employed. The term "retirement" is used to describe this latter point, but retirement is an ambiguous term because of changes in the nature of employment. Any life change can either enhance or diminish health. Our objectives in this paper are to summarize what is known of the health implications of the transition from employment to retirement, and to describe ways to enhance the positive health effects of this transition. To achieve these related objectives, we must clarify the way health is treated in this work, and clarify the changing nature of retirement.

Our approach to health rests on the broad definition of the World Health Organization, which conceives health as "the extent to which an individual or group is able, on the one hand, to realize aspirations and satisfy needs, and, on the other hand, to change or cope with the environment" (WHO 1986, 4; see also Evans and Stoddart 1990). We wish to identify factors associated with economic security, respect for the individual, social integration, and accessibility of resources required to satisfy aspirations and needs. These factors should contribute, not only to the avoidance of disease and trauma, but also to psychological well-being (Marshall et al. 1995). The determinants of health include, not only the biological inheritance and physiological characteristics of the individual, but also the psychological, social and economic resources that help people realize their aspirations, satisfy their needs, and adapt to their environment.

The effects of rapid social and economic change on work and the life course are depicted in figure 1. In the traditional pattern, the life course could be characterized as a relatively orderly sequence of prework, work, and postwork states (Kohli et al. 1991). However, a new pattern is emerging. Following increased years of educational preparation for work, individuals enter the labour force through a series of jobs before finding employment in an organization that offers some stability and progression. This phase is described as the career job. Whereas, under the traditional pattern, the career job ended with retirement and access to state and private pension schemes, in the emerging pattern many people leave a career job long before they are eligible for state or private pensions. Many seek new employment, typically at a lower level of pay, and often part time. This phase of the life course may see the individual retraining to facilitate entry into what has been termed a "bridge job" (Doeringer 1990).

Figure 1

Models of work and the life course

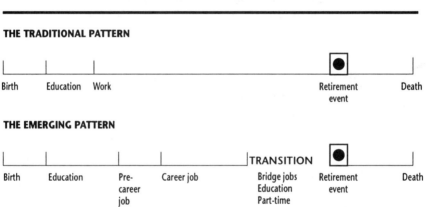

As figure 1 implies, retirement can be seen as an event, as a process, or as a status following the event (Atchley 1976), and each perspective on retirement has different implications in terms of health. Our review focuses on retirement as a process and as an event.

As a starting point, we note that "employment" refers to work for pay or profit (i.e., including self-employment). We shall see that the age at which Canadians are leaving employment is falling, leaving a gap between employment and eligibility for state pensions. We will also show that this gap is filled in many ways. European researchers who are interested in changing age patterns in labour force participation prefer the term "early exit" to describe leaving paid employment without a pension (Kohli et al. 1991). Early exit can be followed by many options: unemployment with support from severance or unemployment insurance while looking for work; unemployment due to illness or disability, with support from disability insurance; full- or part-time reemployment; or "early" retirement with no intention to work (Schmähl 1989). The evidence indicates that older workers have less desirable options than younger workers (Advisory Group 1994; Picot and Wannell 1987).

The elderly are not necessarily the most vulnerable group in the transition from employment to retirement. Rather, some people under the age of 65 may be in danger of unanticipated exit from employment. Displaced older workers, who may choose to describe their situation as "retirement," may be particularly at risk. In response to this problem, our review touches on methods for coping with unemployment, and labour adjustment policies that enhance or imperil health, directly or indirectly. As Frank and Mustard (1994, 9) put it, "An individual's sense of achievement, self-esteem, and control over his or her work and life appears to affect health and well-being."

This is not to say that early exit from the labour force is necessarily or even typically associated with adverse health effects. "Early retirement" is sought by most Canadian workers, who either think it has positive benefits or prefer it to continued employment. Although we can touch only lightly on this issue, in focusing on health in relation to the transition from employment to retirement we must remember that work itself often adversely affects health. We face a complex situation in which some workers are more vulnerable than others to adverse health consequences in their transition from employment to retirement.

The nature of retirement as a process almost certainly influences health outcomes. Although there is little direct literature on this point, inferences can be made from what is known about other social determinants of health that are related to the nature of the retirement process.

The paper is organized as follows: The first section "Introduction: The New Transition from Employment to Retirement in Relation to Health" introduces the new transition. In the section "New Patterns of Transition from Employment to Retirement", we describe the changing patterns of employment and retirement in the industrialized world with particular reference to Canada. In the section "Is Health Change a Cause of Retirement?", we briefly review the evidence concerning health changes as a possible determinant of the timing of retirement. In the section "The Event of Retirement as a Cause of Health Change", we review the literature on the health effects of retirement as an event. In the section "Life Course Instability and Change in Relation to Health", we look at related literature that considers retirement as a life transition process. These sections identify some social determinants of health in the transition from employment to retirement. In the section "Facilitating the Transition from Work to Retirement", we examine some programs and policies that address these social determinants in ways that might influence the health effects of the transition from employment to retirement. In the final section, we address specific policy issues.

NEW PATTERNS OF TRANSITION FROM EMPLOYMENT TO RETIREMENT

We argue that certain social factors affect the timing of the retirement event and the nature of the transition that leads to exit from the labour force; and, in turn, the timing and nature of the process affect health. In this section, we describe how social factors are associated with the timing and process of the transition from employment to retirement.

As in many other countries, the demographics of the Canadian labour force have been changing dramatically. As entry cohorts have become smaller, the average age of the labour force has increased while the 15–24-year-old share of the labour force shrank by 17.4 percent between 1980 and 1993 (Betcherman and Leckie 1995, 1). However, older workers have been leaving the labour force. The average age of retirement in Canada is lowering, and is now 62 for men and 59 for women (Advisory Group 1994; McDonald 1994). (See figure 2)

Despite slight increases in female labour force participation by age, the overall pattern is increasingly one of early exit from full-time employment. Women's labour force participation rates in the 55–64 age category began increasing in the 1950s and reached 30 percent by 1969. After that, increases have been modest; 36 percent was achieved by 1992. Rising rates for women reflect a trend toward gender equality and female activity in the labour force. The rates for men reflect changing patterns of retirement. In 1953, 86 percent of men aged 55–64 were in the labour force. The percentage declined to below 80 percent by 1975, after which the decline accelerated. By 1994, only 61 percent of men aged 55–64 were in the labour force (McDonald 1994). The U.S. and Europe exhibit similar, often stronger, trends toward early exit (Kohli et al. 1991; Schmähl 1989).

Important variations in early exit patterns and the age composition of the labour force are based on industrial sector and occupation. Currently, young workers (age 15–24) are heavily concentrated in the growing service sector, which is characterized by low wages, poor benefits, and high turnover. "Older workers are most prevalent in declining or slow-growth sectors" (Betcherman and Leckie 1995), and thus highly vulnerable to the effects of restructuring and downsizing. As Picot and Wannell note (1987), adjustment following job loss is not necessarily more difficult for the groups most affected by job loss. Younger workers are more likely than older workers to lose their jobs, but they integrate better into new jobs.

Canadian data also suggest variations in retirement patterns by occupation and education. University education is associated with later retirement for men over the age of 65, while men who retire in the 55–64 age group are less likely to be university educated (McDonald 1994). However, Canadian men who retire between the ages of 55 and 64 are more likely to have had middle-range occupational status, to have been in the top end of service industries, and to have been working in the industrial sector. For women, higher-skill occupations are associated with younger retirement age (McDonald 1994).

Similar broad sociological factors also seem to affect women's exit patterns. Because the paid working lives of women tend to be interrupted by child bearing and child rearing, women are less likely than men to accumulate enough pension benefits or other retirement income to permit early exit from the labour force. In an international ecological study of female retirement patterns, including retirement from both paid and unpaid work, Pampel and Park (1986) found that, in developed countries, large families tended to be associated with later retirement, presumably because of more interrupted careers or more dependants to support. Similarly, gender inequality in the labour force, as measured by average level of education attained, was associated with later retirement for women in industrialized societies. Therefore, the unique effects of broad sociological factors for women, such as family size and gender equality in the labour force, may be determinants of early female exit from the labour force.

Figure 2
**Labour force participation rates of men and women
age 55 to 64, Canada**

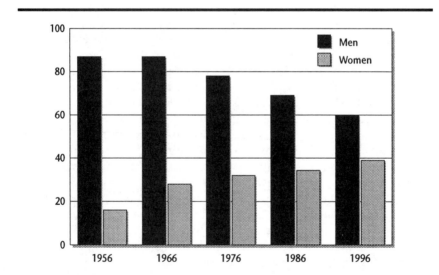

Sources: McDonald 1994; Statistics Labour Force Survey.

Canadian data suggest that married women aged 45–54 are more likely to retire early than single, widowed or divorced women of the same age (McDonald 1994), who presumably lack their financial advantage. However, for women between the ages of 55 and 64, single and widowed women are more likely to leave the labour force (McDonald 1994), perhaps because of the survivor benefits available to the widowed, and because single women may have had more opportunity to have had a stable career path.

Furthermore, as McDonald (1994) has noted, Canadians born in other countries are less likely to retire early, most likely because of restrictions on Old Age Security benefits for immigrants. Canadians living in rural areas, such as the prairie provinces, are also likely to retire later, because presumably there is no mandatory age of retirement from family farming (McDonald 1994).

The Survey on Aging and Independence, conducted in September 1991 with a larger representative sample of Canadians aged 40 and older, produced evidence that many Canadians *expect* to retire early. Two-thirds of respondents not yet retired said they expected to retire; 28 percent of them expected to retire before age 60 and 62 percent expect to retire before age 65 (Seniors Secretariat 1993). The survey did not address whether respondents' expectations were consistent with their wishes. We examine preferences on the timing of retirement in the section "Is Health Change a Cause of Retirement?".

Older workers are caught by a conjunction of demographic and economic factors, with corporate restructuring occurring on an unprecedented scale. As both companies and governments strive to cut their payrolls, the easiest restructuring method has been offering older workers incentives to leave paid employment. These incentives are often backed by threats of layoffs if labour force reduction targets are not met (Hardy and Quadagno 1995).

From a study of 406 large American companies, Useem (1994) concludes that older workers experience both the costs and the benefits of restructuring more intensely than younger workers because older workers are concentrated in industrial sectors that experience certain forms of restructuring. Companies with older workers were more likely to be manufacturers and to be very large; they were also twice as likely to be unionized. These types of companies were most extensively restructured in the U.S., and probably in Canada. Companies with higher proportions of workers aged 50 or older were more likely to sell off business units, lay off large numbers of employees, reduce management staff, offer early retirement, and impose hiring freezes. Conversely, companies with younger workers were more likely to shut down operations, merge units, or shift full-time workers to part-time employment. Useem cites a Louis Harris survey that showed an increase in the proportion of companies that use early retirement schemes to avoid laying off workers, and declines in the percentage of companies using hiring freezes, salary reductions and voluntary separations to avoid layoffs (Useem 1994).

Many transitions from employment to retirement are constrained by employer policies, corporate restructuring and downsizing, plant shutdowns, or the family and personal health situation of the employee or retiree. From the Survey on Aging and Independence, Schellenberg estimates that the incidence of involuntary retirement is increasing (1994, 70). This estimate is consistent with Lowe's analysis of survey data on persons not in the labour force, which showed that, from 1990 to 1992, 211,000 Canadians retired earlier than they had planned, up from 190,000 in a similar period three years earlier. About 88,000 people retired earlier than expected for economic reasons, up from 54,000 (Lowe 1991). As a result, many workers leave full-time, long-term jobs, not for full-time retirement, but for bridge jobs. These are often part time, with lower pay and benefits, and often contractual (Advisory Committee 1994, 47; Doeringer 1990).

The transition between employment and retirement is, thus, often a sequence of moves in and out of the paid labour force and to different positions in the labour force. However, we have little data on this transition sequence. In the Survey on Aging and Independence, almost one in five (17 percent) retirees over the age of 45 reported having returned to paid employment. Men were almost twice as likely as women to do so (Schellenberg 1994, 50). The earlier the retirement and, for men but not women, the higher the retiree's education and skill level of the last job before retirement, the more likely the retiree was to return to work. This study did not provide information about the nature or number of jobs following retirement, other than that 76 percent of men and 45 percent of women who returned to paid employment did so through part-time work. We also know from other survey data (for 1993) that 41 percent of men and 27 percent of women aged 55–64 who work part time do so from necessity and not choice (Schellenberg 1994).

In summary, the transition from employment to retirement is actually a set of possible transitions that vary in timing and nature. This transition for some occurs at age 65, when state and private pensions are likely to be available. For others it occurs later or earlier, creating a disjunction between the transition and the move from employment income to pension income. For some it is a smooth process, for others it is much more disruptive. Some retirees are able to control the process, while for others it is involuntary. This complexity must be borne in mind when assessing research findings about the health implications of the transition from employment to retirement.

IS HEALTH CHANGE A CAUSE OF RETIREMENT?

Popular views about retirement and health tend to emphasize that retirement leads to poorer health. Everyone has an anecdote about someone who retired and died within six months. It is important to recognize that adverse health following retirement is not necessarily due to retirement but in some instances reflects the fact that workers with poor health opt to retire. Here we briefly discuss health as a factor leading to retirement but, to do so, we also discuss factors not related to health that influence the decision to retire.

Voluntary Factors

In reviewing seven major American studies, Palmore (1985) found that most early retirement was caused not by formal policies but by perceptions of health problems, the attractiveness of retirement life, and low job commitment. The distinction between voluntary and involuntary retirement is vague, but we consider health reasons involuntary. Some of the more common reasons for early retirement, such as the attractiveness of retirement life and low job commitment, are personal, and we will consider them voluntary.

As noted above, many Canadians want to retire early. The Survey on Aging and Independence found that 56 percent of retired Canadians said they wanted to stop working, only 18 percent cited mandatory retirement policies and only 14 percent cited early retirement policies (Schellenberg 1994, 55). On the other hand, Schellenberg estimates that 465,000 retirees were forced out of their jobs by health factors, mandatory retirement policies or similar constraints (Schellenberg 1994, 55–6), and 25 percent said their retirement was involuntary. Semiskilled and unskilled workers are affected by socioeconomic factors; less educated people are more likely to describe their retirement as involuntary. Almost half of involuntary retirees cite health as a reason for retirement, more than one-third cite mandatory retirement policy, almost 9 percent cite early retirement policy, and about 15 percent cite lack of work (Schellenberg 1994, 68).

Lowe (1991) presents an analysis of the 1989 General Social Survey indicating that although 34 percent of Canadians aged 15 years or older do not know when they plan to retire, 43 percent say they plan to retire before they reach age 65. Just 14 percent say they plan to retire at age 65, and 1 percent after 65. To the extent that plans measure desires, these data may now be somewhat dated, since corporate restructuring has accelerated. A more recent survey of 1,034 Canadian companies by Murray Axmith and Associates, noted early in 1995 in the *Globe and Mail* (Gibb-Clark 1995), reported that companies that did offer early retirement incentive packages found that only 44.8 percent of eligible employees took them. The news story suggests that "The low acceptance rate could be tied to fear of the unknown or the generosity of the offer" (Gibb-Clark 1995). When people hear that the Canada Pension Plan might be in trouble, or that pension or annuity income might be taxed heavily or "clawed back," they decide not to retire early.

Economic Factors

Canadian data suggest that economic factors, including plant shutdowns, and situations that are only partially voluntary, such as early retirement incentive programs (Statistics Canada 1993), have more influence on the decision to retire early than purely voluntary factors (Marshall 1995a). Analyses from the Survey on Aging and Independence (McDonald 1994) indicate that lack of available work was a significant independent predictor of early retirement for Canadian men.

Several studies have found that sufficient financial resources, such as employer- and government-provided pensions, influences the decision to retire early (see Boaz and Muller 1990). The Survey on Aging and Independence (McDonald 1994) suggests that a sufficient income influences the decision to retire for Canadian men and women. Canadian men who retire between the ages of 45 and 54 have less debt than those who continue to work, whereas men who continue to work past the age of 65 tend to have financial obligations such as mortgages and personal debt. Similar findings from the 1989 General Social Survey are reported by LeBlanc (1995).

An increasingly poor fit, whether real or perceived, between the skills of older workers and rapidly changing requirements may also be a subtle involuntary factor precipitating exit from the labour force (CARNET 1995a, b; Towers Perrin 1991).

Health as a Factor in Itself

It is argued that health is an important influence on the decision to retire, but the data are far from clear. Health may make a difference to retirement timing for very early retirees and very old workers, but be relatively unimportant for other workers (Ruchlin and Morris 1992). For very early retirees, Canadian data indicate that health is a strong predictor of early retirement for men, while responsibility for caring for others in poor health is an important influence on women's retirement. However, when considering a broad span of ages, health is a relatively minor predictor of age of retirement for both men and women, as judged from self-reports in the Survey on Aging and Independence (McDonald 1994).

Determining the significance of health to retirement timing is partly a methodological problem. One difficulty is that health is often reported in cross-sectional studies of retirees as the reason for retirement because it is a more acceptable reason to retire than layoff or failure to find a job (Boaz 1990; Myers 1982). Using a longitudinal approach, Bazzoli (1985) found that, although health-related reasons tend to be inflated after retirement, they still explained a significant proportion of the probability of retirement and, therefore, could not be discounted as a legitimate motivation to retire. Similarly, Boaz and Muller (1990), using data from an American longitudinal survey, compared mortality and hospitalization rates for those who did not report health problems either before or after retirement with rates for those who reported health problems only after retirement, on the assumption that, if health problems were simply a retrospective rationalization for deciding to retire early, mortality and morbidity statistics for the two groups would be similar. However, individuals who reported health problems retrospectively were more likely to be hospitalized and to die earlier than those who did not report health problems. Furthermore, people who retired before the age of 65 years of age because of health concerns were more likely than later retirees without health concerns to die within two years after retirement and more likely to be hospitalized at the time of their retirement.

Factors Linking Health with Class, Gender and Ethnicity

These results suggest that poor health may be an important cause of early retirement, even when reported after exit from the labour force. However, Boaz and Muller (1990) also found that people who retired early due to illness were less educated than later retirees, were less likely than later retirees to be managers or professionals, and were more likely to be in physically demanding jobs. Therefore, although the literature tends to focus on issues such as financial stability and health as predictors of early retirement, other social factors, such as level of education and occupational status, may, in fact, underlie early exit. In the Survey on Aging and Independence, people in low-status occupations reported health more often as a reason for retirement. For example, 19 percent of male professionals and senior managers listed health as the reason for retiring, compared with 33 percent of semiskilled and unskilled workers. The same pattern was observed for women (Schellenberg 1994).

In a paper controversial in its day, Kingson (1981) anticipated a social determinants of health perspective by arguing that by concentrating on the events immediately surrounding the decision to retire early, we overlook a broad range of life events, such as racial and class factors, that are key predictors of early withdrawal from the labour force. In his study, Kingson examined the characteristics of a representative sample of American men who retired before the age of 62 and found that higher education was more likely to be associated with voluntary exit from the labour force and with higher retirement incomes. Therefore, lifelong factors such as educational opportunities and social position may be more important determinants of early exit than the more immediate factors such as health and available pension income.

THE EVENT OF RETIREMENT AS A CAUSE OF HEALTH CHANGE

The effects of retirement on health have long been debated. Some studies suggest that retirement has adverse health effects, some maintain that it has neutral effects, and others suggest that the health effects of retirement are positive. The debate has been fuelled by several issues: the difficulty in distinguishing secular age patterns of deteriorating health from retirement-precipitated health changes; problems in measuring health; reliance on cross-sectional studies to infer longitudinal changes; a focus on voluntary retirement at age 65 rather than on the potential effects of involuntary retirement and early retirement; and the fact that most early studies focused exclusively on men. In general, we think the literature supports the conclusion that voluntary retirement has positive or at worst neutral effects, but that involuntary retirement, often at early ages, has negative effects.

The Argument for Adverse Effects of Retirement on Health

Palmore and associates (1985) reanalysed six American longitudinal studies and found that all recorded at least one significant negative relationship between retirement status and a health indicator. However, these relationships were only modest.

The Argument for No Effects of Retirement on Health

Changes in health status following retirement may be simply a result of deteriorating health with age, and disentangling retirement effects on health and well-being from the effects of other age-related changes in health itself, or in determinants of health such as income or social contacts, has posed major challenges for researchers (Minkler 1981). For example, one early major study of a representative sample of American men aged 65 and older demonstrated that the negative effects of retirement on men's morale are explained away when controlling for age, perception of health, disability and income (Thompson 1973).

Minkler's 1981 literature review concluded that many investigators found that retirement had no adverse effects on the health of individuals. However, she noted, the issue remained unresolved because of the cross-sectional nature of these studies, unmeasured potential effects of subject attrition (e.g., Streib and Schneider 1971), and conceptual and measurement problems in differentiating retirement-related health effects from other health conditions. On the other hand, a recent cross-sectional survey of Americans 25 years of age and older (Herzog et al. 1991) found that retirees reported no more decline in their health and well-being than employed people, when individuals who retired for health reasons were excluded.

The Argument for Positive Effects of Retirement on Health

Some studies suggest that health improves with retirement, particularly in blue-collar workers. Thompson and Streib (1958) found that retired men reported improved health over the follow-up period, measured by subjective report and objective examinations. This finding held even for those who retired for health reasons. A recent U.S. survey comparing the mental health and health-promoting behaviours of almost 600 retirees with employed people found that retired men reported less stress than employed people. However, no differences were found between retired and employed women. Retired people were more likely to regularly exercise, and retired women were less likely to report alcohol problems than employed women (Midanik et al. 1995).

From a review of the literature on work, retirement and mental health, Warr (in press) says that good mental health in later life does not depend on having a job, and that the mental health of retired people is not significantly different from that of employed people. However, Warr says that it has been repeatedly shown that people who experience early involuntary unemployment are "psychologically harmed," although older unemployed people tend to exhibit less distress than younger unemployed people.

Unscheduled and Early Retirement

The negative health effects of involuntary and early retirement may be understood in light of what is known about the importance of predictability and control over life events. A great deal of literature concerns the negative effects of stressful events on health, particularly when perceived demands outweigh individuals' perceived response capability (Selye 1982). Typical examples of stressful events are widowhood, relocation and divorce, and evidence suggests that these events are associated with decreased well-being.

Certain factors may predispose retirement to be a stressful life event (Minkler 1981): poor timing, unexpectedness, lack of control over the event, or potential for economic problems. People feel threatened by events that they feel are out of their control. Herzog et al. (1991) argue that retirement has only negative effects when individuals are forced to retire against their personal preferences. They found that individuals over the age of 65 who retired voluntarily reported significantly higher life satisfaction than those who had retired involuntarily. Other studies have found that early, involuntary retirement decreases retirement satisfaction (Beck 1984) and overall well-being (Peretti and Wilson 1975).

Whether motivated by health problems or company restructuring, involuntary retirement involves a loss of personal control (Reis and Gold 1993). This may explain why individuals who feel little control over their impending retirement have been found to exert little control over their lives after retirement (Fletcher and Hansson 1991). Warr (in press) identifies the opportunity for control as one of nine environmental variables associated with greater job-related well-being.

Since work is a central activity and source of identity for adults, the loss of work may have ramifications similar to those of other stressful life events. Some evidence suggests that older people may have more difficulty adapting to the role loss associated with retirement (Eisdorfer and Wilkie

1977; Elwell and Maltbie-Crannell 1981). The more frequent role losses that occur with age (including widowhood, divorce and retirement) have a negative impact on life satisfaction (particularly for men), in part due to the simultaneous losses of social supports, income and health that also tend to occur as a result of these events.

Canadian research suggests that, in general, retirement is not a serious life event. Martin Matthews and Brown (1988) asked a sample of 300 retired men and women in southern Ontario to indicate the extent to which 34 life events affected them. Retirement ranked twenty-seventh on their list—death of a spouse ranked first and birth of a child second. Those who said they retired when they wanted to were significantly more likely to rate the event of retirement positively. This relationship was particularly strong for women, whose retirement timing, according to Martin Matthews and Brown, may be dictated by circumstances beyond their control, such as the retirement of their husbands. This interpretation may require qualification because labour force patterns are changing, in part because of retirement incentives used to reduce workforces. Retirement incentive packages for men are generally more attractive than those for women because men tend to have had more stable work histories and, thus, more opportunity to accumulate pension credits. Anecdotal evidence suggests that in many couples, the wife continues to work and the husband takes the retirement incentive package.

Unscheduled and early retirement probably influence health more directly by affecting income, which has been shown to be an important predictor of life satisfaction in retirement (Fillenbaum, George, and Palmore 1985). However, income may depend partly on health. Although some evidence suggests that older people may be satisfied with fewer economic resources than young or middle-aged adults (see George 1992 for a detailed review), insufficient income may not only reduce life satisfaction, it may also adversely affect health if there is not enough money to purchase necessary aids and devices, home care, or adequate nutrition.

Some American studies have found that people who have involuntarily retired early because of health or layoffs are at greater risk of poverty than voluntary retirees (Boaz and Muller 1990; Hausman and Paquette 1987). Women, in particular, have been shown to have smaller retirement incomes (Ballantyne and Marshall 1995), which may compromise their life satisfaction and health. Similarly, some evidence suggests that blue-collar workers are less likely than white-collar workers to receive pension benefits and other financial incentives to retire early (Schellenberg 1995).

In summary, unscheduled and early exit from employment can influence health and well-being in several ways. The stress of any life event increases when it is unexpected, leading to a loss of the sense of control. Identity may suffer as the individual loses familiar social contacts. Because loss of employment usually means loss of income, health may be at risk by the individual's reduced ability to obtain the prerequisites for health and health care. Women may be particularly threatened by unscheduled or involuntary loss of employment, both because of their economic dependence on men, and because they have less control over the transition from employment to retirement.

LIFE COURSE INSTABILITY AND CHANGE IN RELATION TO HEALTH

Following Atchley (1976), Minkler (1981) interprets retirement as a process. Drawing on her review, first we will examine health in relation to the process of retirement in the traditional pattern. We will then examine health as it is influenced by the transition from employment to retirement as a process (see figure 1).

The Traditional Pattern of Work and Retirement

Retirement has always been more than simply an event marking the boundary between employment and pensioned unemployment. The retirement experience tends to be a process on a continuum, in which the perception and experience of events, and the health effects of these events, may vary throughout the retirement process. As outlined by Minkler (1981), individuals first experience the anticipation of retirement, then the actual event. This is typically followed by a "honeymoon" phase characterized by a positive view of retirement, to be followed by a "disenchantment" period in which retirees face the realities of their new lives. Next comes a period of reorientation and stability, in which retirees adapt to and begin to cope with their new lives. Although this process is not universal—we will shortly contrast it with the emerging pattern—it helps to conceptualize retirement as a series of stages, rather than a static event, influenced at different times by factors such as health and income.

The process perspective is supported by studies that demonstrate variations in morbidity and mortality rates at different periods throughout the retirement process (Martin and Doran 1966; Haynes et al. 1977). It is interesting to note that these effects were more pronounced among blue-collar workers. In fact, blue-collar workers may be less likely to experience the honeymoon phase perhaps because of limited financial resources, generally poorer health, and reduced social contacts.

Szinovacz and Wasko (1992) argue that the retirement transition should be viewed as a process that includes awareness of other life events, such as widowhood, that occur at the same time as retirement. Women, in particular, experience more life events around retirement, and are consequently more vulnerable to maladjustment. This may be because women tend to be more emotionally involved in their social networks, in which life events tend to occur, and they are also frequently asked to support others during these life events (Kessler and McLeod 1984) The importance of the postretirement adaptation process is confirmed by the greater degree of adaptation seen in longer-term retirees (retired for four to five years) with better income, health and social supports (Szinovacz and Wasko 1992).

The Emerging Pattern of Work and Retirement

In contemporary Canada, increasing numbers of middle-aged people are experiencing unanticipated, nonnormative, involuntary loss of employment. The health effects of this loss have been explored (although not in depth) in relation to the health effects of unemployment in another paper in this series. However, we are not interested in the health effects of unemployment caused by loss of a career job, but in the health effects of an emerging transitional phase of life between loss of the career job and entry into full retirement (i.e., a self-definition as not in the labour force, accompanied by a desire not to seek employment; receipt of formal and, perhaps, private pension income). We noted in figure 1 that this transitional period may be characterized by bridge jobs or searching for bridge jobs or education. Unfortunately, there are no data from which to extract evidence of the health effects of this emerging transitional period. We must speculate from more general knowledge of the social determinants of health and from very limited data concerning career disruption earlier in life.

In the American context, Elder and Pavalko (1993) have described different patterns of the retirement transition process in men born between 1900 and 1920, focusing on differences between the 1900–1909 and 1910–1920 generational cohorts. The sample is overrepresentative of white, middle-class people. The younger cohort retired earlier and followed a more complex transition; the older cohort retired later and was more likely to exit from employment to retirement in a single transition. Elder and Pavalko state (1993, S187):

> Men born between 1900 and 1909 (the older cohort) tended to retire at a later age, even with other relevant factors controlled. As expected, men subject to mandatory retirement tended to retire at an earlier age, while those who identified work as the major factor in their lives tended to begin retirement at a later age. Not surprisingly, being self-employed in one's fifties also influences the age at which men retire, with the self-employed tending to retire at later ages.

Most of the sample retired gradually (46 percent), while many exited in a single transition (30 percent). Elder and Pavalko (1993, S188) summarize their findings as follows:

> ... net of other factors, men in the older cohort are still more likely to retire in a single transition. Compared to professionals, men in sales, clerical, or

technical occupations were more likely to retire abruptly.... It may be that these workers, particularly those who are not self-employed, have fewer options for partial retirement than professionals or high-level managers and executives, many of whom did some kind of consulting or teaching on a part-time basis.

The health consequences of these transition patterns are described in a companion paper using the same data (Pavalko, Elder, and Clipp 1993). Two main effects of employment histories on mortality were described. Career patterns up to 1960 were taken as the independent variables in relation to mortality after 1960. Career patterns were differentiated according to overall progression and the extent of unrelated job shifts. Of interest for our purposes is the striking finding that "men who experienced a period of several unrelated job shifts have a mortality risk that is 57 percent higher than those who do not have such a period" (Pavalko, Elder, and Clipp 1993, 374). This relationship is not adequately accounted for by several explanatory factors measured in this study: physical health, alcoholism, anxiety and depression measured in 1960; or variability in occupational status in 1959. Much of the observed effect was due to unrelated job moves early in the individual's career, suggesting, the authors say, that later entry into career jobs has negative implications for health. The authors take the position that more than just the nature of the job is important; rather, it is "the pattern and order of those jobs as they form a worklife" (375). A work-stress model does not explain the observed relationships between employment pattern and mortality. The authors then investigate a social class model in which orderly career progression, rather than many shifts among unrelated jobs, might be associated with economic advantages leading subsequently to better health. This hypothesis could not be tested with their data. However, the authors speculate that an interrupted career path may not provide the opportunity to accumulate adequate pension or other economic benefits for a secure retirement, which may affect health adversely.

The applicability of this important longitudinal study to the Canadian context and the specific situation of the transition from employment to retirement requires theoretical development and merits subsequent research. First, the study used a highly delimited sample of intellectually gifted[1], middle-class American males, and its broader applicability to other social classes is questionable. Second, this study found that early worklife instability was important for mortality, whereas we are interested in unstable employment in the years before full retirement. However, this may not be a serious limitation, as the age of exit from career jobs is falling, and as the

---

1. IQ as measured by intelligence tests is, of course, highly biased against lower–social status people. IQ scores may not indicate intelligence so much as socioeconomic privilege.

general effects of instability may apply regardless of the position of this instability in the life course. The following sections attempt to explain why a disruptive transition from employment to retirement might affect health adversely.

Economic Security

The nature of the specific socioeconomic context of retirement may also influence the degree of stress caused by retirement (Minkler 1981). Retirement is likely to be more stressful during a recession or depression (Minkler 1981, 120), when workers experience more pressure to retire early within a context of reduced economic security and higher inflation. Elder and Pavalko (1993) note that the two cohorts they studied retired under substantially different economic circumstances, which may explain why the younger cohort retired earlier.

The economic insecurity that Pavalko, Elder, and Clipp (1993) suggest results from disruptive early labour force experiences is now being experienced not only by young cohorts struggling to find work, but also by older cohorts struggling to remain in the labour force. If younger people have difficulty finding the stable jobs that bring pensions and allow them to acquire wealth, older workers are losing pension entitlements when their jobs disappear because of plant closings or downsizing (Lowe 1991).

Identity, Self-Esteem and Control

Because retirement can be perceived as the beginning of the "role-less role" (Minkler 1981, 119), retired people must create a new identity for themselves in the absence of socially defined roles. According to a report on Seniors in Service (discussed in the section below), 70 percent of adults over the age of 65 report missing the contacts they enjoyed before retirement, and many experience profound loneliness (Danzig and Szanton 1987) and a feeling of idleness (Freedman 1994). If retirement per se can have these effects, early involuntary retirement probably has worse effects because it also involves a loss of control. Research shows that workers prepare for retirement by reducing their commitment to their jobs (Ekerdt and DeViney 1993). When retirement is unscheduled or accelerated, however, workers may not get the opportunity for this anticipatory adaptation.

FACILITATING THE TRANSITION FROM WORK TO RETIREMENT

In this section, we present several "nonmedical" initiatives to enhance physical and mental health during the transition from work to retirement. Each case study is presented and discussed in standard form. First, we outline the values underlying the project, including the reasons for the initiative and a description of the participants in the project. The project is then analysed in terms of the extent that the goals and objectives were achieved, including a discussion of the replicability of the initiative in other contexts, and funding issues are described and discussed. Finally, the evaluation of each project is documented.

Little information is available on the success rate of initiatives designed to enhance health in the transition from work to retirement, particularly in Canada. Nevertheless, secondary sources provide information on projects that were designed to enhance the well-being of retiring individuals in the workplace itself or during the transition period. Few initiatives have been formally evaluated or even described in detail. However, we have endeavoured, wherever possible, to assess the viability of these programs. First, we provide a general overview, then present some case studies.

Overview of Strategies to Assist in the Transition from Employment to Retirement

The previous sections reinforced the significance of control to the well-being of retirees. Programs that use part-time work to make the transition gradual may facilitate this sense of control. Continuing to work at least part time may also promote well-being in seniors by providing income or an enhanced sense of purpose. Transitional jobs also generate a pool of active and productive individuals who will be needed as the proportion of younger workers decreases.

Polaroid Corporation of Cambridge, Massachusetts, has several "retirement rehearsal" programs that give workers up to six months unpaid leave or allow them to taper their work schedules gradually (Jack and Axelrad 1995). The company also offers its employees temporary or permanent part-time work, flextime and consulting contracts and a retiree job bank, all of which allow workers to control their retirement transition by adjusting slowly to less work. Travellers Companies also has a retiree job bank that permits its retirees to work up to 960 hours in any 12-month period without losing pension benefits (Rix 1990).

Under its Community Service Career Program, IBM offers qualified retirees two years of guaranteed, full-time employment in a nonprofit community organization at a salary of at least $10,000 per year (Rix 1990). Although IBM's stated objective for this program is to help meet community needs as well as the postretirement needs of its employees, the contract also keeps participants from working for a competitor for at least two years, by which time it is assumed that any proprietary knowledge the employee would bring to a competitor would be outdated. Therefore, the program benefits both retirees and the company. A similar program is offered by Nova Corporation, a Calgary-based company, which pays up to half the retiree's salary for two years. Workers of any age in designated business units are eligible for this program as part of a campaign to reduce the payroll without targeting older workers.

It is ironic that, while many companies downsize by retiring older workers, others hire older workers because they face labour shortages. In the fast-food industry, McDonald's and Kentucky Fried Chicken have turned to older workers in response to rapid industry growth and the simultaneous decrease in the number of young workers (Rix 1990). McDonald's "McMasters Program" has a four-week training program, tailored specifically for workers over the age of 55, featuring part-time work schedules, higher wages, and a more attractive benefits package. Company managers are also trained to work with older workers, in part to abolish myths and prevent biases against older workers (Rix 1990). However, employment in the fast-food industry can be exhausting, entailing hours of standing, which may not be particularly attractive or beneficial to older people.

Days Inns Case Study

Actions on Nonmedical Determinants of Health

One of the best-known success stories in the older worker literature is the Days Inns case study (McNaught and Barth 1992). Days Inns of America, the third largest U.S. hotel chain, decided to hire older workers for its reservations centre. Although this initiative was motivated by a staff shortage and not by any desire to benefit older workers, it improved the health and well-being of retirees while benefitting the business.

Reasons for the Initiative

In 1986, the hotel chain had trouble staffing its Atlanta reservation centre, mostly because of a high turnover rate with younger workers. The company did not believe that raising wages would significantly reduce turnover (McNaught and Barth 1992). It decided instead to hire workers over the age of 50 to manage the 9,000 daily calls for information and reservations.

Actors

Workers were recruited from senior citizen centres when advertisements in the general print media received a poor response. Younger workers are usually recruited through advertisements in local newspapers or by sending recruiters to schools, but these methods were not effective with older workers. Days Inns had more success recruiting older workers by making personal visits to senior citizen centres and by arranging for interested individuals to speak with older workers who had already joined the company (McNaught and Barth 1992).

Little information is available on the characteristics of project participants apart from a brief demographic profile of the 187 workers who staffed the reservations centre from 1987 through 1990 (McNaught and Barth 1992). Of the 187 workers, 18 percent were over the age of 60 and 26 percent were over the age of 50. Most of those over 50 were women.

Analysis of the Results

McNaught and Barth (1992) conducted a comparative analysis of Days Inns' older and younger workers from 1987 to 1990. The company was concerned that the older workers would not be as cost effective as the younger workers because older workers were thought to work more slowly than younger workers and have difficulty picking up new skills, particularly in computer technology (CARNET 1995a,b). As McNaught and Barth (1992) state, the job of the reservation agent is not easy. "Each agent must simultaneously engage in a conversation with the prospective client, query the reservations system for information, report on data appearing on the system's CRT screen, and obtain local amenity and environmental information from a five-inch-thick binder" (McNaught and Barth 1992, 55).

Initially, the older workers required an extra week of training than the younger workers, adding costs. However, it was discovered that the problem lay with the training program itself, not with the workers' ability to learn. Once the company changed its training programs to accommodate the fears and insecurities of older workers, there was no longer any difference between the training times of younger and older workers.

Furthermore, and of considerable importance to the company, older workers had substantially higher retention rates than younger workers; 87 percent of them remaining for a full year, compared with 30 percent of younger workers (McNaught and Barth 1992). This higher retention rate reduced training costs and increased the number of experienced workers on the job. But perhaps most important, although the older workers tended to spend more time on each call (usually in only the first six months of work), the study also found that older workers made more reservations (success in 43 percent of calls, compared with 38 percent for younger workers).

Part of the success of this initiative was due to the company's ability to recognize and understand the particular training needs of older workers and that older workers use different strategies, such as longer telephone conversations, to complete their job tasks. But, apart from an effective business strategy, the Days Inns case study demonstrates the potential benefits to older retirees and workers of receiving the opportunity to continue to work. Similar projects may benefit older individuals by supplementing their retirement incomes (especially important for women), and by offering social contacts. Furthermore, employment opportunities for workers approaching or reaching retirement may offer a much-needed choice and, consequently, a sense of control over the options and decisions in the retirement years for older people who are not sure they want to retire at a designated age.

Replicability of the Initiative

The Days Inns project could be replicated quite easily. In fact, several similar projects have been implemented with comparable benefits. For instance, the Hot House Flowers initiative provided employment opportunities for older workers in a British retail firm (James 1994). Like Days Inns, this retail company was experiencing labour shortages due to high staff turnover and a recent expansion. In 1987, the company hired 50 people over the age of 55 for their stores in London and southeast England. It found that older workers had a higher rate of retention than younger workers, and were reliable and conscientious. The initiative was so successful that the retail company now makes a point of hiring older workers, reporting that 18 percent of its workforce is over the age of 50 (James 1994). Most of these older workers are women, working part time in customer service, where the company believes their skills lie.

The company recently conducted an evaluation of the 300 employees over the age of 40 and found benefits for the health and well-being of older workers. The work provided extra income to those on reduced retirement incomes and the subsidized staff meal plan provided a nutritious three-course meal for less than a dollar. The work also provided companionship. Thirty-six percent of the older workers surveyed said they returned to work because they wanted the social interaction (James 1994). This social component may be particularly important for people who have lost a spouse or close relative or who have lost contact with friends and coworkers following retirement.

Funding

Since the Hot House Flowers project involved only regular company recruiting and training activities, funding and resources were not difficult to obtain. Any costs specifically associated with the older workers were offset by their higher productivity and retention rates. Although Days Inns initially had to spend more on training their older workers, the subsequent changes in training equalized the costs of the program. Also, recruiting methods for older and younger workers cost the same (McNaught and Barth 1992). Despite expectations to the contrary, the study found that health insurance costs for older and younger workers were relatively equal, perhaps in part because older workers who can work tend to be in better health, and because their additional expenses tend to be offset by the larger number of dependants younger workers typically insure under the health plan.

Evaluation

The project has not been formally evaluated, apart from an assessment of productivity and finances. No testimony is available from participants.

Silver Human Resource Centres in Japan

Actions on Nonmedical Determinants of Health

It can also be insightful to look to other countries for policy initiatives designed to facilitate the transition from work to retirement. In Japan, fully 71.4 percent of men aged 60–64 are employed compared with only 54.2 percent of U.S. men of that age (Bass and Oka 1995). This finding suggests that older workers in Japan may have more favourable resources and programs. One such program, the Silver Human Resource Centres (SHRC), was designed to improve the lives of older workers while enhancing the contributions of older people in the community (Bass and Oka 1995).

Reasons for the Initiative

The first SHRC was established in Tokyo in 1975 to expand the job prospects of retirees. The SHRCs are a collaboration between industry, government and local communities that contract for services provided by retired workers. SHRCs are similar to employment agencies for temporary workers where the agency solicits work from companies and dispatches workers. However, SHRCs employ only retired workers, and they do only work that will benefit the local community. Retirees typically do tasks such as proofreading and translation; gardening and simple carpentry; sorting and filing papers; addressing letters and making simple calculations; maintaining or collecting admission fees at parks and other public places; inspecting gas and water meters; making deliveries and collecting bills; cleaning streets; packing and wrapping; and providing home help and other services for older people (Bass and Oka 1995). Hourly wages range from $7 to $10, depending on the task, and earnings are not deducted from pensions (Bass and Oka 1995).

Actors

Created by the local community or municipality, each SHRC negotiates services contracts with businesses, agencies or individuals for older people. The average age of the members of the SHRCs is 68.5 years; 69.1 years for men and 67.4 years for women (Bass and Oka 1995). Most members are men, with almost twice as many men as women partly because older women are Japan's traditional caregivers and Japanese society is reluctant to have older women working outside the home. However, more than 20 percent of women employed through SHRCs have not previously held a job, indicating that the centres do provide job opportunities for older women who desire to work. The type of work offered may also restrict the ability of women to participate in the centres, since many tasks, such as gardening, maintenance and carpentry, are traditional male jobs that require physical labour. Broadening the range of positions to match the needs and skills of more people is currently being discussed. In future, as more highly skilled people retire, there will be a need to contract out more specialized labour.

Analysis of the Results

The number of SHRC centres has grown tremendously. In 1994, there were 661 centres in Japan, employing 310,000 people over the age of 60. They have given older workers the opportunity to earn additional income and remain in contact with and contribute to society. As discussed earlier, these roles and contacts may prove to be a source of overall well-being. The SHRCs have also become permanently established in Japanese society, which may reinforce the presence and importance of older people. They also demonstrate how collaboration between different levels of government and industry can successfully benefit both older workers and the community.

Replicability of the Initiative

To what extent can such an initiative be replicated in Canada? As outlined by Bass and Oka (1995), there is nothing intrinsic to the program that cannot be initiated elsewhere, apart from the commitment from local and federal governments to employ older people. It is not clear whether Canadian government policies could provide the funding commitment necessary to initiate such a program, nor whether the public would accept the redirection of financial resources to older people. Furthermore, as recognized by Bass and Oka (1995), such a program may be opposed by unions who may view participants as cheap labour potentially taking jobs from younger workers.

Bass and Oka (1995) offer alternatives to the SHRCs that might fit better in the North American situation, such as small private cooperatives of older workers who contract out their skills.[2] Funding could come from existing small business loan programs.

Funding

Each SHRC may apply for federal funding to cover its administrative costs. Local governments must match federal funds in cash. However, if local

---

2. There are some Canadian examples, such as Senior Talent Bank of Ontario.

governments contract work to the SHRC, the federal government reimburses them one dollar for every three dollars paid to the SHRC for services.

In 1993, the Japanese Ministry of Labour provided $93,104,720 (all figures in U.S. dollars) (Bass and Oka 1995) in infrastructure support to the SHRCs, and $53,777,930 in reimbursements to local governments for contracting with SHRCs. The 1993 total public sector funding of $349,646,000 was used to create more than $1 billion in jobs for older people. More than two-thirds of the work contracts came from private companies.

The SHRC initiative has been so successful that the Japanese government has had to reduce its contribution to the program. There are plans for the gradual elimination of reimbursable funds for SHRCs that are at least 10 years old. The original intent of the program was to encourage the centres to become self-supporting in the longer term.

Evaluation

The SHRC program has not been formally evaluated in terms of its effect on the health and well-being of older people.

Seniors in Service

Actions on the Nonmedical Determinants of Health

Seniors in Service is a U.S. initiative to direct the resources of a growing elderly population toward community service. Seniors in Service currently employs 100,000 seniors, most of them low income, in its various programs. The programs offer a stipend to seniors willing to do various kinds of community service, including education, child care, elder care, public safety, and environmental and human service assignments. School systems suffering from funding restraints and overburdened teachers benefit from seniors who provide teaching assistance, tutoring, counselling and clerical work, as well as maintaining and repairing school facilities (Freedman 1994). The growing number of single-parent households and working parents also increases the need for child care in the community and institutions.

Reasons for the Initiative

The Seniors in Service initiative sprang from the National Service ideal launched by the Clinton administration through the *National and Community Service Trust Act* of 1993 (Freedman 1994). Although the initiative was directed mainly at youth, growing numbers of older people prompted the expansion of the program to include older Americans, and this component came to be called Seniors in Service.

Actors

Because the programs focus on education, child care and elder care, most participants are women. For instance, only 11 percent of the Foster Grandparents and 15 percent of Senior Companions are men, and only 34 percent of the participants in the Senior Community Service Employment Program are men (Freedman 1994, 51). The contrast with the Japanese SHRCs initiative is dramatic.

Analysis of the Results

One component of Seniors in Service is the Foster Grandparent Program, in which low-income seniors over the age of 60 work five half-days a week with young people with special needs in schools, daycare centres and institutions (Freedman 1994, 26). Foster Grandparents care for abused and neglected children, counsel teenage mothers, and help children with disabilities. Foster Grandparents receive a tax-exempt stipend of $2.45 an hour.

The program clearly benefits the younger recipients, since older individuals are able to provide guidance, care and knowledge learned through many years of raising children. But the program also benefits the Foster Grandparents. As one 70-year-old women commented on her work with school children:

> It does me as much good, because we have needs, too, we want to be wanted, to be loved, to give our love. If we don't have a chance to do that, then it takes something away. That's where a lot of older people are lonely... (Freedman 1994, 7).

Another component is the Community Service Program, which employs seniors over the age of 55 to work in local services, such as education, public safety, human services and the environment (Freedman 1994, 31). Participants work 20 hours a week for a minimum wage of $4.25 an hour plus minimal benefits. Seventy-five per cent of participants must have incomes below the poverty level; the rest can be at 125 percent of poverty level. A retired school principal in his middle 60s, who took a position in the program supervising a food bank, a senior citizen centre and a volunteer clearing house, commented:

> You know, when I retired they gave me a bunch of fishing equipment. Said, "Now here, you get on your boat, do some fishing." Well I went fishing three times and I thought, if this is what it's all about, I'll go back to work... By the time you retire, you're programmed to get up and go to work, then all of a sudden you have to get up and think, "what am I gonna do today?" That's probably the hardest thing to adjust to in retirement.

You have to figure out what each day's gonna be. That's why I like the Corps, because I've got something to do every day...to get involved and have some things to get up in the morning and look forward to doing. I'm a people person, like to help people, get a good feeling out of putting something back into a society that I've taken a lot from these 60 years (Freedman 1994, 17).

Another component of Seniors in Service is the Seniors Companion Program, which provides social contact to housebound elderly people and people with Alzheimer's disease, and respite care to families caring for elderly people. Companions provide a range of services, including light house-keeping, meal preparation and transportation to medical appointments. The program often matches people with similar history and background. Veterans are matched with veterans, recovering addicts with seniors recovering from alcohol and drug problems. Most (88 percent) companions are women; they receive a stipend of $2.45 an hour.

One man in the program, a 65-year-old retired cab driver and prison guard, visits frail seniors in the community to help them live independently and delay institutionalization. He comments:

I guess it's kind of corny, but I feel good if I can help somebody else... Partly, it's because of the independence. The flexibility. I don't punch a clock. It's also fun... And you get close to the other Companions (Freedman 1994, 34).

The program is both a vital resource to the community and a source of well-being for older people. It provides income support for seniors who live near or below the poverty level and a much-needed source of social contact for older adults. Postretirement work can offset loneliness and loss of purpose. Volunteers have been found to have more life satisfaction and a stronger will to live, with fewer somatic, anxious and depressive symptoms than similarly aged individuals who do not do volunteer work (Freedman 1994, 13).

Despite these demonstrated benefits, there are limitations to the programs (Freedman 1994, 50). The programs are limited to seniors on low incomes so most working-class and middle-class seniors cannot participate, even if they are only slightly above the eligibility line. Because the programs revolve around caregiving, support or clerical work, most participants are women.

Furthermore, the program falls far short of its potential. Many needy communities do not benefit from these programs since the initiative is available in only a small fraction of the counties in the U.S. (Freedman 1994, 50). At the same time, many seniors willing to serve remain on waiting lists or do not know about the service possibilities (Freedman 1994, 57). This is partly because many potential program sponsors do not believe that seniors are sufficiently skilled for public service (Freedman 1994, 50) and that many organizations lack the infrastructure required to employ older workers.

Replicability of the Initiative

To replicate Seniors in Service in Canada would certainly involve major financial and structural commitment from the government. The Government of Canada is well positioned to assess need for services that can be provided through this type of program because of long involvement in supporting community programs through the New Horizons Program, the Seniors Independence Program and the Health Promotion Directorate.

Funding

Seniors in Service demonstrates the benefits that can be achieved through government policy initiatives to support locally controlled programs. However, such programs are expensive (Freedman 1994). The Foster Grandparents program has a budget of $95 million, $65 million from federal and $30 million from nonfederal sources; and the Seniors Companion Project receives $29.5 million in federal funding and $16.8 million from nonfederal sources (Freedman 1994, 27). Each program needs adequate training, supervision and recruitment resources as well as transportation and other support services. Overall, the U.S. federal government contributes $483.8 million annually to the programs, while $115.7 million comes from nonfederal resources (Freedman 1994, 47). Most of the federal money, 70 percent, goes to the more than 90,000 senior participants (Freedman 1994, 47).

   The costs of such a program are substantial, but as Freedman (1994, 49) points out, more needs to be done to clarify the cost-benefits. The initiative may prevent many costly outcomes such as crime and social maladjustment, extensive health care usage by older adults and institutionalization, and may reduce welfare rates. All these benefits may more than offset the costs of the program.

Evaluation

A series of studies has been conducted to evaluate the success of the various programs of the Seniors in Service initiative. Over 20 years, 35 evaluations of the Seniors Companion Program have been done; one found that the program had "an important impact on alleviating the loneliness of the adults it serves, increasing their level of activity, and meeting other basic needs" (Booz, Allen, and Hamilton 1975). Seniors are a growing and valuable resource for these unmet needs, and recent studies suggest that they are skilled and eager for paid or volunteer work (Commonwealth Fund 1993; Marriott Senior Volunteerism Study 1991). A 1977 U.S. study found that the greatest unmet needs are in human services (Yarmolinsky 1977), where older individuals tend to perform better because they have more patience and experience. A 1988 study found that the Companion Program served a truly needy population by supplementing existing services (Research Triangle Institute 1988). Similar findings were observed in evaluations of other programs of the initiative (see Freedman 1994, 35–40 for a review).

Evaluations also highlight the benefits seniors receive as workers in the programs. A five-year study comparing Companion Program participants with seniors on the waiting list found that participants demonstrated greater improvement in their mental health (SRA Technologies 1985). A three-year longitudinal study of 14 Foster Grandparents found that participants in that program displayed an improvement in their mental health and social resources, while people on the waiting list deteriorated in these areas. Furthermore, 83 percent of participating Grandparents reported being "more satisfied" with their life, and only 52 percent of people on the waiting list made similar claims (Litigation Support Services 1984).

Retirement Planning Programs for Women

Actions on Nonmedical Determinants of Health

As outlined earlier, the transition from work to retirement may be particularly difficult for women. Because their careers are more likely to be interrupted, women are less likely than men to develop the financial resources necessary for a secure retirement and are, therefore, at greater risk of lower income in retirement (Ballantyne and Marshall 1995). Also, because their life expectancy is longer, women are more likely to be widowed or to become responsible for the care of a spouse in their retirement years (Houlihan and Caraballo 1990).

Retirement planning programs may alleviate anxiety surrounding this transition and help women prepare adequately for this process. Participation in such programs has been shown to foster a sense of control and a positive attitude (Abel and Hayslip 1987) and is also predictive of a happier retirement (Ekerdt 1987). Counselling should be given well in advance, and raise awareness of the possibility of sudden early retirement (Reis and Gold 1993).

However, few studies have successfully demonstrated the benefits of retirement planning programs. Studies frequently lack an adequate control group, have insufficient follow-up and biased samples, since most study subjects are male volunteers. For instance, a longitudinal study comparing an intensive discussion group retirement planning program with a self-directed module and a control group (Glamser 1981) found that the intensive program did little to improve retirees' self-reported adjustment to and preparation for retirement. However, the study used only male retirees and the postprogram assessment was conducted almost four years after retirement. As the author acknowledges, the benefits of retirement preparation programs may be seen only in the preretirement stage or in the period immediately after retirement, when the transition is the most traumatic (Glamser 1981). Moreover, the benefits of such a program for women retirees are not addressed.

Current retirement preparation programs emphasize financial and legal issues of interest to middle- and upper-management executives (Houlihan and Caraballo 1990) who are usually male; therefore, the content of such programs is of little benefit to women. Women are, therefore, less likely to participate in retirement preparation programs (Szinovacz and Washo 1992), even though they may be at greater risk of economic and personal difficulties in the retirement transition (Beck 1984).

Reasons for the Initiative

To address this problem, some retirement planning programs are specifically directed to the needs and concerns of middle-aged women. Future Connections, Inc. was developed by the Gerontology Institute of the University of Massachusetts at Boston (Houlihan and Caraballo 1990). Female students at the Institute, the majority of whom were retired, expressed difficulty in their transition to retirement. Through a number of population surveys and analyses of retirement preparation programs in the Boston area, the researchers realized that many people, especially women, do not plan for their retirement, nor do they appreciate the problems they will face. The Institute then surveyed existing retirement planning programs and discovered that retirement programs do not consider women's gender, income and class issues adequately. Subsequently, they developed a program to address these specific needs.

Actors

This program is unique in many ways. The students who run it are mostly retired women with an average age of 60 (Houlihan and Caraballo 1990) who are highly aware of the needs of retiring women and act as strong role models for participants. A dozen students staff the program, either as members of the board of directors or as administrators working part time from 6 to 20 hours per week. The Institute provides one full-time employee for training, technical assistance and fundraising support.

The retirement programs are marketed to organizations employing large numbers of women and to community groups, such as churches and community centres, frequented by women. Each 12-hour program is offered either as six two-hour weekly sessions or as an intensive two-day retreat. This structure was designed to accommodate the extensive domestic demands on women's time outside working hours. The sessions are tailored to the specific needs of program participants to ensure that examples are drawn from the group's specific situation, such as nursing or clerical work.

Analysis of the Results

The program addresses an identified need for information on economic, health care and supportive resources that women require as they age. It also teaches prospective retirees to help themselves through the retirement transition by recognizing their vulnerabilities and directing them to appropriate resources.

However, the program faced obstacles along the way. Because the retirees employed by the Institute in the program were not required to have specific experience in administration or organization, they needed specialized training and technical assistance. Also, because many retired employees hesitated to promote or sell the program, particularly in a reluctant market, marketing specialists were needed to help program leaders develop employees' skills and confidence.

The program also encountered obstacles from companies requesting the program. Many companies wanted only the financial and legal presentations, preferring not to pay for the sessions on personal development. The organizers decided to sell the program in its entirety or not at all, even at the risk of declining business, to maintain the original program objective, particularly since participants evaluated the "softer" components of the program highly (Houlihan and Caraballo 1990).

Finally, Future Connections may have weaknesses similar to those of other retirement preparation programs. Because participation is voluntary, participants may be predisposed to help themselves through the transition to retirement. Such a program, therefore, may be of little help to people who are not actively considering the implications of retirement—precisely those who may need assistance most. Short of making such programs mandatory, it is difficult to reach this reluctant group.

Replicability of the Initiative

Can a program like Future Connections be developed in Canada? Houlihan and Caraballo (1990) point out that such an initiative is useful only if a need for such a program is identified in a particular geographical area. Given the aging Canadian population and the increase in the trend toward early exit from the labour force, it may be useful to establish a similar program, considering its potential benefits not only for those facing retirement, but also for retirees interested in continuing to work. Other seniors or retiree organizations may provide a pool of labour to administer and run the program, just as students of the Gerontology Institute did for the Future Connections program.

Funding

Program funding came from two sources: grants from private foundations and fees from participants. As a nonprofit enterprise, the program was eligible for charitable funding. The sessions were priced to compete with other programs, but were kept low enough to encourage women with limited incomes to attend.

Evaluation

The effects of the program on the well-being of women in the transition to retirement have not been formally evaluated. However, postsession evaluations by participants were favourable (Houlihan and Caraballo 1990).

POLICY IMPLICATIONS

The literature on the health effects of the transition from employment to retirement indicates certain areas of concern. Specifically, although the retirement event per se does not carry health risks, some phases of the retirement process are associated with elevated risks to health and, most important, involuntary retirement has significant negative health effects, whether viewed as an event or as a process.

Policies would be most effective if directed to: instilling a sense of control over the transition, either in the anticipatory phase of the transition or following exit from paid employment; lowering the risk of economic insecurity resulting from job loss and loss of the opportunity to accumulate adequate pension benefits; and supporting programs to facilitate social support and maintenance of self-esteem, which is often threatened by retirement and probably placed at greater risk by early, involuntary retirement. We recommend policy initiatives in several areas.

Support gradual and phased retirement

The research evidence quite strongly supports the benefits of gradual and phased retirement, yet many Canadian workers have no opportunity to move into retirement through part-time or less demanding work. Part-time jobs have benefits in job creation (Foot 1994), but among the barriers to introducing part-time work as a career stage are inflexible pension regulations and union resistance (Marshall 1995a, b). Many of the model programs we have described provide options for partial and flexible retirement.

Develop and support retiree service programs

Given that the recent trend toward early exit is not likely to be reversed in the near future, it is important to develop programs that will allow those who still wish to contribute to society to do so. Retiree service programs such as we have described do this while enhancing self esteem and providing supportive social contact. The programs need not conflict with the currently employed. As we showed with the Companion Program of Seniors in Service, services provided by retirees can complement rather than replace existing services.

Support retirement education programs that recognize the diversity of transitions from employment to retirement

We noted that retirement education programs have found little support in evaluation studies. This may reflect the failure of such programs to address the changing nature of the transition from employment to retirement. Given that control is such an important determinant of a good transition to retirement, individuals forced to retire early may benefit from counselling to help them adapt to losses in control and formulate goals for life in retirement. Retirement education and counselling programs should deal explicitly with a host of issues that follow midlife departure from career jobs, such as changing family relationships, seeking bridge employment, and income security.

Develop and support programs explicitly directed to training and placing older workers and early retirees in bridge jobs

Two of the case studies we presented, Days Inns and Hot House Flowers, describe bridge job opportunities for people who have made an early exit from career jobs. Both cases included a strong training component that resulted in high productivity and substantial benefits to the sponsoring companies. The development of similar programs in Canada should be fostered through public policy initiatives in collaboration with business. Publicly funded demonstration programs incorporating strong evaluations could provide information to help generate such collaborations. Human Resources Development Canada might fund the training component of such programs and assist with evaluation costs and the dissemination of evaluation study results.

Promote positive images and counter negative stereotypes of older workers through social marketing and educational programs

Several of the case studies demonstrate the productivity of older workers. However, negative stereotypes about the productivity of older workers, and their ability to adapt to technological and organizational change, persist in Canada (CARNET 1995a, b; Marshall 1995b). Social marketing and public education programs can have an impact in this area. Some of the programs we have described, such as Seniors in Service, can foster intergenerational solidarity by bringing older and younger people together. The experience of the Division of Aging and Seniors in this area gives it the expertise to support such initiatives in collaboration with provincial seniors directorates and offices of senior affairs.

Recognize the greater vulnerability of women and those of lower socioeconomic status to career disruption

Since women are so much more vulnerable than men in the transition from employment to retirement, and as Canada has the policy structure to focus on women's issues, we recommend that policy initiatives in this area should highlight gender differences. Similarly, the greater impact of career disruption, interrupted work histories and abnormal retirement patterns on those of lower socioeconomic status call for attention. For managers and professionals, threats to self-esteem and identity might be the major issues linking the retirement transition to health; for blue-collar workers, the major health-related issue is likely to be loss of income security.

Foster research on the health effects of disruptive work careers

Throughout this review, we have emphasized that the evidential basis for understanding the health effects of disrupted work histories is very thin. The changing nature of work over the life course warrants a concerted effort to understand its health effects. Seen in the broad framework of the social determinants of health, these research efforts should explicitly address the relationships between career characteristics, economic security issues, and social-psychological factors such as coping, sense of control, and identity maintenance.

CONCLUSION

Many of the case studies we have reviewed are based on the assumptions that retaining older workers in the labour force and encouraging the re-entry of displaced older workers are positive. Currently this view is not widely held in Canada, as both governments and corporations seem to be trying hard to reduce their workforces. However, some European countries have responded with alarm to the move to early exit, and have introduced policies to reverse that trend. They recognize the dangers of having too few people working, with too many people at risk economically and socially. This is partially a question of who pays for the social safety net, and partially a question of the kind of society we want.

Our policy recommendations are framed within the context of an aging society in which older workers are devalued—as indicated by the willingness and even eagerness of employers to be rid of them. However, the case studies represent several examples of programs that simultaneously benefit older workers, early retirees, on-time retirees, employers and the community. Many of these programs seem cost effective.

The case studies represent initiatives that address many of the general social determinants influencing the relationship between health and the transition from employment to retirement. Some of these initiatives, and others for which we have not found examples, can be launched or supported by government policy. We argue that the most productive policy directions place the government in partnership with the corporate sector (public and private, owners, managers and unions), community organizations, older workers and seniors.

Victor W. Marshall *is director of the Institute of Human Development, Life Course and Aging, and professor of Behavioral Science at the University of Toronto. He was network director of CARNET: The Canadian Aging Research Network from 1990 to 1995, and served as editor-in-chief of the* Canadian Journal on Aging *for five years. He is currently vice-president of the Canadian Association of Gerontology and a member of the Canada Pension Plan Advisory Board. His current research focuses on social, labour force and health policy issues in relation to aging.*

BIBLIOGRAPHY

ABEL, B. J., and B. HAYSLIP. 1987. Locus of control and retirement preparation. *Journal of Gerontology* 42: 165–167.

ADVISORY GROUP ON WORKING TIME AND THE DISTRIBUTION OF WORK. 1994. *Report of the Advisory Group on Working Time and the Distribution of Work.* Ottawa: Human Resources Development Canada.

ATCHLEY, R. G. 1976. *The Sociology of Retirement.* New York: Halstead Press.

BALLANTYNE, P.J., and V. W. MARSHALL. 1995. Wealth and the life course. In *Contributions to Independence over the Life Course*, eds. V. W. MARSHALL, J. A. MCMULLIN, P. J. BALLANTYNE, J. DACIUK and B. T. WIGDOR. Toronto: Centre for Studies of Aging, University of Toronto. pp. 49–83.

BASS, S. A., and M. OKA. 1995. An older worker employment model: Japan's Silver Human Resource Centers. *The Gerontologist* 35 (5): 679–682.

BAZZOLI, G. J. 1985. The early retirement decision: New empirical evidence on the influence of health. *The Journal of Human Resources* 20 (2): 215–234.

BECK, S. H. 1984. Retirement preparation programs: Differentials in opportunity and use. *Journal of Gerontology* 39: 596–602.

BETCHERMAN, G., and N. LECKIE. 1995. Age structure of employment in industries and occupations. Working Paper Series, *Issues of an Aging Workforce: A Study to Inform Human Resources Policy Development.* Toronto: Centre for Studies of Aging, University of Toronto.

BOAZ, R. F., and C. F. MULLER. 1990. The validity of health reasons as a reason for deciding to retire. *Health Services Research* 25 (2): 361–386.

BOOZ, A. and HAMILTON. 1975. *Senior Companion Program Study.* Washington (DC): ACTION.

CANADA. STATISTICS CANADA. 1993. *Survey of Persons not in the Labour Force.* Ottawa: Ministry of Supply and Services Canada.

CARNET: THE CANADIAN AGING RESEARCH NETWORK. 1995a. *Issues of an Aging Workforce: A Case Study of the Sun Life Assurance Company of Canada.* Toronto: Centre for Studies of Aging, University of Toronto.

_____. 1995b. *Issues of an Aging Workforce: A Case Study of the Prudential Life Insurance Company of America.* Toronto: Centre for Studies of Aging, University of Toronto.

COMMONWEALTH FUND. 1993. *The Untapped Resource: The Final Report of the Americans over 55 at Work Program.* New York: The Commonwealth Fund. pp. 14–28.

DANZIG, R., and P. SZANTON. 1987. *National Service: What Would It Mean?* Lexington (MA): Lexington Books. pp. 63–68.

DOERINGER, P. B. (Ed.) 1990. *Bridges to Retirement.* Ithaca (NY): IRL Press of Cornell University.

EISDORFER, C., and F. WILKIE. 1977. Stress, disease, aging and behavior. In *Handbook of the Psychology of Aging*, eds. J. E. BIRREN, and K. W. SCHAIE. New York: Van Nostrand Reinhold. pp. 251–275.

EKERDT, D. J. 1987. Retirement planning. In *The Encyclopedia of Aging*, ed. G. L. MADDOX. New York: Springer. pp. 583–584.

EKERDT, D. J., and S. DEVINEY. 1993. Evidence for a preretirement process among older male workers. *Journal of Gerontology: Social Sciences* 48 (2): S35–S43.

ELDER, G. H., and E. K. PAVALKO. 1993. Work careers in men's later years: Transitions, trajectories, and historical change. *Journal of Gerontology: Social Sciences* 48 (4): S180–S191.

ELWELL, F., and A. D.MALTBIE-CRANNELL. 1981. The impact of role loss upon coping resources and life satisfaction of the elderly. *Journal of Gerontology* 36: 223–232.

EVANS, R. G., and G.L. STODDARD. 1990. Producing health, consuming health care. *Social Science and Medicine* 31 (2): 1347–63. Reprinted in *Why Are Some People Healthy and Others Not? The Determinants of Health of Populations*, eds. R. G. EVANS, M. L. BARER, and T. R. MARMOR. New York: Aldine de Gruyter, 1994.

FILLENBAUM, G. G., L. K. GEORGE, and E. B. PALMORE. 1985. Determinants and consequences of retirement among men of different races and economic levels. *Journal of Gerontology* 40: 85–94.

FLETCHER, W. L., and R. O. HANSSON. 1991. Assessing the social components of retirement anxiety. *Psychology and Aging* 6: 76–85.

FOOT, D. 1994. David Foot discusses career paths. Interviewed by Doreen Duchesne. *Perspectives on Labour and Income* 6 (winter): 13–21.

FRANK, J., and J. F. MUSTARD. 1994. The determinants of health from a historical perspective. *Daedalus* 123 (4): 1–19.

FREEDMAN, M. 1994. Seniors in national and community service. A report prepared for the Commonwealth Fund's Americans over 55 at Work Program. Philadelphia: Public/Private Ventures.

GEORGE, L. K., 1992. Economic status and subjective well-being. In *Aging, Money, and Life Satisfaction*, eds. N. E. CUTLER, D. W. GREGG, and M. P. LAWTON. New York: Springer. pp. 69–99.

GIBB-CLARK, M. MARCH 25, 1995. Many workers shun retiring early. *The Globe and Mail.*

GLAMSER, F. D. 1981. The impact of preretirement programs on the retirement experience. *Journal of Gerontology* 36 (2): 244–250.

GWYTHER, L. P. 1992. Generation: A corporate-sponsored retiree health care program. *The Gerontologist* 32 (2): 265–269.

HARDY, M. A., and J. QUADAGNO. 1995. Satisfaction with early retirement: Making choices in the auto industry. *Journal of Gerontology: Social Sciences* 50B (4): S217–S228.

HAUSMAN, J. A., and L. PAQUETTE. 1987. Involuntary early retirement and consumption. In *Work, Health and Income among the Elderly*, ed. G. BURTLESS. Washington: Brookings Institute.

HAYNES, S. G., A. J. MCMICHAEL, and H. A. TYROLER. 1977. The relationship of normal, involuntary retirement to early mortality among U.S. rubber workers. *Social Science and Medicine* 11: 105–114.

HERZOG, A. R., J. S. HOUSE, and J. N. MORGAN. 1991. Relation of work and retirement to health and well-being in older age. *Psychology and Aging* 6 (2): 202–211.

HOULIHAN, P. and E. CARABALLO. 1990. Women and retirement planning: The development of Future Connections, Inc. In *Preretirement Planning for Women: Program Design and Research*, eds. C. L. HAYES and J. M. DEREN. New York: Springer. pp. 63–76.

JACK, L., and S. AXELRAD. 1995. The aging workforce. *Occupational Health and Safety Canada* (Sept.–Oct.): 28–37.

JAMES, L. 1994. Hot House Flowers—a U.K. retailer's response to older workers. In *Investing in Older People at Work: Contributions, Case Studies and Recommendations*. London: Health Education Authority. pp. 118–122.

KESSLER, R. C., and J. D. MCLEOD. 1984. Sex differences in vulnerability to undesirable life events. *American Sociological Review* 49: 620–631.

KINGSON, E. R. 1981. Retirement and circumstances of very early retirees: A life cycle perspective. *Aging and Work* 4 (1): 11–22.

KOHLI, M., M. REIN, A.-M. GUILLEMARD, and H. VAN GUNSTEREN (Eds.) 1991. *Time for Retirement: Comparative Studies of Early Exit from the Labour Force*. Cambridge: Cambridge University Press.

LEBLANC, L. S. 1995. The influence of structural factors on the early retirement plans and expectations of older workers. Doctoral thesis, Department of Sociology, University of Toronto.

LITIGATION SUPPORT SERVICES. 1984. *Impact Evaluation of the Foster Grandparent Program on the Foster Grandparents*. Washington (DC): ACTION.

LOWE, G. S. 1991. Retirement attitudes, plans and behavior. *Perspectives, Statistics Canada* (fall): 8–17.

Marriott Senior Volunteerism Study. 1991. Washington (DC): Marriott Senior Living Services.

MARSHALL, V. W. 1995a. Rethinking retirement: Issues for the twenty-first century. In *Rethinking Retirement*, eds. E. M. GEE, and G. M. GUTMAN. Vancouver: Gerontology Research Centre, Simon Fraser University. pp. 31–50.

_____. 1995b. The older worker in Canadian society: Is there a future? In *Rethinking Retirement*, eds. E. M. GEE, and G. M. GUTMAN. Vancouver: Gerontology Research Centre, Simon Fraser University. pp. 51–68.

MARSHALL, V. W., J. A. MCMULLIN, P. J. BALLANTYNE, J. F. DACIUK, and B. T. WIGDOR. 1995. *Contributions to Independence over the Adult Life Course.* Toronto: Centre for Studies of Aging, University of Toronto.

MARTIN, J., and A. DORAN. 1966. Evidence concerning the relationship between health and retirement. *Sociological Review* 14: 329.

MARTIN MATTHEWS, A., and K. H. BROWN. 1988. Retirement as a critical life event: The differential experiences of men and women. *Research on Aging* 9 (4): 548–571.

MCDONALD, P. L. 1994. Retirement revisited: A secondary data analysis. *Working Paper: Issues of an Aging Workforce: A Study to Inform Human Resources Policy Development.* Toronto: Centre for Studies of Aging, University of Toronto.

MCDONALD, P. L., and M. Y. T. CHEN. 1993. The youth freeze and the retirement bulge: Older workers and the impending labour shortage. *Journal of Canadian Studies* 28 (1): 75–101.

MCNAUGHT, W., and M. C. BARTH. 1992. Are older workers "good buys"? A case study of Days Inns of America. *Sloan Management Review* 33 (3): 53–63.

MIDANIK, L. T., K. SOGHIKIAN, L. J. RANSOM, and I. S. TEKAWA. 1995. The effect of retirement on mental health and health behaviors: The Kaiser Permanente Retirement Study. *Journal of Gerontology* 50B (1): S59–S61.

MINKLER, M. 1981. Research on the health effects of retirement: An uncertain legacy. *Journal of Health and Social Behaviour* 22 (June): 117–130.

MYERS R. J. 1982. Why do people retire from work early? *Aging and Work* 5 (2): 83–91.

PALMORE, E. B., B.M. BURCHETT, G. G. FILLENBAUM, L. K. GEORGE, and L. M. WALLMAN (Eds.) 1985. *Retirement: Causes and Consequences.* New York: Springer.

PAMPEL, F. C., and S. PARK. 1986. Cross-national patterns and determinants of female retirement. *American Journal of Sociology* 91 (4): 932–955.

PAVALKO, E. K., G. H. ELDER, and E. C. CLIPP. 1993. Worklives and longevity: Insights from a life course perspective. *Journal of Health and Social Behavior* 34 (Dec.): 363–380.

PERETTI, P. O., and C. WILSON. 1975. Voluntary and involuntary retirement of aged males and their effect on emotional satisfaction, usefulness, self-image, emotional stability, and interpersonal relationships. *International Journal of Aging and Human Development* 6 (2): 131–138.

PICOT, G., and T. WANNELL. 1987. *Job Loss and Labour Market Adjustment in the Canadian Economy.* Ottawa: Analytical Studies Branch Working Paper Series. Social and Economic Studies Division. Statistics Canada.

REIS, M., and GOLD, D. P. 1993. Retirement, personality, and life satisfaction: A review and two models. *The Journal of Applied Gerontology* 12(2): 261–282.

RESEARCH TRIANGLE INSTITUTE. 1988. *Senior Companion Program: Homebound Elderly Demonstration Projects.* Washington (DC): ACTION.

RUCHLIN, H. S., and J. N. MORRIS. 1992. Deteriorating health and the cessation of employment among older workers. *Journal of Aging and Health* 4 (1): 43–57.

RIX, S.E. 1990. Employment opportunities for older workers. In *Older Workers: Choices and Challenges,* S. E. RIX, California: ABC–CLIO, Inc. pp. 97–120.

SCHELLENBERG, G. 1994. *The Road to Retirement: Demographic and Economic Changes in the '90s.* Ottawa: Centre for International Statistics. Canadian Council on Social Development.

SCHMÄHL, W. (Ed.) 1989. *Redefining the Process of Retirement: An International Perspective.* Berlin: Springer-Verlag

SELYE, H. 1982. History and present status of the stress concept. In L. GOLDBERGER and S. BREZNITZ (Eds.), *Handbook of Stress: Theoretical and Clinical Aspects.* New York: The Free Press. pp. 7–17.

SENIORS SECRETARIAT. 1993. *Aging and Independence: Overview of a National Survey.* Ottawa: Minister of National Health and Welfare. Cat. H88-3/13-1993E.

SRA TECHNOLOGIES. 1985. *Senior Companion Program Impact Evaluation.* Washington (DC): ACTION.

STANFORD, E. P., C. J. HAPPERSETT, D. J. MORTON, C. A. MOLGAARD, and K. M. PEDDECORD. 1991. Early retirement and functional impairment from a multi-ethnic perspective. *Research on Aging* 13 (1): 5–38.

STATISTICS CANADA. 1993. *Survey of Persons Not in the Labour Force.* Ottawa (ON): Ministry of Supply and Services Canada.

STREIB, G. F., and C. J. SCHNEIDER. 1971. *Retirement in American Society.* Ithaca: Cornell University Press.

SZINOVACZ, M., and C. WASKO. 1992. Gender differences in exposure to life events and adaptation to retirement. *Journal of Gerontology* 47 (4): S191–S196.

THOMPSON, G. B. 1973. Work versus leisure roles: An investigation of morale among employed and retired men. *Journal of Gerontology* 28 (3): 339–344.

THOMPSON, W. E., and G. F. STREIB. 1958. Situational determinants, health and economic deprivation in retirement. *Journal of Social Issues* 14 (2).

TOWERS PERRIN. 1991. *Workforce 2000: Competing in a Seller's Market: A Survey Report on Organizational Responses to Demographic and Labour Force Trends in Canada.* Toronto: Author.

USEEM, M. 1994. Business restructuring and the aging workforce. In *Aging and Competition: Rebuilding the U.S. Workforce*, eds. J. A. AUERBACH, and J. C. WELSH. Washington: National Planning Association. pp. 33–57.

WARR, P. In press. Age, work and well-being. In *Impact of Work on Older Adults*, eds. K. W. SCHNIE and C. SCHOOLER. New York: Springer Publishing Company.

WORLD HEALTH ORGANIZATION. 1986. Health promotion: Concept and principles in action, a policy framework. Discussion document. Copenhagen: WHO Regional Office for Europe.

YARMOLINSKY, A. 1977. National Service Program. In *National Compulsory Service.* West Point: U.S. Military Academy. p. 101.

Encouraging the Wise Use of Prescription Medication by Older Adults

DR. ROBYN TAMBLYN

Epidemiologist, Professor at McGill University
Director of the Quebec Research Group on Medication Use in the Elderly
(USAGE)

DR. ROBERT PERREAULT

Psychiatrist, Professor at Université de Montréal
Chief of Preventive Medicine (HMR)
Direction de la santé publique de Montréal-Centre

SUMMARY

Health problems in the elderly are becoming of increasing concern as the population ages. Seventy-eight percent of the elderly have at least one chronic disease and the use of medication increases with age. Drug expenditures are responsible for an increasing proportion of Canadian health care costs, an increase which is partly attributable to the use of new drugs by physicians and partly due to increased utilization rates. The increased utilization rates by the elderly are, in turn, attributable to the increased number of prescriptions.

Drugs are prescribed to a greater proportion of the senior population than is indicated by the prevalence of indications for drug therapy. In contrast, many patients who may benefit from drug therapy do not appear to be receiving it. Furthermore, among patients who receive drug treatment, 23–29 percent are prescribed therapy that is potentially inappropriate. Lastly, prescriptions are often written for drugs that are more costly than equally effective, less expensive alternatives. The challenges in prescribing for the elderly are substantial, particularly for physicians who are providing primary care management to a variety of problems in all age groups. These challenges are potentiated by the number of drugs (20,600) available for use.

Patient behaviour also influences drug prescribing. As noncompliance accounts for the majority of drug-related illnesses, priority needs to be placed on identifying better methods of involving patients in the process of making decisions about their medication, reducing the number of drugs and the complexity of the drug regimen, and having more accessible and concise information on how to take their medications properly.

Four levels of intervention have been identified as effective in addressing the problem of drug prescribing for the elderly: health care system interventions (prescription caps, physician clawbacks, etc.), physician-level interventions, pharmacist-level interventions, and patient-level interventions.

One example of a successful patient-based intervention is that of a research project that aroused considerable interest. The objective of the project, which was conducted in England, was to assess the efficacy of a computer-generated reminder chart in increasing compliance in patients incapable of taking their medication correctly. The reminder chart was determined to be practical and cost effective.

Of the physician-based interventions, personalized visits to physicians by pharmacist educators were studied in greater depth. The objective was to counterbalance the "glossy" presentations of the pharmaceutical industry and to provide physicians with neutral, objective information on new drugs. Personalized visits to physicians by pharmacist educators have a significant positive effect on the prescribing habits of physicians.

In conclusion, the large number of studies conducted on the subject allows the various elements of the problem to be organized into "microdeterminants" (physicians, patients, pharmacists, drugs) and "macrodeterminants" (government policy, drug industry, society). The present review of the research literature shows that no single cure exists for the problems of medication use in the elderly because no single problem exists. A variety of policy approaches must therefore be instituted, both at the patient, physician, pharmacist and public health organization levels, and in government-industry relations and medical education.

TABLE OF CONTENTS

FIGURE

LIST OF TABLES

PRESCRIPTION DRUG USE

The Epidemiology of Drug Use in the Elderly

Health problems in the elderly are becoming of increasing concern as the proportion of those over the age of 65 in the population increases. Seventy-eight percent of the elderly have at least one chronic disease, and 30 percent have three or more (Williams and Rush 1986). Seniors who use health care services during the year (90 percent; Gouvernement du Québec 1992) will make nine physician visits (Tamblyn et al. 1996), will fill an average of 29.8 prescriptions, and will be dispensed seven different drugs (Tamblyn, Lavoie, Abrahamowicz, et al. 1994). The 5 percent of the elderly who are frequent users of health and social services have, on average, seven health problems and take an average of 11.1 drugs (Beland 1989). Use of prescribed and over-the-counter medication increases with age (Health and Welfare Canada 1985, 1981; Williams and Rush 1986; Carruthers et al. 1987). Although seniors represent 12 percent of the Canadian population, they are the main consumers of prescription drugs, accounting for 28–40 percent of all prescriptions (Gordon 1987; Sova 1989; Quinn, Baker, and Evans 1992). It is estimated that by the year 2025, 18.1 percent of the population will be elderly (Larochelle et al. 1986; Sova 1989). This change in the age distribution of the population is expected to have a major impact on health care expenditures (Roch, Evans, and Pascoe 1985).

Prescription Drug Costs

Drug expenditures are responsible for an increasing proportion of Canadian health care costs. In Canada in 1991, $9.9 billion of the $66.8 billion spent on health care was attributable to prescription drug costs, a 53 percent increase in the proportion of health care costs devoted to this sector of expenditure over the past decade (Health and Welfare Canada 1993). Similar trends are evident at the provincial level. In Ontario, prescription drug expenditures rose from $59 million in 1976/77 to $400 million in 1986/87 (Lexchin 1992). British Columbia's prescription reimbursement costs for elderly registrants increased from $21 million in 1981/82 to $90 million in 1988/89 (Anderson et al. 1993). In more recent years (1986–1992), the Quebec government has reported an average annual increase in prescription drug costs of 16 percent in comparison to a 5 percent increase for medical service (Gouvernement du Québec 1990, 1991, 1992). By 1992, the Quebec government was spending $650 million for the 1,466,498 Medicare registrants who were eligible for coverage in the provincial drug plan, and 73 percent of these expenditures were for persons 65 years of age and older (Gouvernement du Québec 1992). Anderson et al. (1993) demonstrated that one-third (34 percent) of the increase in prescription drug expenditures was due to the use of new drugs by physicians, and 24 percent was due to increased utilization rates by patients. Increased utilization rates by elderly patients have also been documented in Quebec (Gouvernement du Québec 1992), a change that is attributable to an increasing number of prescriptions per patient rather than an increase in the proportion of patients who receive prescriptions.

Prescription Drug Expenditures: Are We Getting Good Value for Our Dollar?

Optimally, the burden of increasing costs for prescription drugs should be offset by the benefits of reduced morbidity and mortality and/or improvements in the quality of life. These benefits have been dramatically demonstrated in some diseases. For example, in 1920, the incidence of tuberculosis was 250 per 100,000. Treatment involved a prolonged stay in sanitariums; even then, only 50 percent of patients survived (Comstock 1994). With the advent of antituberculosis drugs such as isoniazid and rifampin, the incidence of tuberculosis fell to 9 per 100,000, and case fatality rates fell to 1 percent (Comstock 1994). Similar success stories are evident in many other conditions: the development of insulin for the treatment of diabetes, antibiotics for the treatment of pneumonia and meningitis, chemotherapy for the treatment of cancer, AZT for the treatment of AIDS, antipsychotic drugs for the management of schizophrenia, and antihypertensive medication for the prevention of stroke, kidney disease, and cardiac problems. For individuals, drug treatment has often offered the opportunity for a better, longer, and more productive life and, for some, a cure. For society, we have reaped the benefits of a healthier and more productive workforce and a better life expectancy.

Although the development of new drugs has provided unquestionable benefits, the question remains as to whether the rapid growth in prescription drug expenditures over the last two decades has actually translated into equivalent health benefits. To answer this question, we need to examine the conditions under which prescription drug use would be cost effective. In this respect, four criteria are relevant:

- *Is drug treatment necessary (overuse and underuse of prescription drugs)?* Drug treatments, like other forms of medical therapy, have documented risks, expected benefits, and known costs. A drug is considered to be necessary when the expected benefits of drug treatment outweigh the risks and when the cost can be justified by the absence of an effective and less expensive alternative form of therapy. Unnecessary prescriptions add to avoidable costs and, most importantly, contribute to the risk of adverse outcomes that are not justified by the expected benefits of drug treatment. On the other hand, the failure to prescribe a drug when one is needed contributes to avoidable morbidity, mortality, and health service costs.

- *Is the drug therapy selected appropriate for the patient's problem (clinically appropriate vs. inappropriate drug therapy)?* The clinical "correctness" of a physician's choice of drug therapy may not influence the cost of a prescription, but it does influence the outcome of drug treatment for a patient. Suboptimal drug treatment can reduce or negate the potential benefit of a drug (e.g., subtherapeutic doses of an antibiotic) and/or result in an unnecessary increase in the risk of an adverse drug-related event (e.g., prescription of a long-acting benzodiazepine for insomnia in the elderly). Ultimately, the costs of suboptimal drug treatment may be considerable, because it can have a direct impact on the burden of avoidable morbidity in the population.

- *Is the drug selected the most cost-effective choice, or could alternative drugs of equal efficacy and lower cost have been prescribed (cost-justified vs. cost-unjustified prescribing)?* In many clinical situations, a variety of different drugs is available to treat the same condition, with no one drug being clearly superior to the others for most patients. However, available treatment options may differ considerably in cost, and this has implications for prescription expenditures. For example, to treat bacterial pneumonia, a physician may choose a seven-day course of generic ampicillin at a cost of $4.97 or one of the new quinolone antibiotics such as ciprofloxacin at a cost of $68.60 (Medical Letter 1992c). Although quinolone antibiotics are superior for a limited number of infections, the marked differences in therapy costs are not justified by the available clinical evidence (Medical Letter 1992c).

- *Is the prescribed medication taken correctly (compliance vs. noncompliance)?* If benefits are to be derived from drug treatment, the medication needs to be taken at the prescribed dose (and time) and for the appropriate duration. If prescribed drugs are dispensed but not taken, then expenditures are made with no possibility of benefit. Undercompliance with prescribed medication will lead to suboptimal therapeutic benefits (treatment failures) and, as a result, medical services and hospitalizations related to poor disease control. It may also lead to the prescription of additional drugs or substitution of more expensive therapies to achieve optimal therapeutic benefits. Overcompliance with prescribed medication increases the risk of drug toxicity and drug-related illness and, for some drugs, leads to problems of habituation and dependency.

If drugs were prescribed to individuals who need them and not to those who do not, if prescribed drug treatments were clinically appropriate and cost effective, and if patients took needed and appropriate prescriptions correctly, then rising prescription expenditures would be a justified and appropriate response to changes in available treatments. However, if prescription drug use deviates substantially from this ideal, patients may be placed at unnecessary risk, and rising prescription expenditures may not be compensated by improved health status. In this sense, two questions are relevant: Does prescription drug use deviate from the ideal? If yes, what is the magnitude of the problem?

National (Brook et al. 1989; Hine, Gross, and Kennedy 1989; Sanz, Bergman, and Dahlstrom 1989; Cusson et al. 1990; Grasela and Green 1990; Wessling, Boethius, and Sjoqvist 1990; Wysowski, Kennedy, and Gross 1990; Garrard et al. 1991; Rawson and D'Arcy 1991; Medical Letter 1992a; Lipton and Bird 1993), regional, (Bellamy et al. 1989; Review Committee 1989; Clary, Mandos, and Schweizer 1990; Ferguson and Maling 1990; Pharmaceutical Inquiry of Ontario 1990; Wessling, Boethius, and Sjoqvist 1990; Williams and Cockerill 1990; Ministère de la Santé et des Services sociaux 1993; Davidson, Malloy, and Bédard 1994), and local (Skegg, Doll, and Perry 1977; Murdoch 1980; Alexander, Goodwin, and Currie 1985; Freer 1985; Portenoy and Kanner 1985; Nolan and O'Malley 1988b; Beers et al. 1989; Katz et al. 1990; Molstad et al. 1990; Pullar et al. 1990; Ekedahl et al. 1993) drug review programs have been initiated to answer these questions. The elderly are usually the target group of interest, because seniors account for approximately 40 percent of all prescription drug use (Quinn, Baker, and Evans 1992), and in many jurisdictions governments or third-party insurance agencies provide partial or complete coverage for their prescription drug costs. Physician prescribing behaviour is an issue that emerges in all drug utilization reviews. It is the physician who controls access to prescription medication and who decides the drug, dose, and duration of therapy required for a patient.

Evidence of Overuse and Underuse of Prescription Drugs

Overuse

It is difficult to obtain definitive estimates of the rate of unnecessary prescribing, because consensus guidelines for prescribing do not exist for most clinical ailments and because, in drug reviews, the precise clinical circumstances that led to the prescription are often not known (Sleator 1993; Bogle and Harris 1994; Gurwitz 1994; Tamblyn, McLeod, et al. 1994). For this reason, estimates of unnecessary prescribing tend to be limited to smaller-scale studies of certain conditions or to indirect evidence from eco-logical, observational, and intervention studies. Attention has been devoted to drug groups where there is greater potential for unnecessary prescribing either because the drug may be overused to treat common problems (e.g., antibiotics for viral infections) or because clinical indications and end points for therapy have been less well defined (psychotropic drugs, nonsteroidal anti-inflammatory drugs [NSAIDs]).

In the general population, antibiotics are the most commonly prescribed group of drugs, accounting for 16.5 percent of all drugs prescribed (Nelson 1993), and 5–22 percent of these prescriptions are believed to be unnecessary (McConnell et al. 1982; Avorn et al. 1988; Brook et al. 1989; Pitts and Vincent 1989; Katz et al. 1990; DeSantis et al. 1994). Psychotropic drugs have been the subject of considerable attention, because these drugs are commonly prescribed to the elderly (Aoki et al. 1983; Morgan and Gopalaswamy 1984; Grantham 1987; Beardsley et al. 1989; Irvine-Meek et al. 1990; Wysowski and Baum 1991; Beers et al. 1992; Quinn, Baker, and Evans 1992; Van der Waals, Mohrs, and Foets 1993; Tamblyn, McLeod, et al. 1994), particularly elderly women (Copperstock 1971; Hohmann 1989; Cafferata and Meyers 1990; Ashton 1991; Morabia, Fabre, and Dunand 1992; Tamblyn, McLeod, et al. 1994; Tamblyn et al. 1996) and nursing home residents (Gurwitz, Soumerai, and Avorn 1990; Garrard et al. 1991). An estimated 42–75 percent of patients who receive psychotropic medication have no evidence of psychiatric morbidity or documented clinical indication (Raynes 1979; Westerling 1988; Garrard et al. 1991; Weyerer and Dilling 1991). Although mental health problems are more common in the elderly (Salzman 1985; Sheikh 1992), psychiatric problems account for only 15–17 percent of psychotropic prescribing in the elderly (Westerling 1988).

NSAIDs are also commonly prescribed in the elderly (Quinn, Baker, and Evans 1992; Hogan et al. 1994; Tamblyn, McLeod, et al. 1994; Tamblyn et al. 1995), often in conjunction with gastrointestinal drugs used to treat the side-effects of these medications (Hogan et al. 1994). NSAIDs have not been demonstrated to be any more effective than acetaminophen in the treatment of osteoarthritis (Bradley et al. 1991; Liang and Fortin 1991), yet two physician surveys suggest that NSAIDs are frequently used by physicians to treat uncomplicated osteoarthritis (Mazzuca et al. 1991; Holt and Mazzuca 1992). In our own research on NSAID prescribing, we found that unnecessary prescriptions for NSAIDs were provided in one-third of 155 blinded office visits made by standardized patients, and unnecessary gastrointestinal medications for NSAID-related gastritis were prescribed in 80 percent of visits (Tamblyn et al. 1993).

The limited number of studies available suggest that almost all physicians can prescribe an unnecessary drug in some situations (Pitts and Vincent 1989; Mazzuca et al. 1991; Holt and Mazzuca 1992; Tamblyn et al. 1993). What appears to differ among physicians is the extent to which they prescribe unnecessarily. For example, in one study of antibiotic prescribing, the percentage of patients who are unnecessarily treated by their physicians spanned the spectrum from 0 percent to 100 percent (Pitts and Vincent 1989). Equally dramatic differences have been seen between physicians ·in their general propensity to prescribe (Ferguson 1990; Davidson et al. 1994). Some physicians prescribe medications to a greater number of their patients as well as prescribe more medications per patient. It has been suggested that these physicians are more likely prescribing unnecessary medication, but this assumption has not been tested.

Underuse

Only a handful of studies have examined whether individuals who could benefit from drug therapy are actually receiving it. The Canadian Study of Health and Aging provided a recent opportunity to answer this question (Hogan and Ebly 1995). A population of 2,914 Canadian seniors, randomly selected from all regions in Canada, was independently assessed and investigated by a team of physicians (geriatricians, psychiatrists, internists, and family physicians). In independent medical assessments, 204 patients were diagnosed with clinical depression, yet only 31.7 percent were being treated with antidepressant therapy. Nine hundred and fifty-five patients were identified as having a history of hypertension. One-third of this group was not receiving antihypertensive therapy, and 46.1 percent of these (130 individuals) were hypertensive on examination. Hypertension is the most important preventable risk factor for stroke in seniors (Mayo 1993), and stroke is the most disabling chronic condition in older Canadians (Verbrugge, Lepkowski, and Imanaka 1989). Of those 478 seniors with a history of a past stroke, only 191 (40 percent) were receiving drug treatment that has been proven to be effective in reducing the risk of a subsequent episode.

Although many seniors may be unnecessarily prescribed lipid-reducing drugs for primary prevention of cardiovascular disease, there is evidence that many who may benefit from lipid-lowering treatment in the prevention of the recurrence of cardiovascular problems are not being identified or treated. In a recent report of a consecutive series of 3,304 patients admitted for cardiovascular problems in Alberta (Montague et al. 1995), only 28 percent of patients had been investigated for lipid abnormalities, and only 29 percent received lipid-lowering interventions, including diet modification (22 percent), drug treatment (8 percent), and risk factor modification (5 percent).

Evidence of Inappropriate Prescribing

Four criteria are used to judge the appropriateness of drug therapy:
- the *drug selected* was the appropriate choice for the patient's problem and was not contraindicated by allergy, other diseases, patient age, or concurrent medication;
- the *dose and amount prescribed* were appropriate to achieve optimal therapeutic benefit and minimize the risk of toxicity or overdose;
- the *duration of therapy* was appropriate for the problem treated; and

- the *follow-up monitoring* was sufficiently frequent and detailed to assess therapeutic success and adverse drug effects.

There is evidence that prescribing deviates from these criteria in a significant proportion of elderly patients. Results from two U.S. population surveys indicated that 23.5 percent of seniors were taking at least one medication that is contraindicated in the elderly (Wilcox, Himmelstein, and Woolhandler 1994), and 8–29 percent were prescribed at least one inappropriate drug or drug combination (Ferguson 1990). In a database survey of Quebec seniors (Tamblyn, McLeod, et al. 1994), we found that 29 percent received at least one inappropriate drug combination, 36 percent received benzodiazepines for more than the recommended 30 days, and 15.4 percent received long-acting benzodiazepines, drugs that are contraindicated in the elderly because of the risk of traumatic injury (Sorock and Shimkin 1988; Tinetti, Speechley, and Ginter 1988; Ray, Griffin, and Downey 1989; Ray, Fought, and Decker 1992). Similar estimates of the prevalence of inappropriate prescribing are found in clinic-based and institutional reviews of prescriptions (Maronde et al. 1971; Kurfees and Dotson 1987; Beers, Storrie, and Lee 1990; Lesar et al. 1990; Shorr, Bauwens, and Landefeld 1990; Beers et al. 1992, 1993; Bloom et al. 1993). The prevalence of potentially inappropriate prescribing has been estimated to be between 11 percent and 45 percent in elderly clinic patients (Ferguson 1990; Shorr, Bauwens, and Landefeld 1990; Bloom et al. 1993) and between 19 percent and 40 percent in nursing home residents (Svarstad and Mount 1991; Beers et al. 1992).

Studies of inappropriate prescribing have limitations. The precise clinical circumstances that led to the prescribing decision are difficult to evaluate, and, for some patients, "higher-risk" drug therapy may be warranted. Furthermore, there is a lack of consensus on the clinical significance of some "inappropriate medications," because definitive data on the outcome experience of patients prescribed these drugs are not available. To circumvent these problems, we carried out a study on NSAID prescribing, using two cases in which there was definitive evidence about the "inappropriateness" of certain prescribing decisions (Griffin et al. 1991; Tamblyn et al. 1993). Standardized patients were used to present the two cases so that the prescribing decisions made by the 102 physicians who agreed to participate in the study were judged for the exact same cases. In 315 blinded visits in the office practice setting, suboptimal or unsafe prescriptions were written in 31 percent of visits and by 28 percent of physicians. We concluded that "inappropriate prescribing" was probably a significant problem in the elderly, a problem that could not be discounted or explained by limitations in measurement.

Although no information is available on the proportion of physicians who prescribe inappropriately, it has been assumed that prescribing problems are limited to a small number of physicians. This is because "labour-intensive" intervention programs tend to target the outer group of physicians with extremely problematic prescribing (McConnell et al. 1982; Avorn and Soumerai 1983; Schaffner et al. 1983; Ray et al. 1986). However, in preliminary analysis of our own data (Tamblyn, McLeod, et al. 1994), we found that this assumption was not valid. Among the 14,121 physicians who provided care for the 65,349 elderly in this study, 51 percent were directly responsible for writing one or more of the potentially inappropriate prescriptions received by these patients (table 1).

Table 1

Potentially inappropriate prescribing among the 14,121 physicians who provided medical care for a random sample of 65,349 elderly in Quebec in 1990

	Physicians prescribing one or more potentially inappropriate prescriptions	
	Number	Percent of sample
Potentially inappropriate drug combinations		
Psychotropic drugs	3,075	21.8
Cardiovascular drugs	2,370	16.8
Nonsteroidal anti-inflammatory drugs	1,869	13.2
Contraindicated drugs or duration		
Long-acting benzodiazepines	4,171	29.5
Benzodiazepine for >30 days	6,918	49.0
Any potentially inappropriate drug	**7,168**	**50.8**

Evidence of Unjustified High-Cost Prescribing

Research on the cost-effectiveness of prescribing decisions has focused on drug groups that have the highest per prescription costs: antimicrobial drugs, gastrointestinal drugs, and cardiovascular drugs. There are three characteristics of these drug groups that contribute to their cost. First, these drugs are used to treat prevalent medical conditions and therefore are commonly prescribed. Given the large number of persons exposed, even low rates of cost-ineffective prescribing can translate into considerable costs. Second, each of these drug groups is composed of different classes of medications that can be used to treat the same clinical condition but at a substantially different cost. The difference in cost is justified in some conditions because of improved efficacy or decreased side-effects, but not in many others. Third, *unjustified costs* can be created by the prescription of more costly drugs in the same pharmacological class, the "me too drugs," or the prescription of brand name drugs rather than generics.

Studies of prescribing rates for new drugs suggest that prescribing consistently exceeds the expected incidence of health problems for which such drugs would be indicated (Ferguson 1990; Bradlow and Coulter 1993; Inman and Pearce 1993; Maxwell et al. 1993; McGavock et al. 1993; Morton-Jones and Pringle 1993a, 1993b). There are dramatic differences in the rates of prescribing new and more costly drugs among different physicians (Pitts and Vincent 1989; Molstad et al. 1990; Inman and Pearce 1993). When physicians are surveyed with respect to their drug choices for hypothetical cases, unnecessarily costly drugs are selected in 79 percent of prescriptions (Holmes 1992). Controlled intervention trials to reduce unnecessarily costly prescribing have provided the most convincing evidence that room for improvement exists. Dramatic changes in prescribing decisions and a corresponding two- to eightfold reduction in prescription costs have been reported with a variety of interventions (Schaffner et al. 1983; Gehlbach et al. 1984; Ray, Schaffner, and Federspiel 1985; Hershey et al. 1986; Avorn et al. 1988; Kawahara and Jordan 1989; Steele et al. 1989; Zieve and Ciesco 1993). The main mechanisms by which prescription costs are reduced are increasing the rate of generic prescribing (Gehlbach et al. 1984; Hershey et al. 1986; Steele et al. 1989), reducing the use of more expensive classes of drugs for common conditions (Schaffner et al. 1983; Ray, Schaffner, and Federspiel 1985), and encouraging the use of less expensive drugs in the "me too" categories of medication (Kawahara and Jordan 1989; Fudge et al. 1993; Zieve and Ciesco 1993).

Evidence of Noncompliance

The problem of patient compliance is significant. Approximately one-fifth of the prescriptions written are not filled (Saunders 1987; Graveley and Oseasohn 1991). Although some prescriptions may be unnecessary, 20.7 percent of patients who were seen for hypertension in one clinic were reported to have not filled their prescriptions (Graveley and Oseasohn 1991). When a prescription is filled, estimated rates of noncompliance with treatment range from 16 percent to 73 percent (Parkin et al. 1976; Brody 1980; Inui et al. 1980; Cooper, Love, and Raffoul 1982; Kendrick and Bayne 1982; Morrow, Leirer, and Sheikh 1988; Weingarten and Cannon 1988; Col, Fanale, and Kronholm 1990; Graveley and Oseasohn 1991). On average, underuse of prescription medication is more common than overuse, accounting for approximately 80 percent of all compliance problems (Parkin et al. 1976; Brody 1980; Inui et al. 1980; Cooper, Love, and Raffoul 1982; Kendrick and Bayne 1982; Weingarten and Cannon 1988; Col, Fanale, and Kronholm 1990; Graveley and Oseasohn 1991). In seniors, inappropriate discontinuation of a drug may occur up to 40 percent of the time (Jackson et al. 1984). Individuals who are taking several medications will vary in their pattern of adherence to different prescription drugs; drugs of less importance clinically may be taken appropriately, whereas those of greatest importance may not be taken appropriately (Inui et al. 1980). Approximately 23 percent of non-compliance problems are unintentional (Cooper, Love, and Raffoul 1982). The main reasons for unintentional noncompliance are forgetting and mis-understanding, whereas intentional noncompliance is related to perceptions that the drug is unnecessary or that it produces undesirable side-effects (Cooper, Love, and Raffoul 1982).

Summary

There is a mismatch in prescription drug use. Drugs are prescribed to a greater proportion of the senior population than is indicated by the preva-lence of indications for drug therapy. In contrast, many patients who may benefit from drug therapy do not appear to be receiving it. Among patients who receive drug treatment, 23–29 percent are prescribed therapy that is potentially inappropriate, and, in some drug groups, as many as 79 percent of prescriptions are written for drugs that are more costly than equally effective, less expensive alternatives.

Examining the Consequences

Unnecessary prescribing, misuse of medication, and inappropriate prescrip-tions can contribute to the risk of drug-related illness and unwarranted costs in health care delivery. Drug-related illness is a significant health problem (Klein, German, and Levine 1981; Nolan and O'Malley 1988a; Gurwitz and Avorn 1991). It has been estimated to account for about 5–23 percent of hospitalizations (Hurwitz 1969; May, Stewart, and Cluff 1977; Ives, Bentz, and Gwyther 1987; Grymonpre et al. 1988), 1.7–5 percent of ambulatory visits (Mulroy 1973; Hutchinson et al. 1986), and 1/1 000 deaths (Karch and Lasagna 1975); in most studies, the prevalence of drug-related illness is higher in the elderly (Hurwitz 1969; Smidt and McQueen 1972; Klein, German, and Levine 1981; Hutchinson et al. 1986; Lumley et al. 1986; Nolan and O'Malley 1988a; Gurwitz and Avorn 1991). Several studies have attempted to identify the "cause" of drug-related admissions as a means of identifying primary targets for prevention. Patient compliance problems account for the majority of admissions for drug-related illness (Grymonpre et al. 1988; Col, Fanale, and Kronholm 1990), an estimated 40 percent in a recent study of 89 consecutive drug-related admissions in elderly patients (Col, Fanale, and Kronholm 1990). Both intentional and unintentional noncompliance lead to problems of drug-related illness, and, in the elderly, unintended errors in the administration of medication appear to be twice as common as in the general population (i.e., 19 percent vs. 10 percent) (Edwards and Pathy 1984; Col, Fanale, and Kronholm 1990). Coambs et al. (1995), in a recent review, estimated the direct costs of noncompliance in Canada to be $3.53–4.49 billion per year: $1.78–2 billion in avoidable hospital costs, $0.66 billion in avoidable nursing home admissions, and $1.09 billion in ambulatory medical service costs.

Inappropriate choice of a drug, dose, or drug combination has been estimated to account for an additional 19–36 percent of hospital admissions for drug-related events (Bero, Lipton, and Bird 1991; Hallas et al. 1992) and up to 72 percent of drug-related events occurring in a hospital setting (Bates, Leape, and Petrycki 1993). Based on a prevalence study of potentially inappropriate prescribing in a random sample of Quebec seniors, we estimated that 1,942 of the 154,200 hospital admissions in 1990 may have been due to four potentially dangerous drug combinations, and 2,013 admissions for fall-related injuries were likely attributable to the contraindicated use of long-acting benzodiazepines (table 2).

Table 2

Estimated prevalence and impact of potentially inappropriate prescriptions on morbidity in Quebec seniors

Potentially inappropriate prescription	Prevalence (per 1,000)	Potential outcome	Number of hospital admissions/year attributable to exposure*
Potentially inappropriate combinations			
Asthma med. + beta blocker	11.4	Acute respiratory problem	608
K+ sparing diuretic + K+	10.0	Acute cardiac problem	1,260
Warfarin + NSAID	3.3	Bleeding problem	42
Warfarin + sulfonamides	2.5	Bleeding problem	32
Contraindicated drugs			
Long-acting benzodiazepines	121.0	Fall-related injury	2,013

* For potentially inappropriate combinations, the estimated risk used in the calculations was RR=5.0, and for long-acting benzodiazepines, RR=1.8.

The cost of inappropriate prescribing for Canadian hospitals is approximately $256 million if only 5 percent of hospital admissions are due to drug-related illness and $1 billion if the upper rate of 23 percent is used (using Coambs et al.'s [1995] method of calculation). Thus, both misuse of medication by patients and inappropriate prescribing by physicians contribute to adverse drug-related events. Almost half of these events could be prevented by improvements in patient compliance and the clinical appropriateness of prescribing decisions.

Unnecessary medication can potentiate the risk of drug-related problems. The number of medications taken by a patient is the single most important factor influencing the risk of a drug-related event (Klein, German, and Levine 1981; Gurwitz and Avorn 1991). The odds of an adverse drug reaction increase from 2.7 with two to three drugs to 13.7 with more than six drugs (Carruthers et al. 1987). A patient's compliance with his drug regimen is inversely related to the number of drugs he takes (Gordon 1987; Lowenthal 1987; Grymonpre et al. 1988; Harper, Newton, and Walsh 1989; Graveley and Oseasohn 1991): the greater the number of drugs, the more problems the patient has in adequately adhering to the drug regimen. Thus, unnecessary medication contributes indirectly to the risk of drug-related events. Unnecessary medication also contributes directly to prescription costs, not just for the payment for a drug that may not be needed, but also for drugs that may be used to treat the side-effects of the medication. For example, in Alberta, Hogan, et al. (1994) found that 80 percent of prescriptions for gastrointestinal drugs were dispensed to patients who were prescribed NSAIDs, drug therapy that is known to have significant gastrointestinal side-effects.

The consequences of undertreatment, the failure to prescribe medication when needed, have not been quantified for Canadian seniors. Estimates have been produced for some specific drug exposures. For example, estrogen replacement has been advised for postmenopausal women as an effective means of reducing the risk of cardiovascular disease and osteoporosis. The Canadian Health and Aging Survey documented that only 1.5 percent of women screened were using estrogen replacement (Hogan and Ebly 1995). Grady et al. (1992) estimate that untreated women have a lifetime risk of 45 percent for coronary heart disease and 15 percent for hip fracture secondary to osteoporosis. With estrogen replacement, lifetime risk of coronary heart disease falls to 33 percent and of hip fracture to 12 percent, resulting in the net gain of one year in life expectancy (Grady et al. 1992).

NONMEDICAL FACTORS INFLUENCING DRUG USE AND OUTCOMES OF DRUG THERAPY

The relative risks, benefits, and costs associated with drug therapy relate to several factors, including the health care system, the patient, the physician, and the drug (figure 1). Prescription drugs are unusual in some respects because, unlike other forms of medical therapy, the availability of treatment and its use are dynamically influenced by the private sector—namely, the drug industry. The drug industry invests in the development of new drugs and interacts at several levels in the health care delivery process to influence the availability and use of drugs in the health care sector. Although both the drug industry and the health care sector share the common objective of maximizing the benefits and minimizing the risks of drug therapy, tension

Figure 1

**Schematic representation of the factors
that influence the outcome of prescription drug use**

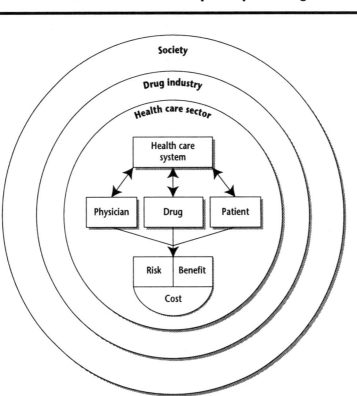

arises because of corporate goals of profit generation and health care sector goals of fiscal restraint. The context for this interaction is set by the values that Canadian society places on investment in the growth and development of the pharmaceutical industry in Canada, on one hand, and the availability of prescription medication for those in need, on the other.

In keeping with the goal of creating a favourable business climate for the drug industry, the Canadian government has instituted extended patent protection (Bills C-22 and C-91) and created a tax incentive structure for investment in Canadian research and development. As illustrated by the Pharmaceutical Manufacturers Association of Canada's summary statistics, this has resulted in a tangible investment in Canada. In 1994, the drug industry accounted for 16,646 jobs in Canada, amounting to $5.5 billion in value-added employment contributions, and invested $536.4 million in drug research and development in the private and public sectors (table 3).

Table 3

The Canadian Pharmaceutical Manufacturers Association Report on Canadian Investment by drug industries

Province	Drug industry employment	1994 StatsCan estimate of employment (value-added) contribution	Research & development expenditures	
			1988	1994
British Columbia	606	$93 M	$5.3 M	$16.6 M
Alberta	700	$107 M	$3.9 M	$24 M
Saskatchewan	106	$16 M	$1.3 M	$3.9 M
Manitoba	264	$40 M	$2.2 M	$7.2 M
Ontario	8,423	$1200 M	$72.2 M	$236.2 M
Quebec	6,128	$1100 M	$71.8 M	$239.8 M
New Brunswick	121	$18.7 M	$0.2 M	$0.5 M
Nova Scotia	225	$34.7 M	$1.2 M	$6.1 M
Prince Edward Island	11	$1.7 M	$0.01 M	$0.11 M
Newfoundland	62	$9.6 M	$0.5 M	$2.0 M
Total	**16,646**	**$2.6 billion**	**$158.6 million**	**$536.4 million**

Source: Pharmaceutical Manufacturers Association of Canada 1994.

Canadians have also placed a value on minimizing financial barriers to prescription drug access. In keeping with this sentiment, all Canadian provinces have instituted a drug benefit plan that covers the costs of prescription drugs for seniors and individuals receiving social assistance; in Saskatchewan, the total population has such coverage. This means that the majority of the expenditures for prescription drug use are borne by the health sector. Thus, extended patent protection creates a more favourable climate for industry, but it prolongs the period in which brand name drugs are prescribed, resulting in a net increase in drug expenditures in the health care system. The dynamic trade-off between industrial development and fiscal restraint in health care is best illustrated by a recent Quebec story:

In 1992, the Quebec government spent approximately $15 million on one drug, omeprazole, a second-line gastrointestinal drug used in the treatment of acid-peptic disease. As the drug was being used as first-line, rather than second-line, treatment, the drug was placed on the restricted formulary list on July 1, 1993. When a drug is placed on the restricted list, a physician must apply for access for his patient to be insured. After this policy was instituted, prescription expenditures for omeprazole fell from $1.3 million per month to $100,000 per month. Astra Pharmaceutical, the manufacturer of the drug, responded by offering to invest $100 million in a new research facility in Quebec and to provide a drug education program for physicians on appropriate omeprazole use, the condition being that omeprazole be placed back on the regular formulary list. The Quebec government agreed, and, six months later, restrictions on the prescription of omeprazole were removed. In the following year, the Régie de l'assurance-maladie du Québec spent $18 million on omeprazole prescriptions.

Additional pressures in the relationship between the health sector and industry relate to the growing number of new drugs that have been approved for marketing in Canada. At the turn of the century, approximately 1,000 drugs were available. They included such "wonder cures" as *columba root* for stomach upset and *extract of cattle arteries* to treat kidney failure (British Pharmacopeia 1910). By 1994, 24,600 drugs had been approved for use in Canada. Not only has the number of drugs changed, but the growth has been exponential. In 1940, three new drugs were added to the list of approved drugs in Canada. By the 1990s, according to the Health Protection Branch of Health Canada, an average of 1,500 new medications were approved each year. Currently in Quebec, approximately $1 million is spent each year to review new drugs for inclusion in the provincial formulary; even then, extensive delays in the process are reported (J. Lelorier, President, Conseil Consultatif Pharmacologie, personal communication, 1996).

The following section outlines how these factors influence the availability of and access to prescription drugs and the additional factors that play a role in the outcome of drug therapy for patients.

Health Care System Influences on Prescription Drug Use and the Outcomes of Drug Therapy

The most direct mechanism by which the health care system influences prescription drug use is through the provincial formulary. Each province lists which drugs will be covered by its insured drug plan. Drugs that are not covered may still be prescribed, but the patient will be required to pay. In practice, this serves as such an economic barrier to access (36 percent of patients will not pay to fill prescriptions because of insufficient funds; Saunders 1987) that the formulary will almost define what drugs are pre-scribed in practice (Soumerai, Avorn, Ross-Degnan, et al. 1987). This means that the government can effectively reduce or remove access to drugs that are considered to be ineffective, potentially dangerous, or cost ineffective.

A variety of health care system policies may have an indirect effect on prescription drug use. For example, health policy influences manpower distribution and access, and physician density is associated with the average number of medical visits per individual and the frequency of medical interventions (Hemenway and Fallon 1985; Wennberg 1985). It has been estimated that drugs are prescribed in 65–75 percent of medical visits (Mapes 1980). As a result, one would suspect that the average drugs prescribed per patient would be higher in regions of greater physician density. In testing this hypothesis, we found that the average number of prescriptions per patient was similar in high and low physician density regions; however, the prevalence of potentially inappropriate prescriptions was not. Montreal, the region with the highest density of physicians, had the lowest prevalence of potentially inappropriate prescribing (Tamblyn, McLeod, et al. 1994), whereas the Quebec region with the second highest density of physicians had the highest prevalence.

Although physician density per se did not have a direct impact on drug prescribing, the number of physicians prescribing for a patient has been identified as one of the most important determinants of drug utilization and inappropriate prescribing (Tamblyn 1996). The number of prescribing physicians was the single most important determinant of the number of medications dispensed to Quebec seniors ($R2=25$ percent) (Tamblyn 1996). Between 10 percent and 66 percent of potentially inappropriate drug combinations were created by prescriptions written by two different physicians. The median number of physicians prescribing for the elderly in 1990 was two, and 5.2 percent of elderly patients had more than six prescribing physicians during the year (Tamblyn 1996). Primary physicians have the potential to play a major role in the coordination of care provided for elderly patients, particularly as it relates to drug therapy. In 1990, 51.9 percent of seniors who visited a physician in Quebec had a single primary physician, and 60.4 percent had a single dispensing pharmacy (Tamblyn 1996). Both of these factors reduce the risk of inappropriate prescriptions (Tamblyn 1996). We suspect that the 20–30 percent reduction in risk of inappropriate prescriptions that we observed in this population may have been greater if primary physicians and pharmacists had better access to information about all drugs prescribed to patients.

Physician reimbursement policy is an important factor in shaping practice patterns (Newhouse et al. 1981; Manning et al. 1984). The time spent with patients and the type of services delivered are influenced by the method of payment (salary vs. fee-for-service) and the fee schedule (Manning et al. 1984; Pineault 1986). Services with low economic return are performed with lower than expected frequency, the reverse being true for services with better economic returns. In keeping with these general observations, shorter patient contact times have been observed among fee-for-service physicians compared with salaried physicians (Renaud et al. 1980). Shorter patient contact times and increased drug prescribing have been found to be strongly correlated in the two studies in which this was investigated (Renaud et al. 1980; Hartzema and Christensen 1983). Furthermore, patient education, a nonbillable service per se, is carried out less frequently by fee-for-service physicians (Renaud et al. 1980). These factors will play an important role in the success of interventions designed to minimize unnecessary drug utilization. In physician-based intervention studies, poorest compliance is observed with recommendations to stop medication (rather than substitute or simplify) (Kroenke and Pinholt 1990). Although patient resistance was cited as one of the main reasons for noncompliance, we found that physicians who stopped medication responsible for a drug-related illness spent twice the time with the patient as did those physicians who did not stop the medication (Tamblyn et al. 1993). Thus, appropriate physician remuneration for drug review and modification may play an important role in minimizing unnecessary prescribing.

Physician Characteristics and Their Influence on Prescription Drug Use and the Outcomes of Drug Therapy

Physicians are the gatekeepers to prescription medication access in the health care system. In this role, they have the responsibility to make judicious use of medication to maximize their patients' health and functional status.

One of the challenges that physicians face in prescribing for the elderly is the relative absence of evidence of the effects of prescription drugs in this age group. Much of the information about the therapeutic doses and effectiveness of current drugs is based on the evaluation of younger adults (Cusson et al. 1990). Yet, with many drugs, the vast majority of users are the elderly, and the validity of generalizations to this age group is unknown. For example, in a 30-year review of the studies used to evaluate the effectiveness of drug treatment for myocardial infarction, Gurwitz, Col, and Avorn (1992) found that 60 percent of trials excluded persons over the age of 75. Prescribing guidelines for physicians have only recently been developed, and, in the absence of evidence, most guidelines are based on clinical opinions, rather than empirical evidence.

Prescribing Propensity

In characterizing physicians' practice patterns, it has been noted that some physicians are more apt to prescribe drugs than others (Hartzema and Christensen 1983; Mokkink et al. 1990; Davidson et al. 1994; Tamblyn et al. 1996). These physicians are more likely to be male (Davidson et al. 1994; Tamblyn et al. 1996), to have a high-volume practice (Hartzema and Christensen 1983; Davidson et al. 1994), to see their patients more often (Davidson et al. 1994; Tamblyn et al. 1996), to refer more of their patients (Mokkink et al. 1990; Tamblyn et al. 1996), and to feel a restricted responsibility for medical tasks (Mokkink et al. 1990). Patients of these physicians are more likely to be prescribed a greater number of drugs (Davidson et al. 1994; Tamblyn et al. 1996), to receive prescriptions for psychotropic drugs, particularly if they are women (Tamblyn et al. 1996), and to perceive themselves as being in poorer health (Mokkink et al. 1990). We have found that a physician's propensity to prescribe drugs to the elderly can be partly predicted by his scores on licensing examinations (Tamblyn 1996). Physicians with lower scores in clinical assessment are more likely to prescribe a greater number of drugs to their elderly patients, particularly symptom relief medications such as anxiolytics, analgesics, and NSAIDs. This finding is important, because it provides the means of identifying physicians who may develop problematic prescribing habits after they enter practice and the means to prevent this from happening.

A greater propensity to prescribe drugs in discretionary circumstances may increase the risk of drug-related morbidity by increasing the average number of drugs taken by patients in the practice; it may also contribute to unjustified drug costs. The New Brunswick study was the first to examine the impact of prescribing patterns on patient outcome (Davidson, Malloy, and Bédard 1994). The investigators found that physicians with a greater propensity to prescribe had higher age-adjusted rates of morbidity and mortality in their practice (Davidson, Malloy, and Bédard 1994); however, these findings could have been explained by differences in the health status of patients in the practice.

Inappropriate Prescribing

Physicians are more likely to prescribe potentially inappropriate medication to the elderly than to middle-aged adults (Miles 1977; Ferguson 1990; Shorr, Bauwens, and Landefeld 1990), possibly because seniors are more likely to take more medications and to have a number of health problems that must be considered in prescribing decisions (Kurfees and Dotson 1987; Nolan and O'Malley 1988b; Beers, Storrie, and Lee 1990; G. Soucy, Directeur d'évaluation, Régie de l'assurance-maladie du Québec, personal communication, 1993). Although studies are limited in this area, physician training appears to have an impact on prescribing appropriateness. There is systematic evidence that general practitioners are more likely than specialists to prescribe inappropriately (Miles 1977; Ferguson 1990; Hallas et al. 1992; Beers et al. 1993; Monette, Tamblyn, et al. 1993) and to use drug detail people as one of their primary sources of drug information (Stolley and Lasagna 1969; Peay and Peay 1990). These trends are an important public health concern, because general practitioners/family physicians are the official primary care physicians in the Canadian health care system (Canadian Medical Association 1994), a general practitioner is the most frequently visited physician for 81 percent of the elderly (Tamblyn 1996), and approximately 80 percent of all drugs dispensed to the elderly are prescribed by general practitioners (Tamblyn, McLeod, et al. 1994). Unlike specialists, primary physicians prescribe medication from many different drug groups in the care of their patients (table 4). This is particularly true for elderly patients, whose primary physicians may be responsible for refilling prescriptions initiated by specialist and general practitioner colleagues. Fifty-one percent of elderly patients will be prescribed more than six different medications during the year (Tamblyn et al. 1996); for this group of patients, general practitioners, in comparison to specialists, prescribe five times as many different types of drugs from four times as many different classes.

Table 4

The average number of drug classes and drugs prescribed by specialists and general practitioners for their elderly patients during 1990

Type of physician	Number of physicians	Number of different drug classes		Number of different drugs	
		Mean ± SD	Median	Mean ± SD	Median
General practitioners	2,539	22.4 ± 11.2	23	43.6 ± 28.0	41
Specialists	2,491	7.3 ± 6.9	6	12.0 ± 13.7	8

The medical school attended by the physician appears to have an impact on the physician's subsequent prescribing patterns. This is an important finding, because changes in medical school training could provide the means of preventing future problems in prescribing. Graduation from a foreign medical school has been associated with higher rates of failure on licensing examinations (W.D. Dauphinee, Executive Director, Medical Research Council of Canada, personal communication, 1994), disproportionately higher prescribing rates for newer high-cost drugs in all categories (Inman and Pearce 1993), and an increased risk of inappropriate benzodiazepine prescribing (Monette et al. 1993). In addition, in the one study that examined differences between graduates of Canadian medical schools, it was noted that graduates from one medical school in Quebec were at significantly greater risk of inappropriate benzodiazepine prescribing than were graduates from the three other schools in the province (Monette et al. 1993).

Physician age and practice setting are other factors that have been linked to prescribing habits. Older physicians who have been in practice for a longer period of time are more likely to be disproportionately heavy prescribers of new high-cost drugs (Inman and Pearce 1993), to be at greater risk of prescribing inappropriately (Beers et al. 1993; Monette et al. 1993), to prescribe psychotropic drugs to a greater proportion of patients, particularly their female patients (Hadsall, Freeman, and Norwood 1982; Tamblyn et al. 1996), to have higher rates of prescribing (Hartzema and

Christensen 1983), to have poorer knowledge of geriatric prescribing (Ferry, Lamy, and Becker 1985), and to use drug detailers as a source of drug information (Ferry, Lamy, and Becker 1985). Older physicians are also more likely to have deficiencies in the quality of care they deliver (McAuley et al. 1990). This is an important issue, because older physicians are more likely to have older patients in their practice (Monette et al. 1993). Thus, the most vulnerable physicians are caring for the oldest patients.

With respect to practice setting, having a greater proportion of elderly patients in a physician's practice is associated with better knowledge about geriatric prescribing (Ferry, Lamy, and Becker 1985), and physicians with larger nursing home practices are less likely to prescribe inappropriate medications for these patients (Beers et al. 1993). Physicians in metropolitan areas and those with teaching hospital affiliations are less likely to prescribe inappropriately (Ferguson 1990; Monette et al. 1993). Teaching hospital affiliation is also noted to be a positive predictor of better quality of care (Palmer and Reilly 1979). Higher rates of psychiatric referral are associated with a lower risk of prescribing inappropriate medications to nursing home residents (Beers et al. 1993). Presumably referral is protective, because it provides the physician with expert advice on drug treatment. Interestingly, we found that recent graduates referred a greater proportion of their elderly patients than physicians who had been in practice for an extended period of time (Tamblyn, Lavoie, et al. 1994). It is possible that the apparent negative effect of years of practice experience on the quality of prescribing decisions is mediated through the "underuse" of expert advice by older physicians.

Costly Prescribing

With respect to prescribing costs, marketing forces rather than empirical evidence appear to be the main factor in a physician's choice of drugs (Greene and Winickoff 1992; Medical Letter 1992b; Safavi, Rodney, and Hayward 1992; Zieve and Ciesco 1993). About 85–90 percent of physicians in Canada see pharmaceutical representatives (Lexchin 1993). Doctors surveyed in Ontario reported attendance at 5.2 drug-sponsored symposia in the past two years in comparison to 1.9 continuing medical education courses (Lexchin 1993). Drug marketing appears to have an important influence on physician prescribing behaviour. Chren and Landefeld (1994) found that physicians who made requests for the addition of specific drugs to the hospital formulary were likely to have met with the pharmaceutical representatives from the companies manufacturing those drugs and to have accepted money from the companies. A study of internists in one academic centre found that 25 percent of faculty and 32 percent of residents reported making at least one change in their practice in the past two years on the basis of a discussion with a detailer (Lurie, Rich, and Simpson 1990). Physician knowledge of the costs of the drugs they prescribe is notoriously poor (Steele et al. 1989; Ryan et al. 1990), so it is not surprising that cost is not an important consideration in prescribing decisions.

Summary

There is some evidence that physicians who prescribe unjustified, high-cost medication may also be more likely to prescribe potentially unnecessary and inappropriate medication. Certain physician and practice setting characteristics are associated with a greater likelihood of cost-ineffective prescribing in the elderly. Physicians who appear to be at higher risk of prescribing problems include general practitioners, older physicians, non-academically affiliated physicians who are practicing in isolated practice settings, and possibly physicians from certain medical schools. The challenges in prescribing for the elderly are substantial, particularly for physicians who are providing primary care management of a variety of health problems in all age groups. The available evidence on drug effectiveness in the elderly is inadequate, and, as a result, evidence-based guidelines for prescribing are difficult to develop. These problems are potentiated by the number of drugs available for use. There are 20,600 drug products that have been approved for marketing in Canada (Health and Welfare Canada 1993). At last count, there were 33,803 drug combinations that should be avoided because of potential drug interactions, 6,962 drug-disease contraindications, and 5,779 drug-allergy combinations to be avoided (Drug Facts and Comparisons 1993; Medical Letter Handbook 1993; USDPDI 1996). It is probably *not realistic* in the 1990s to expect even the most diligent primary physician to keep up-to-date on all current medications.

Patient Characteristics and Their Influence on Prescription Drug Use and the Outcomes of Drug Therapy

Patients' expectations for prescription drugs have an important impact on the rate of drug use. In our society, we have come to view drugs as a way of normalizing behaviour. For example, several studies have found that individuals using psychotropic drugs felt that they needed the medication in order to sustain "normal" relationships with others (Locker 1981; Helman 1984). Some women stated that their drugs enabled them to maintain nurturing roles, whereas men often saw their medication as a means of suppressing somatic discomforts that interfered with their occupational roles. This social acceptance of "chemical coping" (Nichter and Vuckovic 1994), where drugs are used to improve one's personal relationships and emotional well-being and to help abide by social norms and expectations, appears to run counter to any stigma associated with psychological dependency on medication. With so many pharmaceutical products available, it is likely that people are turning to drugs more readily to alleviate physical and psychosocial problems, and people's conceptions of what constitutes a "normal" healthy state have subsequently changed (Nichter and Vuckovic 1994).

In most studies of drug utilization in industrialized countries, women have been found to consume more medication than men (Power, Downey, and Schnell 1983; Verbrugge 1984; Cafferata and Meyers 1990; Ashton 1991; Morabia, Fabre, and Dunand 1992; Quinn, Baker, and Evans 1992; Tamblyn, McLeod, et al. 1994), and in some studies women are disproportionately represented among patents admitted for drug-related illness (Seidl et al. 1966; Bergman and Wiholm 1981; Grymonpre et al. 1988). Differences in drug consumption between men and women are particularly large for psychotropic drugs (Copperstock 1971; Hohmann 1989; Cafferata and Meyers 1990; Ashton 1991; Morabia, Fabre, and Dunand 1992; Tamblyn, McLeod, et al. 1994; Tamblyn et al. 1996), medication that is often used to treat nonspecific complaints. It has been argued that women are socially encouraged in western society to recognize feelings such as depression and anxiety, to perceive themselves as sick, and to be more comfortable playing the sick role (Copperstock 1971; Cafferata, Kasper, and Bernstein 1983). Women are more frequent users of health care services than men (Cafferata and Meyers 1990; Gouvernement du Québec 1992; Van Nostrand, Furner, and Suzman 1993), even after adjustment for services related to child bearing. Women are also more likely to present nonspecific complaints that may lead to drug treatment (Cafferata and Meyers 1990) and to use medication rather than alcohol as a means of stress management (Hohmann 1989). Although differences in health-seeking behaviour between the sexes may explain some of the differences in drug utilization, the situation is more complex. Even when men and women present to a physician's office with social problems, women are still more likely to be prescribed a psychotropic drug by their physician (Fiorio et al. 1989). We demonstrated that there is substantial variation between physicians in differential prescribing of psychotropic drugs to elderly men and women (Tamblyn et al. 1996). These differences were related to physician characteristics and practice patterns, but they may also be attributable to differences in the expectations of male and female patients (Tamblyn et al. 1996) for prescription medication.

The "absence of medical indications" for a prescription does not necessarily translate into the absence of a prescription, nor does it mean that a drug will be stopped when it is no longer needed. A variety of factors influence prescribing decisions, including patient expectations and social circumstances (Raynes 1979; Mapes 1980; Cafferata, Kasper, and Bernstein 1983; Wells et al. 1985; Isacson and Haglund 1988; Hohmann 1989; Pringle and Morton-Jones 1994), physician attitudes (Stolley and Lasagna 1969; Linn 1971; Wallen, Waitzkin, and Stoeckle 1979; Mapes 1980; Melville 1980; Bernstein and Kane 1981; Verbrugge and Steiner 1981; Hadsall, Freeman, and Norwood 1982; Weiss et al. 1983; Verbrugge 1984; Bucks et al. 1990), practice setting (Renaud et al. 1980; Hartzema and Christensen 1983; Beers et al. 1993; Morton-Jones and Pringle 1993b), and health insurance policy (Nelson and Quick 1980; Nelson, Reeder, and Dickson 1984; Leibowitz, Manning, and Newhouse 1985; Reeder and Nelson 1985; Soumerai and Ross-Degnan 1990; Soumerai et al. 1991; Bradlow and Coulter 1993). In a recent survey of older Canadians, 47 percent reported that they expect to receive a medication when they visit their physician, and 37 percent indicated that they would seek another physician if one was not prescribed (Angus Reid Group Inc. 1991). Furthermore, patient resistance to stopping unnecessary medication is responsible for an estimated one-third of failures to reduce the number of medications in a patient's drug regimen (Kroenke and Pinholt 1990). Although patient expectation may play an important role in unnecessary prescribing, it appears that physicians overestimate the extent of their patients' expectations for drug therapy. In one study, physicians reported that 80–90 percent of their patients expected drugs, when in fact only 30–50 percent of patients actually did (Bliss 1981).

There is little doubt that the dialogue between a physician and patient about therapy decisions is inadequate. Patient satisfaction surveys in both the United States (Webster 1989) and Canada (Tamblyn, Abrahamowicz, et al. 1994) find that patients are most dissatisfied with their lack of involvement in decisions about their care. The development of effective patient communication skills has not been a focus in traditional medical training. In fact, with the exception of certification requirements of the Canadian College of Family Physicians, effective communication skills are abilities that are neither tested nor required for a physician to enter the practice of medicine. The physician's overestimation of the patient's desire for drug therapy may, in fact, be related to difficulties in establishing a productive exchange about the available therapeutic options. Some methods of supporting this dialogue are clearly needed, for primary physicians spend, on average, 11.2–12.1 minutes with their elderly patients at each visit (Radecki et al. 1988), and less than one minute of that time is devoted to discussion of prescription medication (Burgess 1989).

If patient expectations are influencing the prescription of medication, then direct consumer prescription drug marketing by the drug industry may have a dramatic effect on prescription drug use. There is no information on the impact of this relatively new approach to disseminating information on prescription drugs. On the positive side, it may increase drug treatment for those who should be treated, and on the negative, it may increase the prescription of unneeded medication. Whatever the case, if effective, it will increase prescription expenditures, and the consequences of these increases on both service costs and patient outcomes should be monitored.

Patient expectations may influence the prescription of unnecessary medication and the number of medications being taken by a patient.

Number of medications is the strongest risk factor for drug-related morbidity (Klein, German, and Levine 1981; Gurwitz and Avorn 1991). However, it is recognized that number of medications may influence the risk of a drug-related illness through a number of routes. It may serve as a more accurate proxy of disease status and reflect the sensitivity of diseased tissues and organs to the toxic effects of drugs (Gurwitz and Avorn 1991; G. Soucy, Directeur d'évaluation, Régie de l'assurance-maladie du Québec, personal communication, 1993). If this were the case, preventive measures would rely on the introduction of drugs with improved risk-benefit ratios. On the other hand, increasing the number of medications may increase the risk of adverse drug effects by increasing the risk of drug interaction (Beers, Storrie, and Lee 1990). Related to this possibility, we have demonstrated that there is a positive linear association between the number of medications and the presence of both rational and questionable combinations of drugs, which could lead to potentially serious adverse effects from drug interaction (Tamblyn 1996). Finally, the number of medications may increase the risk of drug-related illness by posing greater challenges for patient compliance (Stewart and Caranasos 1989; McLane, Zyzanski, and Flocke 1995). The available evidence supports this hypothesis. The number of medications taken by a patient and the complexity of the drug regimen are inversely related to compliance (Gordon 1987; Lowenthal 1987; Grymonpre et al. 1988; Nolan and O'Malley 1988a; Buechler and Malloy 1989; Harper, Newton, and Walsh 1989; Stewart and Caranasos 1989; Graveley and Oscasohn 1991; McLane, Zyzanski, and Flocke 1995). As patient compliance problems account for the majority of preventable adverse drug events, it is important to review other factors that influence compliance and may be potentially amenable to change. Although no consistent relationships have emerged between age, sex, education, or ethnicity and compliance, social isolation appears to be an important contributor to poor compliance (Porter 1969). Seniors who are living alone are more likely to neglect taking their medication.

An individual's belief systems about both health and medications are strong mediators in a individual's ultimate decision to comply with the medication regimen (Amarasangham 1980). Patients who perceive their illness as less severe, who perceive the treatment as less efficacious, and who fail to have insight into the relationship between treatment and illness are more likely to be noncompliant than patients who perceive their disease as severe and the treatment as efficacious (Becker 1976; Foo Lin, Spida, and Fortsch 1979).

The interaction a patient has with his physician is an important factor influencing compliance; the more satisfied the patient is with the medical encounter, the greater the likelihood of compliance (Francis, Dorsch, and Morris 1969; Becker and Green 1975; Cowan 1987). Consistent with these findings, the use of more than one physician or pharmacist is associated with noncompliance (Cooper, Love, and Raffoul 1982). A patient's understanding of the treatment regimen and how to follow it is a more important determinant of compliance than his understanding of the medical condition being treated (Becker, Drachman, and Kirscht 1972; Hulka, Cassel, and Kupper 1976). In this respect, it is important to note that 53–89 percent of patients do not understand what is communicated to them by their physicians on how to take their medication (Ley 1982), and 31–71 percent forget what the doctor said after leaving the office (Ley 1982).

A patient's understanding of how to take his medication is further complicated by poor labelling instructions (Kendrick and Bayne 1982). The more complex the dosing regimen, the more likely a patient will make errors in administering his medication (Stewart and Caranasos 1989; McLane, Zyzanski, and Flocke 1995). One study found dose planning errors to be 22 percent for alternate day dosing of warfarin and 59 percent for graduated dose increases for captopril (Isaac, Tamblyn, and McGill Calgary Drug Research Team 1993). Safety packaging (child-resistant caps) has been shown to reduce compliance in the elderly (Lane et al. 1971), likely because the caps cannot be opened by some patients as a result of poor grip strength and dexterity (Isaac, Tamblyn, and McGill Calgary Drug Research Team 1993). The number of medications and the complexity of the dosing regimen may also demand greater changes in a patient's lifestyle to comply. Compliance is less likely when medication taking is inconvenient or when it requires substantial lifestyle changes (Stewart and Caranasos 1989). Finally, as might be expected, medications to treat asymptotic illnesses (e.g., hypertension) are less likely to be taken than medications that provide symptom relief (e.g., arthritis medications) (McLane, Zyzanski, and Flocke 1995).

Incorporating patient treatment preferences into the therapeutic recommendations can enhance compliance. The success of using patient preferences in the health decision is based on the ability of the patient to communicate his preferences or on the ability of the physician to determine patient preferences and use these to modify therapeutic regimens to improve compliance (Eraker, Kirscht, and Becker 1984). An effective decision is one that is informed, consistent with the decision maker's values, and behaviourally implemented. Decisions that are most satisfactory are those decisions that are consistent with the patient's values, those that are based on issue-specific knowledge, those that are based on confidence in the decision maker's competence (own or others if others are involved), and those that do not involve much decisional conflict. Decisional conflict is influenced by self-perceived level of information about options, risks and benefits, unclear values, lack of support in the decision-making role, and decision-making skills deficits. It is expected that those who are satisfied with their initial decision to take a medication are more likely to adhere to a drug treatment regimen (Holmes-Rovner et al. 1996). These methods may be particularly useful for drug treatments used in asymptomatic conditions, where risk factors are being treated as a means of preventing subsequent disease (e.g., hypertension, lipidemias).

Summary

In summary, patient attitudes and behaviour likely influence whether a drug is prescribed and also whether it is appropriately taken. As noncompliance accounts for the majority of drug-related illnesses, priority needs to be placed on identifying better methods of: involving patients in the process of making decisions about their medication; reducing the number of drugs and the complexity of the drug regimen; and having more accessible and concise information on how to take their medications appropriately.

INTERVENTIONS—WHAT WORKS AND WHAT DOES NOT

Health Care System Interventions

Four main health care system policy approaches have been instituted as a means of influencing prescription expenditures: copayments and caps, physician clawbacks, reference-based pricing, and provincial formularies.

Copayments and Prescription Caps

Prescription copayment plans and caps have been instituted in some jurisdictions as a means of curtailing both the physician's propensity to prescribe unnecessary medication and patient demand for drug treatment (Nelson and Quick 1980; Nelson, Reeder, and Dickson 1984; Leibowitz, Manning, and Newhouse 1985; Reeder and Nelson 1985; Soumerai and Ross-Degnan 1990; Soumerai et al. 1991; Gouvernement du Québec 1992). In the copayment model, the patient is required to pay a fee for each prescription filled; in the cap approach, a maximum number of prescriptions are covered, beyond which the patient is required to pay. These programs uniformly produce a reduction in the number of prescriptions filled per patient, particularly for heavy medication users. Superficially, this change in drug use supports the assumption that 5–30 percent of the prescription drug expenditures may be for unnecessary medication (Nelson and Quick 1980; Nelson, Reeder, and Dickson 1984; Soumerai, Avorn, Ross-Degnan, et al. 1987). However, on closer examination, reductions are evident in both "nonessential" categories of drugs (e.g., benzodiazepines) as well as those that are presumed "essential" for a patient's well-being (e.g., insulin, antihypertensive medication) (Reeder and Nelson 1985; Soumerai, Avorn, Ross-Degnan, et al. 1987). Thus, not all reductions in prescription expenditures are for unnecessary drugs, and cost savings on prescription expenditures may lead to greater costs in the treatment of avoidable morbidity resulting from undertreatment (Soumerai et al. 1991). In New Hampshire, the institution of a three-drug prescription cap was followed by an increase in the rate of nursing home admissions. When the cap was discontinued, admission rates fell to the precap rate. This experience seems to provide convincing evidence that arbitrary caps on prescription drug coverage increase morbidity. Unfortunately, similar outcome information is not available for most of the health care system policies that have been instituted.

Physician Clawbacks

The physician clawback is a variant of the patient prescription cap. The physician is given a prescribing cap that specifies the maximum drug budget for his practice, and expenditures above the cap are deducted from the physician's salary. This policy was used as an indirect method of curtailing a physician's propensity to prescribe unnecessary medication and of encouraging the use of less expensive drug therapy in Germany. When the physician prescription caps were introduced in Germany in 1993, 2 billion deutsche Marks were saved in prescription expenditures during the first six months (Graf and Schulenburg 1993). However, an analysis of the behaviour of 409 general practitioners and internists in the seven months preceding and seven months following the cap revealed a different picture. Physicians responded to the cap by increasing their referral rate (patients with more costly medications were sent to someone else) by 9 percent and by admitting more patients to hospital—an increase of 10 percent (drug expenditures during hospitalization are not included in a physician's prescribing cap) (Graf and Schulenburg 1993). Similar to the New Hampshire cap experience (Broshy, Matheson, and Hansen 1993; Soumerai, McLaughlin, and Ross-Degnan 1994), it is evident that apparent savings in prescription drug costs may mask compensatory increases in other sectors of the health budget, possibly because of the adverse effects of such policies on patient health or simply as a compensatory means of "carrying out business as usual" in another way.

Reference-Based Pricing

Unlike prescription caps and copayments, reference-based pricing is targeted exclusively at expenditures reimbursed for prescriptions, not the rate of utilization of potentially unnecessary drugs. Three forms of reference-based pricing are recognized:

Phase 1   A reference reimbursement price will be set for all drugs with the same active ingredient, the price corresponding to the lowest cost treatment among drugs that are equivalent molecules (e.g., the lowest-priced generic drug).

Phase 2   A reference reimbursement price will be set for all drugs in the same therapeutic class (e.g., histamine$_2$ or H$_2$ blockers, acetylcholinesterase inhibitors), the price corresponding to the least expensive among equally effective, but different, molecules.

Phase 3   A reference price will be set for all drugs used to treat the same clinical condition (e.g., drugs used in the treatment of migraine), the price corresponding to the lowest price for therapy among drugs from different classes that are presumed to have equivalent clinical effectiveness (Zammit-Lucia and Dasgupta 1995).

In Canada, all provinces have phase 1 reference-based pricing—when generic drugs are available, reimbursement is set at approximately the leading generic price. As evidenced in a recent evaluation in Sweden of the introduction of phase I reference-based pricing, there is a fall in prescription expenditures in the initial period after introduction (by about 3 percent), followed within 12–24 months by a return to baseline levels (Zammit-Lucia and Dasgupta 1995). This dip and wave effect may be due to a change in prescribing patterns (i.e., towards categories of drugs where no generics are available) or background increases in utilization rates.

Phase 2 reference-based pricing has recently been instituted in British Columbia, and earlier experience has been gained from Germany and Holland. In Germany, phase 2 reference-based pricing was implemented in July 1991. Medical and legal challenges were raised because of the difficulties in establishing the clinical dose equivalency of drugs that are different molecules within the same therapeutic class. From the perspective of prescription expenditures, expenditures rose by 0.9 percent after the introduction of the policy, in comparison with annual increases of 7.7 percent in the three preceding years (Zammit-Lucia and Dasgupta 1995). However, by 1990/91, annual prescription expenditures rose by 11.8 percent (Zammit-Lucia and Dasgupta 1995). In desegregating different components of pharmaceutical expenditures, it was noted that the short-lived decrease in pharmaceutical expenses after reference-based pricing was implemented was attributable to a significant and unexplained reduction in utilization rates (Zammit-Lucia and Dasgupta 1995). The increase in pharmaceutical expenses one year after reference-based pricing was implemented was primarily due to increasing rates of prescribing in categories not included in the reference-based pricing scheme. In sum, reference-based pricing failed to significantly reduce pharmaceutical expenditures in the long term, because pharmaceutical firms switched their marketing effort to products not targeted by the reference-based pricing, and physicians increased their rate of prescribing in nonreference-based categories of drugs (Graf and Schulenburg 1994; Zammit-Lucia and Dasgupta 1995).

Phase 3 reference-based pricing is designed to minimize the changes in prescribing patterns between therapeutic classes that are observed in phase 2 reference-based pricing. The Netherlands is the only country that has attempted to implement phase 3 reference-based pricing (Rigter 1994). Even greater difficulties were encountered with the attempt to group and equate drugs from different classes with respect to equivalence and efficacy in disease management, and legal challenges ensued after implementation in 1991. Although the annual rate of growth in prescription expenditures was lower in the Netherlands in the year following implementation (1989/90, 11.2 percent; 1990/91, 8.3 percent), the annual growth rate in prescription expenditures returned to the baseline rate in the following year (1991/92, 11.1 percent) (Rigter 1994). The return to the baseline rate of growth of 11 percent was reportedly due to the utilization of new medications that had entered the market in the past five years (25 new drugs accounting for 55 percent of the increase in expenditures), and these drugs were not included in the reference-based pricing (Rigter 1994). Revisions to the policy and reimbursement system are under way; the experiment continues.

Although reference-based pricing seems to be an attractive means of instituting a quick fix to escalating prescription expenditures, it is probably too narrowly focused to reap sustained benefits in prescription drug use. Changes in the behaviour in the health care and private sectors are hard to predict and can substantially modify the expected results. As well, it fails to address the issue of utilization or of the appropriateness of physician prescribing, and both of these characteristics are more centrally related to the expected cost-benefit of prescription drug use than differential expenditures of prescription drugs within the same class.

Provincial Formularies

Each province produces an annual or semiannual list of drugs that will be covered by the insured drug benefit plan (Robinson 1995). Hospitals have also adopted this approach to control the pharmaceutical expenditure component of global institutional budgets. Formularies are such an effective means of controlling what drugs get utilized in a population that there has been little formal analysis (Sloan, Gordon, and Cocks 1993; Chapman 1994; deSmedt 1994; Johnson 1994; Woodhouse 1994; Klapper 1995; Robinson 1995). As provinces are increasingly using their formularies to control prescription expenditures, formal evaluation of the effects of listing and delisting drugs is both timely and overdue. There are two main issues of concern: (1) whether the decision to exclude a drug from the formulary compromises expected health benefits for the population; and (2) whether the decision to delist or restrict access to a drug because of cost or risk has adverse consequences for individuals who were using the medication. The case of the withdrawal of Zomepirac from the U.S. market provides some lessons about the potential consequences of changing drug access without complementary interventions (Ross-Degnan et al. 1993). When Zomepirac (a NSAID) was withdrawn from the market because of reports of drug-related deaths, there was a significant increase in prescriptions of alternative potentially inappropriate analgesics that carry considerable risks for habituation and adverse effects (Ross-Degnan et al. 1993).

Physician-Based Interventions

Physicians are the gatekeepers to prescription medication access, and in this role they have the opportunity to *prevent* exposure to unnecessary and inappropriate medication. This is critical, because existing pharmacological evidence suggests that the risk of adverse outcomes with any drug is most likely within the first few days and weeks of exposure (Hansten and Horn 1989; Schrier 1993). Over the past decade, considerable attention has been devoted to the development of intervention programs to improve physician prescribing. Four main types of interventions have been used to modify physician practice: courses and instructional material, practice aids, one-to-one consultation, and quality monitoring and care delivery systems (Tamblyn and Battista 1993).

Courses and Instructional Material

Continuing medical education courses and mailed instructional material are among the most common forms of physician education. These approaches, when used alone, do not have a significant impact on subsequent practice (Elzarian, Shirachi, and Jonest 1980; Avorn and Soumerai 1983; Ray, Schaffner, and Federspiel 1985; Evans et al. 1986; Soumerai, Avorn, Gortmaker, et al. 1987; Bjornson et al. 1990; Duke et al. 1991) or patient outcome (Evans et al. 1986; Soumerai, Avorn, Gortmaker, et al. 1987). These findings are consistent with the reported lack of effectiveness of these methods for other aspects of medical practice (Haynes et al. 1984). The only exception appears to be in the case of warnings, issued by national drug control agencies, about the use of specific drugs. Dramatic reductions in prescribing rates are observed, and, in some studies, these are accompanied by reductions in the rate of drug-specific adverse effects (Inman and Adelstein 1969; Wade and Hood 1972; Bottiger and Westerholm 1973; Melander et al. 1991). Whether these practice changes are due to the warning per se or to the publicity that typically accompanies this type of problem is impossible to disentangle.

Practice Aids

Practice aids are used to assist physicians in the process of providing care to their patients. Three types of aids have been developed: (1) methods of organizing information so the physician has a more complete and accessible profile on the patient's management; (2) methods of prompting the physician to take certain actions at the time he is making decisions about a patient's therapy; and (3) feedback on the physician's management decisions. Patient drug profiles (with and without drug cost information) have been used to reduce the likelihood of therapeutic duplications, unnecessary prescriptions, and excess cost. Providing information to the physician about current drugs has no significant impact on the number of drugs prescribed or drug cost (Koepsell et al. 1983). The use of computer prompts at the time of ordering has been demonstrated to be effective in reducing cost (Fudge et al. 1993), inappropriate prescriptions (Avorn et al. 1988), and unnecessary prescribing (Barnett et al. 1978). Computerized reminders are also effective in prompting needed follow-up for drug management (Dickinson et al. 1981; Barnett et al. 1983; Tierney, Hiu, and McDonald 1986). Feedback on a patient's drug therapy cost produces significant reductions in prescription costs, through a reduction in the number of prescriptions per patient (Hershey et al. 1986) and through increases in generic prescribing (Gehlbach et al. 1984; Zieve and Ciesco 1993). Feedback on the frequency of prescribing problems is also effective in reducing inappropriate prescribing (Manning et al. 1986; Zieve and Ciesco 1993).

One-to-One and Group Consultation

Avorn and Soumerai (1983) and Soumerai and Avorn (1986, 1987) developed the idea of academic detailing. Borrowing from marketing strategies of the drug industry, they adapted the concept of the drug detailer, a salesperson who visits physicians in their practice setting to educate them about new drugs. Academic pharmacists were trained to provide personalized visits to physicians to target inappropriate use of specific drug groups. In the initial study, a population of 435 physicians was randomly allocated to glossy printed materials alone, personalized prescriber education by a pharmacist or a control group. Three prescription drugs were targeted: peripheral vasodilators (ineffective drugs), oral cephalosporin (an overused and expensive antibiotic), and propoxyphene (an inappropriate medication). Physicians who received visits from the academic pharmacist educator reduced their prescribing of target drugs by 14 percent. Cost-benefit of the intervention was demonstrated (Soumerai and Avorn 1986). The effectiveness of this approach has been replicated in all subsequent studies (Kaufman et al. 1972; McConnell et al. 1982; Schaffner et al. 1983; Ray, Schaffner, and Federspiel 1985; Ray et al. 1986; Steele et al. 1989; Bingle et al. 1991). Variants of this approach have also worked. Stross and Bole (1980) demonstrated that effective change in physician practice could be produced by training the "leader" physician (the educational influential) in a practice community, who in turn influenced the practice of physicians in the community. Inui, Yourtee, and Williamson (1976), Reeder, Horlick, and Laxdal (1991), and Avorn et al. (1992) achieved significant change in physician behaviour by targeting small groups of physicians and discussing the medical management (and drug therapy) for targeted conditions.

Quality Monitoring and Care Delivery Systems

These systems combine several interventions to provide a comprehensive care delivery and quality monitoring system for patients with a specific health problem in a defined geographic area. The philosophy guiding the system is to provide the optimal mix of services (as guided by the available evidence) for a group of patients. Current care and patient outcomes are monitored to identify deficiencies and target interventions, as needed, to physicians, patients, and other health professionals. A pilot model of this approach has been implemented in Alberta for patients with acute myocardial infarction (Montague et al. 1995). Preliminary results suggest that the approach has been successful, particularly in changing the appropriateness of care provided to elderly women (Montague et al. 1995). This approach is appealing, because it targets the broader aspects of medical management and thus has the potential to address the mismatch between overuse and underuse of drugs, as well as the cost and appropriateness of therapy.

Summary

The characteristics of interventions that are effective in changing physician prescribing have been identified. The most effective interventions are those that provide expert advice to physicians in their practice environment, by computer alerts or more typically through one-to-one contact of an expert with the physician (academic detailing) (Avorn and Soumerai 1983; Soumerai, McLaughlin, and Avorn 1990). Despite evidence of efficacy (Soumerai and Avorn 1986; Soumerai, McLaughlin, and Avorn 1990), adoption of one-to-one interventions into regular quality control and intervention programs is not in evidence. Several limitations can be identified. First, one-to-one interventions are costly to introduce, and all interventions require ongoing maintenance for continued effectiveness (Soumerai, McLaughlin, and Avorn 1989). Second, the feasibility of one-to-one interventions rests on the assumption that the majority of prescribing problems are attributable to a small number of physicians and that only one or two target drugs are a problem. The existing evidence suggests that such assumptions are not valid. Potentially inappropriate prescribing is a problem in all major drug groups (Muijen and Silverstone 1987; Beers, Storrie, and Lee 1990; Ferguson 1990; Beers et al. 1992; Bloom et al. 1993; Wilcox, Himmelstein, and Woolhandler 1994; Tamblyn and McLeod 1994). The number of drugs involved appears to be limited only by the number reviewed by each investigator. Third, all existing physician-based prescribing interventions make the assumption that the patient has only one prescribing physician or, alternatively, that each attending physician is fully aware of all medications received by a patient. Among the elderly, this assumption is not valid. We estimated that 70 percent of the elderly had more than one community-based prescribing physician during the year, and 5 percent had more than six (Tamblyn et al. 1996). Furthermore, one-quarter of all potentially inappropriate drug combinations were created because of contemporaneous prescriptions written by two physicians (Tamblyn et al. 1996). These data substantiate earlier speculations about the increased risk of inappropriate prescriptions with multiple prescribing physicians (Maronde et al. 1971), problems that are accentuated by incomplete medication histories (Gurwich 1983) and the difficulty many elderly have in accurately recalling the medication they take (Kendrick and Bayne 1982). In sum, different approaches are needed to optimize prescribing in the elderly. Ideally, a method is needed to accurately track and record drugs currently dispensed, to document current medication in the patient's chart, to review problems with existing and new prescriptions during the office visit, to provide the physician with an up-to-date expert resource that could be used to select a drug treatment, and to provide physicians with ready access to current guidelines on medical management.

Pharmacist-Based Interventions

Pharmacists are responsible for dispensing prescribed medication. In this capacity, they have the opportunity to review a patient's current drug regimen, advise the physician if problems are identified, and counsel the patient on the use of his medication.

The Institutional Pharmacy Consultant

Pharmacy consultants have been used extensively in institutional settings to: (1) assist in the regular review of a patient's current medications, to identify inappropriate, overly costly, and unnecessary medications; (2) provide consultative assistance to physicians on drug therapy problems; and (3) counsel patients about compliance with drug therapy.

Most of the studies of the effectiveness of pharmacy services are uncontrolled comparisons, with unblinded assessment of effectiveness, so it is conceivable that the effects are moderately overestimated. Nevertheless, pharmacy review of medications appears to be an effective means of reducing the total number of drugs per patient (Cheung and Kayne 1975; Hood, Lemberger, and Stewart 1975; Cooper and Bagwell 1978; Strandberg et al. 1980; Cooper and Francisco 1981; Young et al. 1981; Chrymko and Conrad 1982; Cooper 1985; Meyer et al. 1991)—particularly for patients who are taking many medications (Meyer et al. 1991)—reducing medication error rates (e.g., in dose or timing) (Cheung and Kayne 1975; Krstenansky 1993), eliminating inappropriate drug therapy (Wilcher and Cooper 1981; Krstenansky 1993), and reducing drug costs (Williamson et al. 1984). Consultation with physicians and recommendations for changes in a patient's drug therapy regimen appear to be effective in reducing unnecessary and inappropriate medication (Hawkey et al. 1990; Kroenke and Pinholt 1990; McPhee et al. 1991; Gurwitz 1993). Pharmacist counselling of outpatients has been successful in increasing the percentage of prescriptions refilled on time and decreasing the proportion of missed refills (Schwartz 1976). In one study, consultation with a pharmacist before leaving the hospital led to a 75 percent reduction in the patient's previous high rate of noncompliance. The use of a medication counselling program given by a pharmacist was evaluated by Hammarlund, Ostrom, and Kethley (1985). Counselling was given to 183 elderly patients and covered medication compliance, drug regimen, drug interactions, and drug storage. One year after the education intervention, compliance problems dropped by 39 percent, suggesting that pharmacist consultation provides an effective health preventative strategy (Hammarlund, Ostrom, and Kethley 1985).

The Community Pharmacy Consultant

Only a handful of studies have examined the community-based pharmacist's role in drug therapy enhancement. In one study, notification cards to seek medical advice were given to patients who had problems with their drugs (e.g., adverse effects). Half of the patients with significant problems saw their physician; of these, 90 percent had their drugs changed or stopped. Dumas and Matte (1992) examined the effect of introducing a counselling fee for community pharmacies that advised patients or physicians on drug problems. Most fees were paid for patient compliance counselling, rather than physician advice. Patients appeared to comply better with the pharmacist's suggestions than with the physicians' (Dumas and Matte 1992).

Summary

Pharmacist drug review and consultation in institutional settings appears to be an effective means of reducing the overall number of drugs a patient is taking, reducing the number of inappropriate prescriptions, and improving compliance with therapy. The role of the community pharmacist in the optimization of medication therapy for seniors is relatively unexplored.

Patient-Based Interventions

The goals of interventions at the patient level are to modify expectations for drug therapy and to enhance compliance. The majority of interventions reported have addressed the issue of patient compliance; few have addressed the issue of patient expectations.

Interventions to Enhance Compliance

Information Support

Physician counselling – Physician-patient communication is a factor in increasing compliance, especially when it is related to increasing understanding and satisfaction on the part of the patient (Young 1987). Patients have been found to be more compliant when the amount of time spent with their physician is perceived to be sufficient (McLane, Zyzanski, and Flocke 1995). However, it has been found that the time devoted to instructing patients about how to take their medication is a more important determinant of compliance than educating patients about their disease process (Lunden 1978). Scientifically erroneous health beliefs have been shown to impede compliance with a prescribed medical regimen. These erroneous health beliefs, however, are subject to change (Becker 1974). Physician awareness of the health beliefs held by their patients is the first step in trying to alter them. One study addressed this problem. Sixty-two physicians randomly received either a two-hour teaching tutorial on compliance difficulties experienced by patients and possible strategies for altering patients' beliefs and behaviours, or a two-hour "placebo" teaching session on an unrelated topic. Compared with physicians who received the placebo tutorial, physicians who received the experimental tutorial significantly increased the proportion of time they spent on patient education, patient compliance, and patient understanding of disease. Their patients subsequently displayed more appropriate health beliefs and improved compliance with medications (Inui, Yourtee, and Williamson 1976).

Verbal drug education – The effectiveness of patient education given by a clinical pharmacist and nurse clinician on patient compliance among patients attending rheumatology and renal clinics was evaluated (Bond and Monson 1984). Three hundred and fifty-five patients received instruction from a pharmacist or nurse clinician about their medication, adverse side-effects, and potential drug effects. Patient reviews were performed before the intervention (control), nine months after the intervention, and four years, nine months after the intervention. Compliance was estimated by examining prescription refill patterns. Medication compliance was significantly better in both study groups compared with controls, but not significantly different between study groups. This suggests that the close management of outpatient drug treatment by clinical pharmacists can significantly improve patients' compliance with their medication.

Written drug education – The patient's inability to recall verbal explanations about his medication is a hindrance to compliance. The use of written instructions to augment verbal instructions has been proposed as a useful tool in increasing compliance (Coe, Prendergast, and Psathas 1984; Morrow, Leirer, and Sheikh 1988). Written information has been shown to work best when combined with verbal advice and social support of a health care professional. In a review of the effects of written drug information on patients' knowledge and medication compliance (Mazzullo 1976), it was noted that written information improves compliance with short-term use of antibiotic drugs. For long-term drug use, however, written information alone is not sufficient to improve patient compliance. Multifaceted educational and behavioural interventions addressing the patient's specific needs has proven to be more appropriate for long-term medication compliance. Many variations of educational and behavioural compliance strategies have been studied. Medication behaviour problems were evaluated in a group of 58 low-income seniors identified with at least two medication behaviour problems (Hammarlund, Ostrom, and Kethley 1985). Subjects received three one-hour education sessions over the course of one year, plus written information concerning the proper use of medication. A significant 39 percent decrease in medication problems was seen after the one-year period.

Self-Medication Programs

Self-medication programs have been implemented in some hospitals as a method of improving patients' knowledge of their medication regimen before they leave the hospital. Patients move through a series of progressively more involved stages in administering their own medicines while they are in the hospital, with complete self-administration of medicine by the time of discharge (Baxendale, Gourlay, and Gibson 1978; Proos et al. 1992; Lowe et al. 1995). Medication knowledge and compliance were compared between a group of 48 patients randomized to a self-medication program and a group of 45 patients who received written information and counselling but did not administer their own medications (Proos et al. 1992). The investigators found that patients' knowledge of the name of their medication, frequency of dose, reason for taking medication, and potential side-effects improved significantly in patients who were put on a self-medication program. Compliance scores were not significantly improved in the self-medication program patients. In a second study evaluating a self-medication program, improved compliance scores were found in a group of elderly inpatients. Eighty-eight patients were randomized to the self-medication program or standard care while still in hospital. Patients in the self-medication program had a higher mean compliance score (95 percent) than patients receiving standard care (83 percent) and were significantly more knowledgeable about the medications they were taking (Lowe et al. 1995).

Compliance Aids

Dosing formulations – Using a simpler type of dosing formulation has been found to improve compliance. Fifty-eight elderly patients with hypertension were randomized to use either a transdermal patch or standard pill. Compliance rates in patients using the transdermal clonidine patch increased to 96 percent compared with a rate of 50 percent for those taking oral tablets.

Dosing frequencies – Simplifying the medication regimen by replacing multiple daily dosing with single daily dosing has proven to increase compliance (Dwyer, Levy, and Menander 1986; Jacobs, Goldstein, and Kelly 1988; Morgan et al. 1986). One study found that compliance with non-steroidal anti-inflammatory agents given once daily was 65 percent, whereas compliance for drugs requiring dosing four times a day was only 37 percent (Jacobs, Goldstein, and Kelly 1988). The compliance rate of daily, 2 x daily, and 3 x daily doses has been compared with that of 4 x daily doses (Cramer et al. 1989). Compliance improved as the number of daily doses decreased. The mean compliance rate for daily, 2 x daily, and 3 x daily doses was also found to be significantly higher than that for 4 x daily doses (Jacobs, Goldstein, and Kelly 1988). Another study evaluated 192 patients with hypertension and daily, 2 x daily, or 3 x daily doses (Morgan et al. 1986). Compliance with both daily and 2 x daily doses was significantly better than that with 3 x daily doses.

Medication Packaging

The use of pill calendars and blister packages reduces the confusion about dose and frequency of medications and increases compliance. Blister packs were evaluated in one study (Haskitt 1989). Seventy-seven percent of patients using blister packs took 90 percent of their medication, whereas only 28 percent of the control group with regularly dispensed medication were compliant. Wong and Normal (1987) studied the use of a calendar mealtime blister pack in a two-group crossover clinical trial. Average noncompliance with patients using the mealtime blister pack was 2.04 compared with 9.17 from standard pill bottles (Wong and Normal 1987). In another study, improved compliance was sustained at three months postdischarge in 39 elderly patients using a blister calendar pack with foil backing (Ware and Harris 1991). Unit-of-use packaging has also been studied as a compliance strategy (Murray et al. 1993). Unit-of-use packaging is a type of packaging in which all medications to be taken at one time are packaged together in a sealed dose with the date and time to be taken written on it. This decreases the confusion often associated with complex medication regimens. Unit-of-use packaging was compared with standard medication packaging in 36 elderly patients (Murray et al. 1993). Compliance was found to be significantly better in the unit-of-use group compared with the control group.

Medication Reminder Devices

Counter caps – Counter caps, which fit on prescription bottles, indicate the day of the week and the number of doses to be taken. When the patient opens and closes the container, the indicator advances automatically. In a crossover clinical trial of patients with glaucoma, it was found that significantly more refills were requested during the six months patients used the counter cap compared with the six months they used standard pill bottles, and they requested significantly more refills than the control groups (Sclar et al. 1991).

Electronic pillboxes – The electronic pillbox is similar to a counter cap, with the additional feature of an alarm when the medication is due or if a dose has been missed. The electronic pillbox was evaluated on 70 elderly patients with hypertension (McKenney, Munroe, and Wright 1992). Mean compliance rate was 95.1 percent for patients using the electronic pillbox compared with 78 percent for patients using standard pill bottles.

Weekly medication containers – Plastic weekly medication containers enable the patient to organize medication according to indicated times of administration. The device can span up to a one-week period. One hundred and fifty-eight elderly patients were randomized to receive oral instruction alone or in combination with written information, a medication reminder calendar, or a seven-day pill reminder box (Ascione and Shimp 1984). The subjects who used the medication reminder calendar or the seven-day pill reminder box had significantly better self-reported compliance than the subjects who had oral instructions alone or in combination with written instruction. Colour coding patients' pill bottles and pill medication containers has also been used. Significantly improved compliance was found in 103 elderly patients assigned to receive their medications in colour-coded bottles plus colour-coded pill trays compared with patients who received either no intervention or oral and written instructions (Martin and Mean 1982).

Seiko RC wrist terminal – The Seiko RC wrist terminal contains an information storage unit that can be programmed by the pharmacist for one week of medication therapy. An alarm sounds to remind the patient when to take the medication. Another alarm reminds the patient about refilling the prescription. The wrist terminal also has the capability of being programmed to inform the patient about possible side-effects and can display MedicAlert signs to warn health care providers of special conditions, such as allergies, heart problems, and diabetes. The effectiveness of this method has not been evaluated.

Prescription label scratch-offs – Prescription label scratch-offs are labels that have small dots that the patient can scratch off each time the medication has been taken. These are especially useful for patients experiencing confusion and memory impairment. The effectiveness of this method has not been evaluated.

Telephone reminders – Telephone reminders, in the form of computerized voice messages, are meant to remind forgetful patients to take medication at specified times. In one study, computerized voice message reminders were found to reduce noncompliance from 14.2 percent to 2.1 percent, compared with a control group that did not receive voice message reminders (Leirer et al. 1991). This study, however, was based on only eight subjects. Schectman, Hiatt, and Hartz (1994) assessed the use of telephone follow-up calls on compliance of prescription refills on 112 patients from the Lipid Clinic. One-half of the patients were randomized to receive weekly telephone calls for five weeks to counsel them and remind them to continue taking the medications. Compliance in the telephone groups was not significantly higher than in the control group.

Calendar chart – Reminder charts or calendars have been studied as a means of improving compliance. One hundred and ninety-three discharged patients were randomly allocated to receive a combination of counselling, reminder chart, and/or reminder chart with verbal explanation. Mean compliance scores were significantly higher in patients who received the reminder chart vs. no reminder chart, and these patients were more likely to be able to describe their medication regimen than patients who received counselling only (83 percent vs. 47 percent) (Raynor, Booth, and Blenkinsopp 1993). Another study compared the number of medication-taking errors in groups of elderly patients who received verbal instruction alone, verbal instructions plus a calendar detailing their daily medications, or verbal instructions plus a pill identification card that had a picture of the pill and the time to take the pill (Wandless and Davie 1977). Patients using either the pill identification card or medication calendar plus receiving verbal instructions had significantly fewer medication errors than patients who received verbal counselling alone. More recently, the benefits of using a memory aid in a group of 42 elderly inpatients were confirmed (Esposito 1995). Patients were randomized to receive written instruction, written instruction and verbal counselling, medication schedule, or medication schedule plus verbal counselling. Patients who were given the medication schedule attained the highest rates of compliance.

Smart cards – Smart cards, under experimentation in Sweden and Quebec, are credit card–size information storage systems that are carried by the patient and can be read by a computer. Examples of information stored include personal identification, prescription record, and medical history (i.e., blood type, allergies, chronic conditions) (Berg et al. 1993). The effectiveness of this method has not been evaluated.

Package inserts – Eklund and Wessling (1976) included package inserts (small prefolded pamphlets) in alternate patients' prescriptions for antibiotics. Telephone interviews with 360 of 483 patients showed that two-thirds of those who had received the package inserts had read them, and 80 percent gave them a positive evaluation. However, although the package insert patients had better knowledge of side-effects and had reported a better dosage schedule, there was no significant difference between the insert group and the noninsert group on knowledge of the drug name or instructions for use.

Tailoring – A daily routine for taking medications that is "built into" a patient's existing schedule has proven to increase compliance (Fincham 1988; West 1989). For example, if an established routine for a patient involves coffee in the morning, lunch at noon, tea at 3 p.m., and dinner at 6 p.m., then taking medications could be "built into" these activities.

Compliance Surveillance

Continual monitoring of a patient's compliance to the medication regimen is a successful tool used by pharmacists to deter noncompliance. A recent California study found that compliance was increased by 41 percent in patients who were sent a written note reminding them to get their prescriptions refilled (Lachman 1987). Various studies have shown improved patient compliance when frequency of outpatient visits is increased, home visits are added, patients received negative feedback about noncompliance, and continuity of care is provided (Haynes 1976; Smith and Andrews 1983). In one study, elderly patients recently discharged from hospital were visited at home to discuss medication use. During the home visit, patients were counselled about their medications and reasons for taking them. Patients who received the home visits achieved 92 percent compliance, despite the fact that most did not understand the purpose of the medication (Smith and Andrews 1983).

Contingency Contracts

Contingency contracting is a method used to improve compliance among resistant patients. Contingency contracting involves setting treatment goals, establishing time limits, and outlining the responsibilities of both parties (Boudin 1972; Lewis and Michnich 1977; Dapcich-Miura and Hovell 1979). Lewis and Michnich (1977) claim that contingency contracting clarifies what is expected of the patient and provides a power shift, giving the patient a sense of control, rather than being a passive receiver. Contracts provide: (1) written instructions; (2) time for the patient to discuss personal situations and engage in problem solving with the health provider; (3) formal commitment to the treatment regimen; and (4) tangible incentives for compliance (Dapcich-Miura and Hovell 1979). The effectiveness of this method has not been evaluated.

Interventions to Influence Patient Expectations for Drug Therapy

Decision support systems – Patients are dissatisfied with their involvement in the decision making about their care (Webster 1989; Tamblyn, Abrahamowicz, et al. 1994). Decision support systems provide a structure for the patient and physician to discuss therapy options (Holmes-Rovner et al. 1996). These systems assist the patients in evaluating the pros and cons of various therapeutic options for their problem, the value they place on the risks, and the benefits attached to each choice. The objective of the system is to help the patient identify his treatment preferences and to explicitly incorporate these preferences into the choice of treatment regimen. In doing so, it is hypothesized that patients will be more satisfied and more likely to be compliant with their chosen therapy (Eraker, Kirscht, and Becker 1984). Decision support systems have the potential to influence a patient's expectation for drug therapy and minimize intentional underuse of medication once prescribed.

Summary

Patient-level interventions have been primarily focused on methods to improve the patient's compliance with drug therapy, and not on the patient's perception of the need for the prescription in the first place. Noncompliance, in most patients, is intentional (Cooper, Love, and Raffoul 1982), and the most common reason for intentional noncompliance is the belief that the drug is not needed (Cooper, Love, and Raffoul 1982). Decision support systems provide one mechanism for addressing this problem, and further development of this area will address a gap in the health care delivery process. The physician-patient interaction will be central to the success of these methods, for the physician must be willing to respond to the patient's preferences for decision systems to work. A variety of compliance aids are currently available, although no information is present on the prevalence of their use or, in some instances, their effectiveness. Unintentional compliance is often related to forgetting medication or misunderstanding instructions. The most cost-effective means of resolving these problems need to be identified.

SUCCESS STORIES

Patient-Level Intervention

The Problem

It is a well-known fact that noncompliance represents a major problem to individuals, the health care system, and society. Individuals who are hospitalized are often discharged from the hospital with a number of changes or additions to their existing medications. Changing an existing medical regimen by replacing the old medication or adding a new medication puts an individual at a higher risk of not adhering correctly to his prescribed medications and of rehospitalization for drug-related problems associated with noncompliance. Coupled with this problem is the lack of a single successful approach to reduce noncompliance.

The Actors

D.K. Raynor, Ph.D., is the primary investigator for this study. This project was conducted in partial fulfilment of his Ph.D. requirements in the Department of Pharmacy, University of Bradford. T.G. Booth, Head of the Department of Pharmacy at the University of Bradford, acted as D.K. Raynor's thesis supervisor. A. Blenkinsopp, Ph.D., was Dr. Raynor's tutor for this project. He is the Director, Centre for Pharmacy Postgraduate Education, at the University of Manchester.

The Objective

The objective of this research project was to assess the efficacy of a computer-generated reminder chart in increasing compliance with patients who wish to be compliant but fail owing to the complexity of their medical regimen. Patient empowerment was an important issue in the social, psychological, and economic climate of England at this time and thus was a consideration in the development of the reminder chart. The authors believed that the computer-generated reminder chart would increase empowerment in patients who would benefit from it (i.e., patients who wanted to comply but were lacking an efficient method to do so) by providing a means for patients to improve their compliance while maintaining the responsibility of administering their own medications. The use of a computer was felt to be a practical solution to restricted funds, by cutting down on the manpower needed to carry out this project.

The Intervention and Outcome

The intervention evaluated in this project was a computer-generated reminder chart designed to improve patients' compliance with their drug regimen. One hundred and ninety-seven patients discharged from one English hospital with two or more medication prescriptions were randomly allocated to receive a reminder chart, a health professional drug education, or a combination of the two. Patient knowledge and compliance with medications were assessed 10 days after discharge. The computer-generated reminder chart was determined to be a practical and cost-effective aid to compliance. Eighty-six percent of patients given this chart complied with their medication, whereas only 63 percent of patients not given the chart complied with their medication.

Analysis of the Reasons for Success

Success with this approach can be attributed to the use of a combination of established compliance strategies. Tailoring a patient's medical regimen to an existing schedule, personalizing a patient's medical regimen, and taking time to explain how to administer medication are factors that have been shown to increase compliance in other studies. In this study, these strategies were combined in a more simplified manner, and computers were used to remove the labour-intensive aspects of providing personalized information. As a result, this project could be done without the need for significant up-front investment (most pharmacies are computerized), training, or health care professional add-on costs.

The Implications

A wider objective of this study was to implement the use of this computer-generated reminder chart in community pharmacies and hospitals. An official outcome evaluation has not yet been conducted on this intervention. However, to date, 12 pharmacies in the community have been able to integrate this software program into their existing computer successfully. Barriers to its implementation in other pharmacies and/or hospitals have been technical issues, such as the incompatibility of software programs already in place in most pharmacies and hospitals. This project has stimulated an interest in the use of reminder charts as a method of reducing noncompliance. Many of the pharmacies and hospitals that cannot generate a computer-based reminder chart have used the chart detailed in this project as a model and filled it in by hand. The author has subsequently collaborated with the National Pharmaceutical Association of the United Kingdom and produced a reminder chart, based on the computer-generated reminder chart, specifically for use by hand in the community. This handwritten reminder chart is readily available and intended for use in pharmacies, hospitals, and nursing homes. It can be used by the patient and/or caregiver.

Funding

Funding for this project was obtained from the regional health authorities based on a competitive bidding procedure. Sufficient funding was provided for the duration of the project, which constituted the first author's Ph.D. thesis.

Physician-Level Intervention: Academic Detailing

The Problem

Academic detailing was developed by Dr. Gerry Avorn. During his medical school and residency training, he noted that the drug industry was very effective at communicating information through the use of easy-to-read glossy print information and drug detail people who provide personalized visits to physicians. In contrast, medical schools excelled in their ability to provide neutral, objective evaluation of the risks and benefits of drugs but were hopeless when it came to effectively communicating this information to the medical community. The concept of academic detailing arose because of Dr. Avorn's belief that information provided to physicians by the drug industry should be counterbalanced by neutral objective information on the risks and benefits of new drug treatments.

The Actors

Dr. Gerry Avorn is a geriatrician who initiated this project as a young investigator who had just completed his geriatrics training and had been recruited to Harvard University. Dr. Avorn is a charismatic speaker and a very effective writer. It is probably these two characteristics that allowed a very good idea to be carried to its next phase, which was to find funding for its development and evaluation.

Funding

A protocol to develop and evaluate the use of academic detailing among practicing physicians was submitted to the predecessor of the Agency of Health Care Policy and Research in the United States in 1978. Dr. Avorn received $160,000 from this agency to initiate the project. One of the main supporters of this idea, a chief reviewer on the project, was Dr. Joe Newhouse, a medical economist. Dr. Newhouse personally believed in the concept of a marketplace of ideas—the availability and easy access of information to all consumers. His support may have been one of the factors that led to the project's funding during this period.

Analyzing the Results

The first study was carried out in four states: Arkansas, New Hampshire, Vermont, and the District of Columbia. Medicaid data were used to identify physicians who were excessive prescribers of three target drugs that were considered to be relatively inappropriate: propoxyphene, cerebral and peripheral vasodilators, and cephalexin. Four hundred and thirty-five physicians were identified as filling 30 or more prescriptions per year from these drug groups. These physicians were randomized to a control group, a group that would receive only print information, and a group that would receive "face-to-face" detailing by a pharmacist educator. Physicians who received visits from the academic pharmacist educator reduced their prescribing of target drugs by 14 percent. No such effect was observed in the control group or the group that received only printed information. Dr. Steven Soumerai, the coinvestigator on the project, went on to estimate the cost-benefits of academic detailing. He estimated that every dollar spent on academic detailing would result in a $2 savings in prescription drug costs.

In carrying out this project, the investigators developed several methodologies and innovations. The first was to take advantage of the information that was used for pharmacists' reimbursement purposes, the availability of prescription information from Medicaid records. This information had not previously been used by researchers for this purpose. This meant the investigators had to negotiate with Medicaid in each of the states to obtain the information and to learn how to use the millions of prescription records that are usually present to identify physicians that may benefit from the target intervention. The second innovation was in identifying the best methods of providing drug treatment information to physicians in a palatable form that was equivalent in its attractiveness to that of the drug industry. A market research consultant conducted interviews with physicians to identify the physicians' understanding of the drugs that were targeted by intervention and the reason for using them. Information from these interviews was then incorporated into the educational strategy. "Unadvertisements" were prepared for the physicians. In addition, to address the issue of patient demand and its influence on drug prescribing patterns, brochures suitable for the general public were prepared and provided to the physician for distribution to the patients using these drugs.

Evaluation

The results of this study were published in the *New England Journal of Medicine* in 1983. From the perspective of the investigators, the finding that there was a significant positive effect of academic detailing led to a host of other questions, including the cost-effectiveness of the methodology and the relative effectiveness in different subgroups of physicians. Subsequent proposals were submitted to the original funding agency, which continued to provide funds for this next phase.

Replicability of the Initiative

This methodology, and variations on this methodology (e.g., small group detailing, educational influentials, physician detailers vs. pharmacist detailers), have been instituted by a variety of investigators from different countries. The positive and significant effects of this type of intervention have been reproduced systematically in all studies that have been published in the English literature.

According to Dr. Avorn, the concept was adopted by the Kaiser-Permenente Health Maintenance Organization (HMO) on the west coast as part of its regular quality assurance program. Pharmacist educators were hired by this HMO to provide regular and ongoing detailing to physicians who were employed by the organization. At an international level, programs have been initiated in Australia, coordinated by Dr. Frank May, to provide national surveillance and detailing to physicians whose prescribing patterns are deviant. A similar program has been developed in the National Health Service in the United Kingdom by Dr. Steve Chapman at Keele University, Staffordshire. Although adoptions into quality assurance programs have occurred in a number of settings, the process has not been as widespread as one would have expected, given the cost savings potential. Dr. Avorn pointed out that government bodies in the United States, including Medicaid and the Veterans Affairs system, have not incorporated this idea into their quality assurance programs. When asked why this might be the case, he commented that these agencies have a cumbersome bureaucracy and see their role as simply one of paying the bills and not of making or shaping policy decisions. A similar perspective is evident in parts of the Canadian health care system. This is in contrast to HMOs, which possess a more entrepreneurial perspective and have a vested interest in enhancing cost-effectiveness.

Similarly, state boards and provincial colleges of physicians, which have the legal responsibility to review the quality of a physician's practice, have not adopted this process. These self-regulatory bodies have historically adopted the role of granting licenses and rescinding them. They have not taken on the broader role of quality assurance in the education of doctors. This may be changing in Canada. The Federation of Medical Licensing Authorities of Canada has established a policy that they will institute programs of surveillance of medical practice for all physicians in Canada and appropriate remedial programs to address problems that may be evident. An example of the changing role of the colleges in this respect is provided in the next success story.

The Future

Academic detailing, adopted at regional, provincial, and national levels in Canada, has the potential to produce major health care savings. Changes in prescribing have the potential to reduce prescription drug costs and avoidable morbidity.

Physician-Level Intervention: Academic Detailing and the Provincial Colleges of Physicians

The Problem

In 1991/92, the Quebec Ministry of Health (Régie de l'assurance-maladie du Québec) conducted a one-day census survey of potentially inappropriate medication use among Quebec seniors using the prescription claims databases. One region, Quebec City, was identified as having a high prevalence of potentially inappropriate benzodiazepine prescriptions.

The Evolution of a New Partnership

A public health physician in the region, Dr. Philipe Lemieux, decided that action should be taken to reduce the level of benzodiazepine misuse, and he contacted Dr. René Gagnon, Director of Continuing Medical Education at Laval University, for assistance. On the basis of the literature, they decided that academic detailing would be a suitable intervention and proceeded to request the list of names of excessive prescribers of benzodiazepines from the Régie de l'assurance-maladie du Québec. They were advised that only the College of Physicians had the authority to ask for this information. The Director of Continuing Medical Education contacted some persons he knew at the College, Dr. André Jacques and Dr. André Lindon, and a partnership for a joint intervention was planned.

The Production of a Novel Intervention

The College saw this as an opportunity to blend its customary approach of inspection visits (a long-standing program of quality surveillance for hospitals and high-risk physician groups) with an educational intervention. It also provided an opportunity, through data provided by the Régie de l'assurance-maladie du Québec, of enhancing the efficiency of their inspection visits by targeting both specific problems and physicians who were more likely to be in difficulty. Thus, a study was designed to examine three possible methods of intervention: inspection visit alone, inspection visit plus the option of an academic detail visit, and academic detail visit alone.

The Study

Of the 950 physicians in the area, 591 were identified as having potential benzodiazepine prescribing problems. Of these, 161 physicians who had prescribed benzodiazepines inappropriately to 12 or more of their elderly patients were included in the study. Physicians were randomly allocated to the inspection visit alone, inspection visit plus academic detail visit, academic detail visit alone, or a control group. Physicians randomized to the intervention group were sent a letter from the College indicating that their prescriptions for benzodiazepines were sufficiently discrepant from those of their peers to cause concern. Physicians assigned to the inspection visit were told that an inspector would be calling to arrange a time to visit their practice. Physicians assigned to the inspection plus academic detail visit were advised to call the academic detailer and arrange an appointment. During the inspection visit, the inspectors reviewed a selection of the charts of each of the patients who were identified by the Régie de l'assurance-maladie du Québec as having problem benzodiazepine prescriptions, and the physician's rationale for this therapy was discussed. For the academic detail visits, indications and recommended therapy guidelines for benzodiazepine therapy were reviewed, and methods of tapering and discontinuation were suggested. Print material was provided, and a follow-up visit was made six months later. The effectiveness of the interventions will be assessed by evaluating benzodiazepine prescribing by study physicians in the 12 months after the intervention (October 1995 – October 1996).

The Informal Report of the Effects

One of the unexpected effects of the intervention was the snowball effect that was produced by the blitzkrieg of activity in the region. A substantial proportion of the physicians who practiced in the region were targeted by the study, and most of the inspector and detailer visits in the region took place in a condensed period of time. Dr. Jacques comments: "Suddenly everyone knew there was a problem. Courses and seminars on benzodiazepine therapy started to appear in regional newsletters and medical societies. Everyone was talking about it."

Although no data have yet been analyzed, the College believes the project was a success. It found that the Régie de l'assurance-maladie du Québec prescription files could be used for prescribing surveillance. Only 1 of the 46 physicians who had an inspection visit and chart review had clinically justified reasons for using benzodiazepines. The inspection visit and review could be targeted to a specific problem, and the patients who may be affected by this problem could be identified and their charts reviewed. The process seemed more efficient than the usual method of inspection visits, where charts are randomly selected and reviewed, without explicit criteria to judge the acceptability of management. As a result, the College is planning its next intervention, this time in relationship to NSAID prescribing in the Montreal region. The academic detail visit has been abandoned as being too costly. The College is hoping to produce the same snowball effect it obtained in the Quebec City region, perhaps supplemented by the organization of large group sessions. The experiment continues.

Analysis of the Reasons for Success

This project was a story about the right time, the right people, and the right setting. Mr. Gerard Soucy of the Régie de l'assurance-maladie du Québec started the ball rolling by instituting the first quality surveillance survey, because he believed the Régie de l'assurance-maladie du Québec should be doing more than just monitoring expenditures. Dr. Lemieux had the energy and dedication to take action in the region and seek collaboration with the university. Dr. Jacques, who was new at the College, saw the project as a wonderful opportunity to build a partnership between the conventionally independent divisions of inspection and continuing medical education at the College. His interest in creating new partnerships and ways of doing business was supported by the new president (Dr. Roch Bernier) and new executive director (Dr. Joelle Lescop) of the College. Thus, there were at least three visionary people at the College who saw this as an opportunity. Finally, the setting made a difference. The College of Physicians in Quebec has had a long-standing program of surveillance. Unlike other provinces, the College has the legal right to review the activity of any practicing physician in the province, and it has conducted a regular surveillance program for high-risk physicians. The College has also had an ongoing relationship with the Régie de l'assurance-maladie du Québec to evaluate physicians with very deviant billing profiles. The new aspect of this relationship was for the College to make requests to the Régie de l'assurance-maladie du Québec for information.

CONCLUSIONS

The literature provides insight into six broad categories of knowledge relative to medication use in the elderly. These conclusions are taken from a large number of studies conducted in different contexts, but their results can be organized on the basis of the schematic representation of the factors that influence the outcome of prescription drug use presented above (see figure 1). The representation presents the health care system with physicians, patients, and drugs as "microdeterminants" at the centre, with two concentric layers representing the drug industry in the middle circle, and society at the outer circle as "macrodeterminants." The first three conclusions deal with the microdeterminants of the problem—i.e., those related to the immediate environment of the patients, the drugs, the prescribing physicians, and the pharmacists. They are to the effect that:

- Errors made in the patient's use of medication are the single most important and preventable cause of adverse drug effects and suboptimal therapeutic benefit. Drug information and compliance support systems for patients (and families) are inadequate in terms of content and accessibility.

- There is a mismatch between drug expenditures for seniors and maximal health benefit. Overuse, underuse, and misuse of prescription drugs by seniors are documented, and substantial problems are generated by the inappropriate management of prescription drugs, most of which may be associated with problems with the prescription process or compliance issues.
- Improvements in doctor-patient communication may reduce un-necessary prescribing and improve patient compliance. Improvements in physician prescribing will reduce drug-related morbidity and cost. Medical school and postgraduate education play a considerable role in shaping a physician's prescribing patterns, and scores on licensure/certification examinations provide some prediction of a physician's prescribing behaviour.

These conclusions suggest that measures taken in areas such as consumer health information, systems and guidelines for the management of prescriptions at the level of the medical practice and the pharmacy, the creation of conditions that are favourable to the enhancement of compliance and collaboration between patients and physicians, as well as a more systematic approach to nonpharmacological alternatives, would contribute to the reduction of costs and the improvement of care.

At the macro level, the present review identifies three major conclusions that underline the respective role of government policy in the economic, fiscal and health sectors, drug industry practices, and health care system concerns. They are to the effect that:

- Drug marketing has a profound impact on prescription drug use and drug costs. The competing priorities of drug industry development in Canada need to be harmonized with the objective of a fiscally judicious health care system to optimize the cost-benefit of prescription drug use. Failure to do so will compromise the potential success of any intervention.
- There is a paucity of empirical data on the risks and benefits of current drugs and new drugs in the elderly, particularly for seniors who are 75 years of age or older and among those with multiple health problems and medications. Evidence-based guidelines for prescribing cannot be adequately developed until better information is available.
- Revisions in policy should be directed by the common philosophical ground between the drug industry and provincial governments, in order to optimize the effective use of current and new drugs. Incentives or penalties could be instituted to require drug companies to contribute funds to the health care sector to monitor use of prescription medication and to minimize overuse, misuse, and underuse of prescription drugs through the provision of effective physician prescribing aids and patient decision-making and compliance support systems. These incentives or

penalties could be instituted by provinces as part of the formulary application process.

Clearly, the decisions made within the health care system about drugs—e.g., formulary rules—have an impact on other sectors of government, such as industry and commerce or revenue. Ways must be found to transcend present administrative barriers between government sectors if we are to formulate coherent policy. Systems that link services to outcomes and that recognize that efficacy in the field is dependent on more than simple pharmacological efficacy are necessary. Profound revision of drug industry marketing practices is necessary now that the main buyers of drugs are government and insurance companies.

The present review suggests that no single cure exists for the problems of medication use in the elderly, because no single problem exists. Depending upon the level of analysis, problems can be found with patient behaviour, physician and pharmacist behaviour, patient, physician, and pharmacist support systems, drug industry marketing practices and lack of product support to enhance appropriate selection, prescription and utilization of products, health care system inconsistencies, and interdepartmental compartmentalization in government, otherwise known as "stovepiping."

POLICY IMPLICATIONS

The Microdeterminants

Patients

Effective decision and compliance support systems are needed to help patients and their entourage make enlightened decisions about health issues. The technology to provide such information services in a timely and cost-effective manner is available. Fiscal support for their development and evaluation could evolve from changes in regulatory policy governing the application for inclusion in provincial formularies (making participation in the development of such information and systems a precondition to the inclusion of a drug), small business support grants, and Health Canada targeted funding for university-industry partnerships. Collaboration with seniors groups in the development of compliance support systems will facilitate a more rapid dissemination into the seniors community and increase the likelihood that new developments will meet the needs of persons in this age group. Integration of computer technology into the process of providing rapid, personalized access should be pursued. A central objective of this effort would be to improve the match between indication and therapy. A number of strategies could be explored, such as structured methods of assisting seniors in the evaluation of the risks and benefits of drug therapy (for overuse, the risks relative to nonpharmacological therapy; for underuse, the benefits relative to the risks) that are accessible to the public through routes other than the health care system. Decision support systems should be evaluated as one way of providing this assistance. To this effect, we recommend the creation of a National Consumer Health Institute to act as an independent testing and validating facility for patient information and decision support systems.

Physicians and Pharmacists

Because of their powers of influence and the decisions they make every day, physicians and pharmacists are intimately involved in the ways in which medication is dispensed and used. Their behaviour and their practice environment have a crucial impact on utilization. However, in order for their actions to contribute to the overall goal of proper medication use, they must be equipped to face the various challenges generated by the current context of health care services. Among the tools that are needed are clear prescribing guidelines for primary care, and these guidelines should be developed with the constant participation of physicians and pharmacists. However, in order to influence everyday practice, expert support systems to guide prescribing and management decisions in medical practice, to minimize prescribing errors, to provide current drug information, and to provide feedback on prescribing decisions and patient outcomes must be developed and quickly implemented. Primary medical practice is one of the least well endowed environments when it comes to the use of information technology.

We recommend that the primary care and pharmacy settings be identified as a top priority for the application of information technology solutions that link physicians with the appropriate information sources and provide them with access to the pertinent information.

Public Health

One of the major difficulties in monitoring drug utilization lies in the fact that the sources of information are distributed across agencies and are not easily linked. Population databases that allow the linkage of information from varying sources to a patient and to a fairly small geographic area make it possible to ask questions about the impact of various measures on the health of populations. There is a need for multilevel "early alert" population surveillance systems to flag patient, physician, and system problems in prescribing, coordinated with constructive intervention and prevention programs.

We recommend consideration of the realignment of medical services, prescriptions, public health funding, and institutional funding into program-specific budget envelopes as a means of optimizing the package and mix of services delivered to a group of patients while containing costs. This approach would be best tried on a "pilot basis" in provinces that have instituted decentralized health budgets.

The Macrodeterminants

Government-Industry Relations

Revisions in policy should be directed to the common philosophical ground between the drug industry and provincial governments, that being to optimize the effective use of current and new drugs. In this sense, the financial burden of supporting drug utilization beyond the provision of pharmacologically active substances into the behavioural realm should become part of drug makers' responsibilities and shared with the health care system. Drug companies should contribute funds to the health care sector to monitor use of prescription medication and to minimize overuse, misuse, and underuse of prescription drugs through the provision of effective physician prescribing aids and patient decision-making and compliance support systems. This funding could be seen as a component of drug development and could be managed by provinces as part of the formulary application process in collaboration with the National Consumer Health Institute suggested above.

We recommend that such funding become part of the requirement for drug inclusion in the provincial formularies.

Drug Approval Processes

Also, the drug and formulary approval processes provide the logical juncture for redressing the problem of the paucity of empirical data on the risks and benefits of current drugs and new drugs in the elderly, particularly for seniors who are 75 years of age or older and among those with multiple health problems and medications. Evaluation of the effects of new drugs in the elderly could be an added requirement for a drug to be included in the formulary list.

We recommend that a process be instituted for consultation with provincial therapeutic committees, provincial health ministries, the federal Health Protection Branch of Health Canada, and industry to help determine the optimal conditions for the institution of a drug-testing policy in elderly populations.

Medical Education

Improvements in doctor-patient communication may reduce unnecessary prescribing and improve patient compliance. Improvements in physician prescribing will reduce drug-related morbidity and cost. Medical school and postgraduate education play a considerable role in shaping a physician's prescribing patterns, and scores on licensure/certification examinations provide some prediction of a physician's prescribing behaviour.

We recommend that the Association of Canadian Medical Colleges, the Federation of Medical Licensing Authorities of Canada, the Medical Council of Canada, the Canadian College of Family Physicians, and the Royal College of Physicians and Surgeons be encouraged to implement and evaluate a specific plan of action to improve physician prescribing and patient communication skills in undergraduate, postgraduate, and continuing medical education programs. Competence in drug management and patient communication should be evaluated formally on licensure and certification examinations.

We have tried to demonstrate that there is no single or simple solution to the question of appropriate drug utilization in the elderly. The problem has both macro- and microsocial determinants, and these determinants must be seen in an ecological perspective. Failure to do so, as shown by evidence of unforeseen consequences of unilateral decisions and strategies, can lead to distortions of the very goals pursued. The above recommendations touch upon many of the determinants of the problem identified in the literature and are presented as groundwork for a large-spectrum approach to the issue. No single administrative, structural, or behavioural approach will suffice, and a number of traditional practices and relationships will need to be revised if we are to attain any measure of success. The present conditions of fluidity in the health care system and the emerging recognition that the health of the population is an intersectoral concern should furnish the necessary impetus for action.

Dr. Robyn Tamblyn *is an epidemiologist who holds an appointment as a medical scientist in the clinical epidemiology division of the Royal Victoria Hospital and a position as an associate professor in the Department of Medicine and the Department of Epidemiology and Biostatistics at McGill University. She obtained her Ph.D. in epidemiology and biostatistics at McGill in 1989. She has been funded as a Quebec research scholar by the FRSQ, and more recently as a National Research scholar by the NHRDP. She currently leads the Quebec Research Group on Medication Use in the Elderly (USAGE), and a provincial team that is carrying out a research program on the relationships between medical education, medical practice and patient outcome.*

BIBLIOGRAPHY

ALEXANDER, N., J. S. GOODWIN, and C. CURRIE. 1985. Comparison of admission and discharge medications in two geriatric populations. *Journal of the American Geriatrics Society* 33: 827–832.

AMARASANGHAM, L. R. 1980. Social and cultural perspectives on medication refusal. *American Journal of Psychiatry* 137: 353–358.

ANDERSON, G. M., K. J. KERLUKE, I. R. PULCINS, C. HERTZMAN, and M. L. BARER. 1993. Trends and determinants of prescription drug expenditures in the elderly: Data from the British Columbia Pharmacare program. *Inquiry* 30: 199–207.

ANGUS REID GROUP INC. 1991. *Medication Use in Canadians Aged 55 and Older: Opinions and Attitudes.* A Report to the Canadian Coalition on Medication Use and the Elderly, November.

AOKI, F. Y., G. W. LARGE, V. K. HILDAHL, P. A. MITENKO, and D. S. SITAR. 1983. Aging and heavy drug use: A prescription survey in Manitoba. *Journal of Chronic Diseases* 36: 75–84.

ASCIONE, F. J., and L. A. SHIMP. 1984. The effectiveness of four education strategies in the elderly. *Geriatrics and Gerontology* 18: 926–931.

ASHTON, H. 1991. Psychotropic drug prescribing for women. *British Journal of Psychiatry* 158(Suppl. 10): 30–35.

AVORN, J., and S. B. SOUMERAI. 1983. Improving drug therapy decisions through educational outreach: A randomized controlled trial of academically based "detailing." *New England Journal of Medicine* 308: 1457–1463.

AVORN, J., S. B. SOUMERAI, D. E. EVERITT, et al. 1992. A randomized trial of a program to reduce the use of psychoactive drugs in nursing homes. *New England Journal of Medicine* 327(3): 168–173.

AVORN, J., S. B. SOUMERAI, W. TAYLOR, M. R. WESSELS, J. JANOUSEK, and M. WEINER. 1988. Reduction of incorrect antibiotic dosing through a structured educational order form. *Archives of Internal Medicine* 148: 1720–1724.

BARNETT, G. O., R. N. WINICKOFF, M. M. MORGAN, and R. D. ZIELSTORFF. 1983. A computer-based monitoring system for follow-up of elevated blood pressure. *Medical Care* 21(4): 400–409.

BARNETT, G. O., R. WINICKOFF, J. L. DORSEY, M. M. MORGAN, and R. S. LURIE. 1978. Quality assurance through automated monitoring and concurrent feedback using a computer-based medical information system. *Medical Care* 16: 962–970.

BATES, D. W., L. L. LEAPE, and S. PETRYCKI. 1993. Incidence and preventability of adverse drug events in hospitalized adults. *Journal of General Internal Medicine* 8: 289–294.

BAXENDALE, C., M. GOURLAY, and I. I. J. M. GIBSON. 1978. A self-medication retraining programme. *British Medical Journal* 2: 1278–1279.

BEARDSLEY, R. S., D. B. LARSON, B. J. BURNS, J. W. THOMPSON, and D. B. KAMEROW. 1989. Prescribing of psychotropics in elderly nursing home patients. *Journal of the American Geriatrics Society* 37: 327–330.

BECKER, M. H. 1974. *The Health Belief Model and Personal Health Behaviour.* Thorofare (NJ): Charles B. Slack Inc.

———. 1976. *Sociobehavioural Determinants of Compliance.* Baltimore (MD): Johns Hopkins University Press.

BECKER, M. H., and L. W. GREEN. 1975. A family approach to compliance with medical treatment: A selective review of the literature. *International Journal of Health Education* 18: 173.

BECKER, M. H., R. H. DRACHMAN, and J. P. KIRSCHT. 1972. Predicting mother's compliance with pediatric medical regimes. *Journal of Pediatrics* 81(4): 843–854.

BEERS, M. H., J. G. OUSLANDER, S. F. FINGOLD, et al. 1992. Inappropriate medication prescribing in skilled-nursing facilities. *Annals of Internal Medicine* 117: 684–689.

BEERS, M. H., M. STORRIE, and G. LEE. 1990. Potential adverse drug interactions in the emergency room: An issue in the quality of care. *Annals of Internal Medicine* 112: 61–64.

BEERS, M. H., J. DANG, J. HASEGAWA, and I. Y. TAMAI. 1989. Influence of hospitalization on drug therapy in the elderly. *Journal of the American Geriatrics Society* 37: 679–683.

BEERS, M. H., S. F. FINGOLD, J. G. OUSLANDER, D. B. REUBEN, H. MORGENSTERN, and J. BECK. 1993. Characteristics and quality of prescribing by doctors practising in nursing homes. *Journal of the American Geriatrics Society* 41: 802–807.

BELAND, F. 1989. Patterns of health and social services utilization. *Canadian Journal on Aging* 8: 19–33.

BELLAMY, N., P. M. BROOKS, B. T. EMMERSON, J. R. GILBERT, J. CAMPELL, and M. MCCREDIE. 1989. A survey of current prescribing practices of anti-inflammatory and urate-lowering drugs in gouty arthritis in New South Wales and Queensland. *Medical Journal of Australia* 151: 531–537.

BERG, J. S., J. DISCHILER, D. J. WAGNER, J. J. RAIA, and N. PALERM-SHEVLIN. 1993. Medication compliance: A healthcare problem. *Annals of Pharmacotherapy* 27(9): 3–19.

BERGMAN, U., and B. E. WIHOLM. 1981. Drug-related problems causing admission to a medical clinic. *European Journal of Clinical Pharmacology* 20: 193–200.

BERNSTEIN, B., and R. KANE. 1981. Physicians' attitudes toward female patients. *Medical Care* 21(6): 600–608.

BERO, L. A., H. L. LIPTON, and J. A. BIRD. 1991. Characterization of geriatric drug-related hospital readmissions. *Medical Care* 29(10): 989–1003.

BINGLE, G. J., T. P. O'CONNOR, W. O. EVANS, and S. DETAMORE. 1991. The effect of "detailing" on physicians' prescribing behavior for postsurgical narcotic analgesia. *Pain* 45: 171–173.

BJORNSON, D. C., T. S. RECTOR, C. E. DANIELS, A. I. WERTHEIMER, D. A. SNOWDON, and T. J. LITMAN. 1990. Impact of a drug use review program intervention on prescribing after publication of a randomized clinical trial. *American Journal of Hospital Pharmacy* 47: 1541–1546.

BLISS, M. R. 1981. Prescribing for the elderly. *British Medical Journal* 283: 203–206.

BLOOM, J. A., J. W. FRANK, M. S. SHAFIR, and P. MARTIQUET. 1993. Potentially undesirable prescribing and drug use among the elderly: Measurable and remediable. *Canadian Family Physician* 39: 2337–2345.

BOGLE, S. M., and C. M. HARRIS. 1994. Measuring prescribing: The shortcomings of the item. *British Medical Journal* 308: 637–640.

BOND, C. A., and R. MONSON. 1984. Sustained improvement in drug documentation, compliance, and disease control. *Archives of Internal Medicine* 144: 1159–1162.

BOTTIGER, L. E., and B. WESTERHOLM. 1973. Drug-induced blood dyscrasias in Sweden. *British Medical Journal* 3: 339–343.

BOUDIN, H. M. 1972. Contingency contracting as a therapeutic tool in deceleration of amphetamine use. *Behavioral Therapy* 3: 604–608.

BRADLEY, J. D., K. D. BRANDT, B. P. KATZ, L. A. KALASINSKI, and S. I. RYAN. 1991. Comparison of an anti-inflammatory dose of ibuprofen, an analgesic dose of ibuprofen, and acetaminophen in the treatment of patients with osteoarthritis of the knee. *New England Journal of Medicine* 325(2): 87–91.

BRADLOW, J., and A. COULTER. 1993. Effect of fundholding and indicative prescribing schemes on general practitioners' prescribing costs. *British Medical Journal* 307: 1186–1189.

British Pharmacopeia. 1910. Oxford (U.K.): Oxford University Press.

BRODY, D. S. 1980. Physician recognition of behavioral, psychological, and social aspects of medical care. *Archives of Internal Medicine* 140: 1286–1289.

BROOK, R. H., C. J. KAMBERG, A. MAYER-OAKES, M. H. BEERS, K. RAUBE, and A. STEINER. 1989. *Appropriateness of Acute Medical Care for the Elderly*. Santa Monica (CA): RAND Corporation.

BROSHY, E., D. MATHESON, and M. HANSEN. 1993. Want to curb healthcare costs? Manage the disease not each cost component. *Medical Marketing and Media* (September): 76–78, 80, 84, 92.

BUCKS, R. S., A. WILLIAMS, M. J. WHITFIELD, and D. A. ROUTH. 1990. Towards a typology of general practitioners' attitudes to general practice. *Social Science Medicine* 30(5): 537–547.

BUECHLER, J. R., and W. MALLOY. 1989. Drug therapy in the elderly: How to achieve optimum results. *Postgraduate Medicine* 85: 87–99.

BURGESS, M. M. 1989. Ethical and economic aspects of non-compliance and overtreatment. *Canadian Medical Association Journal* 141: 777–780.

CAFFERATA, G. L., and S. M. MEYERS. 1990. Pathways to psychotropic drugs: Understanding the basis of gender differences. *Medical Care* 28: 285–300.

CAFFERATA, G. L., J. KASPER, and A. BERNSTEIN. 1983. Family roles, structure, and stressors in relation to sex differences in obtaining psychotropic drugs. *Journal of Health and Social Behavior* 24 (June): 132–143.

CANADIAN MEDICAL ASSOCIATION. Working Group on Primary Care. 1994. *Strengthening the Foundation: The Role of the Physician in Primary Health Care in Canada.* Ottawa: Canadian Medical Association.

CARRUTHERS, G., T. GOLDBERG, H. SEGAL, and E. SELLERS. 1987. *Drug Utilization. A Comprehensive Literature Review.* Toronto: University of Toronto, Department of Health Administration.

CHAPMAN, S. 1994. Drug formularies—good or evil? A view using prescribing analyses and cost trends data. *Cardiology* 85(Suppl. 1): 46–53.

CHEUNG, A., and R. KAYNE. 1975. An application of clinical pharmacy services in extended care facilities. *California Pharmacy* 23: 22–43.

CHREN, M., and S. LANDEFELD. 1994. Physicians' behavior and their interactions with drug companies: A controlled study of physicians who requested additions to a hospital drug formulary. *Journal of the American Medical Association* 271: 684–689.

CHRYMKO, M. M., and W. CONRAD. 1982. Effect of removing clinical pharmacy input. *American Journal of Hospital Pharmacy* 39: 641.

CLARY, C., L. A. MANDOS, and E. SCHWEIZER. 1990. Results of a brief survey on the prescribing practices for monoamine oxidase inhibitor antidepressants. *Journal of Clinical Psychiatry* 51: 226–231.

COAMBS, R. B., P. JENSEN, M. HAO HER, et al. 1995. *Review of the Scientific Literature on the Prevalence, Consequences, and Health Costs of Non-compliance and Inappropriate Use of Prescription Medication in Canada.* Ottawa (ON): Pharmaceutical Manufacturers Association of Canada.

COE, R. M., C. G. PRENDERGAST, and G. PSATHAS. 1984. Strategies for obtaining compliance with medical regimens. *Journal of the American Geriatrics Society* 32: 589–594.

COL, N., J. E. FANALE, and P. KRONHOLM. 1990. The role of medication non-compliance and adverse drug reactions in hospitalizations of the elderly. *Archives of Internal Medicine* 150: 841–845.

COMSTOCK, G. W. 1994. Variability of tuberculosis trends in a time of resurgence. *Clinical Infectious Diseases* 19(6): 1015–1022.

COOPER, J. K., D. W. LOVE, and P. R. RAFFOUL. 1982. Intentional prescription nonadherence (noncompliance) by the elderly. *Journal of the American Geriatrics Society* 30(5): 329–333.

COOPER, J. W. 1985. Effect of initiation, termination, and reinitiation of consultant clinical pharmacist services in a geriatric long-term care facility. *Medical Care* 23(1): 84–89.

COOPER, J. W., and G. BAGWELL. 1978. Contribution of the consultant pharmacist to rational drug usage in the long-term care facility. *Journal of the American Geriatrics Society* 26 (11): 513–520.

COOPER, J. W., and G. E. FRANCISCO. 1981. Psychotropic usage in long-term care facility geriatric patients. *Hospital Formularies* (April): 407–419.

COPPERSTOCK, R. 1971. Sex differences in the use of mood-modifying drugs: An explanatory model. *Journal of Health and Social Behavior* 12: 238–244.

COWAN, P. F. 1987. Patient satisfaction with an office visit for the common cold. *Journal of Family Practitioners* 24(4): 412–413.

CRAMER, J., R. H. MATTSON, M. L. PREVEY, R. D. SCHEYER, and V. L. OUELLETTE. 1989. How often is medication taken as prescribed? A novel assessment technique. *Journal of the American Medical Association* 261: 3273–3277.

CUSSON, J., C. PEPLER, P. TOUSIGNANT, et al. 1990. *Drug Utilization Related Problems in Elderly Canadians.* Ottawa: Canadian Coalition on Medication Use and the Elderly.

DAPCICH-MIURA, E., and M. F. HOVELL. 1979. Contingency management of adherence to a complex medical regime in an elderly heart patient. *Behavioral Therapy* 10: 193–201.

DAVIDSON, W., W. MALLOY, and M. BÉDARD. 1994. Physician practice characteristics and prescribing behavior: Effects on morbidity and mortality among their elderly patients in New Brunswick. *New England Journal of Medicine* (under review).

DAVIDSON, W., W. MALLOY, G. SOMERS, and M. BÉDARD. 1994. Relationships between physician practice characteristics and prescribing behavior for the elderly in New Brunswick. *Canadian Medical Association Journal* 150: 917.

DeSANTIS, G., K. J. HARVEY, D. HOWARD, M. L. MASHFORD, and R. F. W. MOULDS. 1994. Improving the quality of antibiotic prescription patterns in general practice. *Medical Journal of Australia* 160: 502–505.

DeSMEDT, M. 1994. Drug formularies—good or evil? A view from the EEC. *Cardiology* 85(Suppl. 1): 41–45.

DICKINSON, J. C., G. A. WARSHAW, S. H. GEHLBACH, J. A. BOBULA, L. H. MUHLBAIER, and G. R. PARKERSON. 1981. Improving hypertension control: Impact of computer feedback and physician education. *Medical Care* 19(8): 843–854.

DUKE, T., A. KELLERMANN, R. ELLIS, and T. SELF. 1991. Asthma in the emergency department: Impact of a protocol on optimizing therapy. *American Journal of Emergency Medicine* 9:432–435.

DUMAS, J., and J. MATTE. 1992. Characteristics of pharmaceutical opinions written in a Québec community pharmacy. *Annals of Pharmacotherapy* 26: 835–839.

DWYER, M. S., R. A. LEVY, and K. B. MENANDER. 1986. Improving medication compliance through the use of modern dosage forms. *Journal of Pharmacology Technology* 2: 166–170.

EDWARDS, M., and J. PATHY. 1984. Drug counselling in the elderly and predicting compliance. *Practitioner* 228: 291–300.

EKEDAHL, A., J. LIDBECK, T. LITHMAN, D. NOREEN, and A. MELANDER. 1993. Benzodiazepine prescribing patterns in a high-prescribing Scandinavian community. *European Journal of Clinical Pharmacology* 444: 141–146.

EKLUND, L. H., and A. WESSLING. 1976. Evaluation of package enclosures for drug page. *Lakaridningen* 73: 2319–2320.

ELZARIAN, E. J., D. Y. SHIRACHI, and J. K. JONEST. 1980. Educational approaches promoting optimal laxative use in long-term care patients. *Journal of Chronic Diseases* 33: 613–626.

ERAKER, S. A., J. P. KIRSCHT, and M. H. BECKER. 1984. Understanding and improving patient compliance. *Annals of Internal Medicine* 100: 258–268.

ESPOSITO, L. 1995. The effects of medication education on adherence to medication regimens in an elderly population. *Journal of Advanced Nursing* 21: 935–943.

EVANS, C. E., R. B. HAYNES, N. J. BIRKETT, et al. 1986. Does a mailed continuing education program improve physician performance? Results of a randomized trial in antihypertensive care. *Journal of the American Medical Association* 255(4): 501–504.

FERGUSON, J. A. 1990. Patient age as a factor in drug prescribing practices. *Canadian Journal on Aging* 9: 278–295.

FERGUSON, R. I., and T. J. B. MALING. 1990. The Nelson general practice prescribing project. Part I: A pilot audit of the regional prescribing profile. *New Zealand Medical Journal* 103: 558–560.

FERRY, M. E., P. P. LAMY, and L. A. BECKER. 1985. Physicians' knowledge of prescribing for the elderly. *Journal of the American Geriatrics Society* 33: 616–625.

FINCHAM, J. E. 1988. Patient compliance in the ambulatory elderly: A review of the literature. *Journal of Geriatric Drug Therapy* 2: 31.

FIORIO, R., C. BELLANTUONO, E. ARREGHINI, M. LEONCINI, and R. MICCIOLO. 1989. Psychotropic drug prescription in general practice in Italy: A two-week prevalence study. *International Clinical Psychopharmacology* 4: 7–17.

FOO LIN, I., R. SPIDA, and W. FORTSCH. 1979. Insight and adherence to medication in chronic schizophrenics. *Journal of Clinical Psychiatry* 40: 430.

FRANCIS, V., B. M. DORSCH, and M. J. MORRIS. 1969. Gaps in doctor-patient communication: Patients' response to medical advice. *New England Journal of Medicine* 280: 535.

FREER, C. B. 1985. Study of medicine prescribing for elderly patients. *British Medical Journal* 290: 1113–1116.

FUDGE, K. A., K. A. MOORE, D. N. SCHNEIDER, T. P. SHERRIN, and G. S. WELLMAN. 1993. Change in prescribing patterns of intravenous histamine$_2$-receptor antagonists results in significant cost savings without adversely affecting patient care. *Annals of Pharmacotherapy* 27: 232–237.

GARRARD, J., L. MAKRIS, T. DUNHAM, et al. 1991. Evaluation of neuroleptic drug use by nursing home elderly under proposed medicare and medicaid regulations. *Journal of the American Medical Association* 265(4): 463–467.

GEHLBACH, S. H., W. E. WILKINSON, W. E. HAMMOND, et al. 1984. Improving drug prescribing in a primary care practice. *Medical Care* 22(3): 193–201.

GORDON, M. 1987. Principles in prescribing for the older patient. *Drug Protocol* 2:15–24.

GOUVERNEMENT DU QUÉBEC. 1990. *Statistiques annuelles 1990.* Québec (QC): Régie de l'assurance-maladie du Québec.

_____. 1991. *Statistiques annuelles 1991.* Québec (QC): Régie de l'assurance-maladie du Québec.

_____. 1992. *Statistiques annuelles 1992.* Québec (QC): Régie de l'assurance-maladie du Québec.

GRADY, D., S. M. RUBIN, D. B. PETITTI, et al. 1992. Hormone therapy to prevent disease and prolong life in postmenopausal women. *Annals of Internal Medicine* 117 (12): 1016–1036.

GRAF, J. M., and O. S. SCHULENBURG. 1993. *Implications of the Structural Reform of Healthcare Act (Gesundheitsstrukturgesetz) on the Referral and Hospital Admission Practice of Primary Care Physicians. An Economic Evaluation from the Viewpoint of Third-Party Insurers and the Economy.* Discussion paper no. 34. University of Hanover Institute of Insurance Science, November.

_____. 1994. The German health care system at the crossroads. *Health Economics* 3: 301–303.

GRANTHAM, P. 1987. Benzodiazepine abuse. *British Journal of Hospital Medicine* 37(4): 292–300.

GRASELA, T. H. Jr., and J. A. GREEN. 1990. A nationwide survey of prescribing patterns for thrombolytic drugs in acute myocardial infarction. *Pharmacotherapy* 10: 35–41.

GRAVELEY, E. A., and C. S. OSEASOHN. 1991. Multiple drug regimens: Medication compliance among veterans 65 years and older. *Research in Nursing and Health* 14: 51–58.

GREENE, J. M., and R. N. WINICKOFF. 1992. Cost-conscious prescribing of NSAIDs. *Archives of Internal Medicine* 152: 1995–2002.

GRIFFIN, M. R., J. M. PIPER, J. R. DAUGHERTY, M. SNOWDEN, and W. A. RAY. 1991. Non-steroidal anti-inflammatory drug use and increased risk for peptic ulcer disease in elderly persons. *Annals of Internal Medicine* 114(4): 257–263.

GRYMONPRE, R. E., P. A. MITENKO, D. S. SITAR, F. Y. AOKI, and P. R. MONTGOMERY. 1988. Drug-associated hospital admissions in older medical patients. *Journal of the American Geriatrics Society* 36: 1092–1098.

GURWICH, E.L. 1983. Comparison of medication histories acquired by pharmacists and physicians. *American Journal of Hospital Pharmacy* 40: 1541–1542.

GURWITZ, J., N. F. COL, and J. AVORN. 1992. The exclusion of the elderly and women from clinical trials in acute myocardial infarction. *Journal of the American Medical Association* 268 (11): 1417–1422.

GURWITZ, J. H. 1993. Effects of pharmacists' consultations on drug prescribing. *ACP Journal Club* (January/February): 29.

_____. 1994. Suboptimal medication use in the elderly: The tip of the iceberg. *Journal of the American Medical Association* 272: 316–317.

GURWITZ, J. H., and J. AVORN. 1991. The ambiguous relation between aging and adverse drug reactions. *Annals of Internal Medicine* 114: 956–966.

GURWITZ, J. H., S. B. SOUMERAI, and J. AVORN. 1990. Improving medication prescribing and utilization in the nursing home. *Journal of the American Geriatrics Society* 38(5): 542–552.

HADSALL, R. S., R. A. FREEMAN, and G. J. NORWOOD. 1982. Factors related to the prescribing of selected psychotropic drugs by primary care physicians. *Social Science and Medicine* 16: 1747–1756.

HALLAS, J., L. F. GRAM, E. GRODUM, et al. 1992. Drug-related admissions to medical wards: A population-based survey. *British Journal of Clinical Pharmacology* 33: 61–68.

HAMMARLUND, E. R., J. R. OSTROM, and A. J. KETHLEY. 1985. The effects of drug counseling and other educational strategies on drug utilization of the elderly. *Medical Care* 23(2): 165–170.

HANSTEN, P., and J. HORN. 1989. *Drug Interactions*, 6th ed. Philadelphia (PA): Lea & Febiger.

HARPER, C. M., P. A. NEWTON, and J. R. WALSH. 1989. Drug-induced illness in the elderly. *Postgraduate Medicine* 86: 245–256.

HARTZEMA, A. G., and D .B. CHRISTENSEN. 1983. Nonmedical factors associated with the prescribing volume among family practitioners in an HMO. *Medical Care* 21: 990–1000.

HASKITT, R. L. 1989. Patient compliance: Tapping into a billion-dollar drug market. *Pharmaceutical Executive* 9(7): 46, 48, 52.

HAWKEY, C. J., S. HODGSON, A. NORMAN, T. K. DANESHMEND, and S. T. GARNER. 1990. Effect of reactive pharmacy intervention on quality of hospital prescribing. *British Medical Journal* 300: 986–990.

HAYNES, R.B. 1976. *A Critical Review of the "Determinants" of Patients' Compliance with Therapeutic Regimes.* Baltimore: Johns Hopkins University Press.

HAYNES, R. B., D. DAVIS, A. MCKIBBON, and P. TUGWELL. 1984. A critical appraisal of the efficacy of continuing medical education. *Journal of the American Medical Association* 251:61–64.

HEALTH AND WELFARE CANADA. 1985. *National Health Expenditures in Canada–1985.*

_____. 1981. *Canada Health Survey.* Report No. 82–538E.

_____. 1993. *National Pharmaceutical Strategy Discussion Document.* Ottawa, (ON): Health and Welfare Canada, Health Protection Branch, Drugs Directorate, National Pharmaceutical Strategy Office.

HELMAN, C. 1984. *Culture, Health and Illness.* Bristol (U.K.): Wright-PSG.

HEMENWAY, D., and D. FALLON. 1985. Testing for physician-induced demand with hypothetical cases. *Medical Care* 23(4): 344–349.

HERSHEY, C. O., D. K. PORTER, D. BRESLAU, and D. I. COHEN. 1986. Influence of simple computerized feedback on prescription charges in an ambulatory clinic. *Medical Care* 24(6): 472–481.

HINE, L. K., T. P. GROSS, and D. L. KENNEDY. 1989. Outpatient antiarrhythmic drug use. *Archives of Internal Medicine* 149: 1524–1527.

HOGAN, D. B., and E. M. EBLY. 1995. Regional variations in use of potentially inappropriate medications by Canadian seniors participating in the Canadian Study of Health and Aging. *Canadian Journal of Clinical Pharmacology* 2(4): 167–174.

HOGAN, D. B., N. R. C. CAMPBELL, R. CRUTCHER, P. JENNETT, and N. MACLEOD. 1994. Prescription of nonsteroidal anti-inflammatory drugs for elderly people in Alberta. *Canadian Medical Association Journal* 151(3): 315–322.

HOHMANN, A.A. 1989. Gender bias in psychotropic drug prescribing in primary care. *Medical Care* 27:478–490.

HOLMES, J. K. 1992. Patterns of prescribing in Irish general practitioners. *British Medical Journal* 85(4): 154–156.

HOLMES-ROVNER, M., J. KROLL, M. L. ROTHERT, et al. 1996. Patients satisfaction with health care decision. *Medical Decision Making* 16(1): 58–64.

HOLT, W. S., and S. A. MAZZUCA. 1992. Prescribing behaviors of family physicians in the treatment of osteoarthritis. *Family Medicine* 24(7): 524–527.

HOOD, J. C., M. LEMBERGER, and R. B. STEWART. 1975. Promoting appropriate therapy in a long-term care facility. *Journal of the American Pharmaceutical Association* 15(1): 32–37.

HULKA, B. S., J. C. CASSEL, and L. KUPPER. 1976. Disparities between medications prescribed and consumed among chronic disease patients. In *Patient Compliance*, ed. L. LASAGNA. Mt. Kisco: Futura Publishing Co.

HURWITZ, N. 1969. Predisposing factors in adverse reactions to drugs. *British Medical Journal* 1: 536–539.

HUTCHINSON, T. A., K. M. FLEGAL, M. S. KRAMER, D. G. LEDUC, and H. Ho PING KONG. 1986. Frequency, severity and risk factors for adverse drug reactions in adult outpatients: A prospective study. *Journal of Chronic Diseases* 39: 533–542.

INMAN, W., and G. PEARCE. 1993. Prescriber profile and post-marketing surveillance. *Lancet* 342: 658–661.

INMAN, W. H. W., and A. M. ADELSTEIN. 1969. Rise and fall of asthma mortality in England and Wales in relation to use of pressurised aerosols. *Lancet* 2(615): 279–285.

INUI, T. S., E. L. YOURTEE, and J. W. WILLIAMSON. 1976. Improved outcomes in hypertension after physician tutorials: A controlled trial. *Annals of Internal Medicine* 84: 646–651.

INUI, T. S., W. B. CARTER, R. E. PECORARO, R. A. PEARLMAN, and J. J. DOHAN. 1980. Variations in patient compliance with common long-term drugs. *Medical Care* 18: 986–993.

IRVINE-MEEK, J., W. DAVIDSON, G. SOMERS, and D. OLMSTEAD. 1990. *Benzodiazepine Use in the Senior Citizen and Income Assistance Populations in New Brunswick: Preliminary Report.* Fredericton: New Brunswick Department of Health.

ISAAC, L. M., R. M. TAMBLYN, and THE MCGILL CALGARY DRUG RESEARCH TEAM. 1993. Compliance and cognitive function: A methodological approach to measuring unintentional errors in medication compliance in the elderly. *Gerontologist* 33(6): 772–781.

ISACSON, D., and B. HAGLUND. 1988. Psychotropic drug use in a Swedish community–The importance of demographic and socioeconomic factors. *Social Science and Medicine* 26(4): 477–483.

IVES, T. J., E. J. BENTZ, and R. E. GWYTHER. 1987. Drug-related admissions to a family medicine inpatient service. *Archives of Internal Medicine* 147: 1117–1120.

JACKSON, J. E., J. W. RAMSDELL, M. RENVALL, et al. 1984. Reliability of drug histories in a specialized geriatric outpatient clinic. *Journal of General Internal Medicine* 4: 39–43.

JACOBS, J., A. G. GOLDSTEIN, and M. E. KELLY. 1988. NSAID dosing schedule and compliance. *Drug Intelligence and Clinical Pharmacy* 22: 727.

JOHNSON, J. A. 1994. Pharmacoeconomic analysis in formulary decisions: An international perspective. *American Journal of Hospital Pharmacy* 51(20): 2593–2598.

KARCH, F. E., and L. LASAGNA. 1975. Adverse drug reactions: A critical review. *Journal of the American Medical Association* 234: 1236–1241.

KATZ, P. R., T. R. BEAM, JR., F. BRAND, and K. BOYCE. 1990. Antibiotic use in the nursing home: Physician practice patterns. *Archives of Internal Medicine* 150: 1465–1468.

KAUFMAN, A., P. W. BRICKNER, R. VARNER, and W. MASHBURN. 1972. Tranquilizer control. *Journal of the American Medical Association* 221:1504–1506.

KAWAHARA, N. E., and F. M. JORDAN. 1989. Influencing prescribing behavior by adapting computerized order-entry pathways. *American Journal of Hospital Pharmacy* 46: 1798–1801.

KENDRICK, R., and J. R. D. BAYNE. 1982. Compliance with prescibed medication by elderly patients. *Canadian Medical Association Journal* 127: 961–962.

KLAPPER, J.A. 1995. Toward a standard drug formulary for the treatment of headache. *Headache* 35(4): 225–227.

KLEIN, L. E., P. S. GERMAN, and D. M. LEVINE. 1981. Adverse drug reactions among the elderly: A reassessment. *Journal of the American Geriatrics Society* 29: 525–530.

KOEPSELL, T. D., A. L. GURTEL, P. H. DIEHR, et al. 1983. The Seattle evaluation of computerized drug profiles: Effects on prescribing practices and resource use. *American Journal of Public Health* 73(8): 850–854.

KROENKE, K., and E. M. PINHOLT. 1990. Reducing polypharmacy in the elderly: A controlled trial of physician feedback. *Journal of the American Geriatrics Society* 38: 31–36.

KRSTENANSKY, P. M. 1993. Ketorolac injection use in a university hospital. *American Journal of Hospital Pharmacy* 50: 99–102.

KURFEES, J. F., and R. L. DOTSON. 1987. Drug interactions in the elderly. *Journal of Family Practitioners* 25: 477–488.

LACHMAN, B. G. 1987. Increasing patient compliance through tracking systems. *California Pharmacist* 35: 54.

LANE, M. F., R. V. BARBARITE, L. BERGNER, and D. HARRIS. 1971. Child-resistant medicine containers: Experience in the home. *American Journal of Public Health* 61: 1861–1868.

LAROCHELLE, P., M. J. BASS, N. J. BIRKETT, J. DE CHAMPLAIN, and M. G. MYERS. 1986. Recommendations from the Consensus Conference on Hypertension in the Elderly. *Canadian Medical Association Journal* 135: 741–745.

LEIBOWITZ, A., W. G. MANNING, and J. P. NEWHOUSE. 1985. The demand for prescription drugs as a function of cost-sharing. *Social Science and Medicine* 21: 1063–1069.

LEIRER, V. O., D. G. MORROW, E. D. TANKE, and G. M. PARIANTE. 1991. Elders' non-adherence: Its assessment and medication reminding by voice mail. *Gerontologist* 31(4): 514–520.

LESAR, T. S., L. L. BRICESTAND, K. DELCOURE, J. C. PARMALEE, V. MASTA-GARNIC, and H. POHL. 1990. Medication prescribing errors in a teaching hospital. *Journal of the American Medical Association* 263(17): 2328–2334.

LEWIS, C. E., and M. MICHNICH. 1977. Contracts as a means of improving patient compliance. In *Medication Compliance: A behavioural Management Approach*, ed. I. BAROFSKY. Thorofare: Charles B. Slack Inc.

LEXCHIN, J. 1992. Prescribing and drug costs in the Province of Ontario. 1992. *International Journal of Health Services* 22(3): 471–487.

————. 1993. Interactions between physicians and the pharmaceutical industry: What does the literature say? *Canadian Medical Association Journal* 149(10): 1401–1407.

LEY, P. 1982. Satisfaction, compliance and communication. *British Journal of Clinical Psychology* 21: 241–254.

LIANG, M. H., and P. FORTIN. 1991. Management of osteoarthritis of the hip and knee. *New England Journal of Medicine* 325(2): 125–127.

LINN, L. S. 1971. Physician characteristics and attitudes toward legitimate use of psycho-therapeutic drugs. *Journal of Health and Social Behavior* 12: 132–140.

LIPTON, H. L., and J. A. BIRD. 1993. Drug utilization review in ambulatory settings: State of the science and directions for outcomes research. *Medical Care* 12: 1069–1082.

LOCKER, D. 1981. *Symptoms and Illness: The Cognitive Organization of Disorder.* London (U.K.): Tavistock.

LOWE, C. J., D. K. RAYNOR, E. A. COURTNEY, J. PURIVS, and C. TEALE. 1995. Effects of self-medication programme on knowledge of drugs and compliance with treatment in elderly patients. *British Medical Journal* 310: 1229–1231.

Lowenthal, D. T. 1987. Drug therapy in the elderly: Special considerations. *Geriatrics* 42(11): 77.

LUMLEY, L. E., S. R. WALKER, C. G. HALL, et al. 1986. The underreporting of adverse drug reactions seen in general practice. *Pharmaceutical Medicine* 1: 205.

LUNDEN, D. W. 1978. Medication-taking behavior of the elderly: A pilot study. *Drug Intelligence and Clinical Pharmacy* 12: 518.

LURIE, N., E. C. RICH, and D. E. SIMPSON. 1990. Pharmaceutical representatives in academic medical centers: Interaction with faculty and housestaff. *Journal of General Internal Medicine* 5: 240–243.

MANNING, P. R., P. V. LEE, W. A. CLINTWORTH, T. A. DENSON, P. R. OPPENHEIMER, and N. J. GILMAN. 1986. Changing prescribing practices through individual continuing education. *Journal of the American Medical Association* 256: 230–232.

MANNING, W. G., A. LEIBOWITZ, G. A. GOLDBERG, W. H. ROGERS, and J. P. NEWHOUSE. 1984. A controlled trial of the effect of a prepaid group practice on use of service. *New England Journal of Medicine* 310: 1505–1510.

MAPES, R. 1980. *Prescribing Practice and Drug Usage.* London (U.K.): Croom Helm.

MARONDE, R. F., P. V. LEE, M. M. MCCARRON, and S. SEIBERT. 1971. A study of prescribing patterns. *Medical Care* 9: 383–395.

MARTIN, D. C., and K. MEAN. 1982. Reducing medication errors in a geriatric population. *Journal of the American Geriatrics Society* 30(4): 258–260.

MAXWELL, M., D. HEANEY, J. G. R. HOWIE, and S. NOBLE. 1993. General practice fundholding: Observations on prescribing patterns and costs using the defined daily dose method. *British Medical Journal* 307: 1190–1194.

MAY, F. E., R. B. STEWART, and L. E. CLUFF. 1977. Drug interactions and multiple drug administration. *Clinical Pharmacology and Therapeutics* 22: 322.

MAYO, N. 1993. Epidemiology and recovery of stroke. In *Long-Term Consequences of State-of-the-Art Reviews in Physical Medicine*, ed. R. W. TEASELL. Philadelphia: Hanley & Belfus. pp. 1–27.

MAZZUCA, S. A., K. D. BRANDT, S. L. ANDERSON, B. S. MUSICK, and B. P. KATZ. 1991. The therapeutic approaches of community based primary care practitioners to osteoarthritis of the hip in an elderly patient. *Journal of Rheumatology* 18(10): 1593–1600.

MAZZULLO, J. 1976. Methods of improving patient compliance. In *Patient Compliance*, ed. L. LASAGNA. Mt. Kisco: Futura.

MCAULEY, R., W. M. PAUL, G. H. MORRISON, R. F. BECKETT, and C. H. GOLDSMITH. 1990. Five year results of the peer assessment program of the College of Physicians and Surgeons of Ontario. *Canadian Medical Association Journal* 143 (11): 1193–1199.

MCCONNELL, T. S., A. H. CUSHING, A. D. BANKHURST, J. L. HEALY, A. MCILVENNA, and B. J. SKIPPER. 1982. Physician behavior modification using claims data: Tetracycline for upper respiratory infection. *Western Journal of Medicine* 137(5): 448–450.

MCGAVOCK, H., C. H. WEBB, G. D. JOHNSTON, and E. MILLIGAN. 1993. Market penetration of new drugs in one United Kingdom region: Implications for general practitioners and administrators. *British Medical Journal* 307: 1118–1120.

MCKENNEY, J. M., W. P. MUNROE, and J. T. WRIGHT. 1992. Impact of an electronic medication compliance aid on long-term blood pressure control. *Hypertension* 32: 277–283.

MCLANE, C. G., S. J. ZYZANSKI, and S. A. FLOCKE. 1995. Factors associated with medication non-compliance in rural elderly hypertensive patients. *American Journal of Hypertension* 8(2): 206–209.

MCPHEE, J. A., C. P. WILGOSH, P. D. ROY, D. M. MILLER, and M. G. KNOX. 1991. Effect of pharmacy-conducted education on prescribing of postoperative narcotics. *American Journal of Hospital Pharmacy* 48: 1484–1487.

Medical Letter. 1992a. Enoxacin–A new fluoroquinolone. *Medical Letter* 34(883): 103–105.

———. 1992b. Pravastatin, simvastatin, and lovastatin for lowering serum cholesterol concentrations. *Medical Letter* 34(872): 57–58.

———. 1992c. The new fluoroquinolones. *Medical Letter* 34(872): 58–60.

Medical Letter Handbook of Adverse Drug Interactions. 1993. New York: The Medical Letter Inc.

MELANDER, A., K. HENRICSON, P. STENBERG, et al. 1991. Anxiolytic-hypnotic drugs: Relationships between prescribing, abuse and suicide. *European Journal of Clinical Pharmacology* 41: 525–529.

MELVILLE, A. 1980. Job satisfaction in general practice: Implications for prescribing. *Social Science and Medicine* 14A: 495–499.

MEYER, T. J., D. VAN KOOTEN, S. MARSH, and A. V. PROCHAZKA. 1991. Reduction of polypharmacy by feedback to clinicians. *Journal of General Internal Medicine* 6: 133–136.

MILES, D. L. 1977. Multiple prescriptions and drug appropriateness. *Health Services Research* 12: 3–10.

MINISTÈRE DE LA SANTÉ ET DES SERVICES SOCIAUX. 1993. *L'utilisation des médicaments chez les personnes agées.* Québec (QC): Association Canadienne de l'Industrie du Médicament.

MOKKINK, H., A. SMITS, R. GROL, W. MEYBOOM, J. VAN SON, and UNIVERSITY OF NIJMEGEN. 1990. *Practice Performance and Quality of Care: Practice Styles of Family Physicians.* Ottawa (ON): Can-Heal Publications Inc.

MOLSTAD, S., B. HOVELIUS, L. KROON, and A. MELANDER. 1990. Prescription of antibiotics to outpatients in hospital clinics, community health centres and private practice. *European Journal of Clinical Pharmacology* 39: 9–12.

MONETTE, J., R. M. TAMBLYN, P. MCLEOD, et al. 1993. Profile of long-acting benzodiazepine drug prescribers. *Journal of Clinical Investigative Medicine* 16 (Suppl. 4): B59.

MONTAGUE, T., L. TAYLOR, S. MARTIN, et al. 1995. Can practice patterns and outcomes be successfully altered? Examples from cardiovascular medicine. *Canadian Journal of Cardiology* 11(6): 487–492.

MORABIA, A., J. FABRE, and J.-P. DUNAND. 1992. The influence of patient and physician gender on prescription of psychotropic drugs. *Journal of Clinical Epidemiology* 45(2): 111–116.

MORGAN, R., and A. K. GOPALASWAMY. 1984. Psychotropic drugs: Another survey of prescribing patterns. *British Journal of Psychiatry* 144: 298–302.

MORGAN, T. O., C. NOWSON, J. MURPHY, and R. SNOWDON. 1986. Compliance and the elderly hypertensive. *Drugs* 31(Suppl. 4): 174–183.

MORROW, D., V. LEIRER, and J. SHEIKH. 1988. Adherence and medication instructions: Review and recommendations. *Journal of the American Geriatrics Society* 36: 1147–1160.

MORTON-JONES, T., and M. PRINGLE. 1993a. Explaining variations in prescribing costs across England. *British Medical Journal* 306: 1731–34.

———. 1993b. Prescribing costs in dispensing practices. *British Medical Journal* 306: 1244–1246.

MUIJEN, M., and T. SILVERSTONE. 1987. A comparative hospital survey of psychotropic drug prescribing. *British Journal of Psychiatry* 150: 501–504.

MULROY, R. 1973. Iatrogenic disease in general practice: Its incidence and effects. *British Medical Journal* 2: 407–410.

MURDOCH, J. C. 1980. The epidemiology of prescribing in an urban general practice. *Journal of the Royal College of General Practitioners* 30: 593–602.

MURRAY, M. D., J. A. BIRT, A. K. MANATUNGA, and J. C. DARNELL. 1993. Medication compliance in elderly outpatients using twice-daily dosing and unit-of-use packaging. *Geriatrics and Gerontology* 27: 616–621.

NELSON, A. A., and M. R. QUICK. 1980. Co-payment for pharmaceutical services in a medicaid program. *Contemporary Pharmacy Practice* 3(1): 37–42.

NELSON, A. A., C. E. REEDER, and M. DICKSON. 1984. The effect of a medicaid drug co-payment program on the utilization and cost of prescription services. *Medical Care* 22(5): 724–736.

NELSON, C. R. 1993. Drug utilization in office practice. National Ambulatory Medical Care Survey, 1990. *Advance Data* 232: 1–12.

NEWHOUSE, J. P., W. G. MANNING, C. NORRIS, et al. 1981. Some interim results from a controlled trial of cost-sharing in health insurance. *New England Journal of Medicine* 305: 1501.

NICHTER, M., and N. VUCKOVIC. 1994. Agenda for an anthropology of pharmaceutical practice. *Social Science and Medicine* 39(11): 1509–1525.

NOLAN, L., and K. O'MALLEY. 1988a. Prescribing for the elderly. Part I: Sensitivity of the elderly to adverse drug reactions. *Journal of the American Geriatrics Society* 36: 142–49.

———. 1988b. Prescribing for the elderly. Part II: Prescribing patterns: Differences due to age. *Journal of the American Geriatrics Society* 36: 245–254.

PALMER, R. H., and M. C. REILLY. 1979. Individual and institutional variables which may serve as indicators of quality of medical care. *Medical Care* 17(7): 693–736.

PARKIN, D. M., C. R. HENNEY, J. QUIRK, and J. CROOKS. 1976. Deviation from prescribed drug treatment after discharge from hospital. *British Medical Journal* 2: 686–688.

PEAY, M. Y., and E. R. PEAY. 1990. Patterns of preference for information sources in the adoption of new drugs by specialists. *Social Science and Medicine* 31: 467–476.

PHARMACEUTICAL INQUIRY OF ONTARIO. 1990. *Prescriptions for Health.* Toronto: Pharmaceutical Inquiry of Ontario.

PHARMACEUTICAL MANUFACTURERS ASSOCIATION OF CANADA. 1994. *Provincial Drug Company Investment Profiles.*

PINEAULT, R. 1986. The effect of prepaid group practice on physicians' utilization behavior. *Medical Care* 14: 121.

PITTS, J., and S. VINCENT. 1989. What influences doctors' prescribing? Sore throats revisited. *Journal of the Royal College of General Practitioners* 39: 65–66.

PORTENOY, R. K., and R. M. KANNER. 1985. Patterns of analgesic prescription and consumption in a university-affiliated community hospital. *Archives of Internal Medicine* 145: 439–441.

PORTER, A. M. W. 1969. Drug defaulting in a general practice. *British Medical Journal* 1: 218–222.

POWER, B., W. DOWNEY, and B. R. SCHNELL. 1983. Utilization of psychotropic drugs in Saskatchewan: 1977–1980. *Canadian Journal of Psychiatry* 28: 547–551.

PRINGLE, M., and A. MORTON-JONES. 1994. Using unemployment rates to predict prescribing trends in England. *British Journal of General Practice* 44: 53–56.

PROOS, M., P. REILEY, J. EAGAN, S. STENGREVICS, J. CASTILE, and D. ARIAN. 1992. A study of the effects of self-medication on patients' knowledge of and compliance with their medication regimen. *Journal of Nursing Care Quality* (Special Report): 18–26.

PULLAR, T., B. MURPHY, A. TAGGART, and V. WRIGHT. 1990. Patterns of out-patients non-steroidal anti-inflammatory drug prescribing in two teaching hospital rheumatology units—Implications for post-marketing surveillance. *Journal of Clinical Pharmacy and Therapeutics* 15: 267–272.

QUINN, K., M. J. BAKER, and B. EVANS. 1992. A population-wide profile of prescription drug use in Saskatchewan. *Canadian Medical Association Journal* 146: 2177–2186.

RADECKI, S. E., R. L. KANE, D. H. SOLOMON, R. C. MENDENHALL, and J. C. BECK. 1988. Do physicians spend less time with older patients? *Journal of the American Geriatrics Society* 36: 713–718.

RAWSON, N. S. B., and C. D'ARCY. 1991. Sedative hypnotic drug use in Canada. *Health Reports* 3(1): 33–57.

RAY, M. A., M. R. GRIFFIN, and W. DOWNEY. 1989. Benzodiazepines of long and short elimination half-life and the risk of hip fracture. *Journal of the American Medical Association* 262: 3303–3307.

RAY, W. A., R. L. FOUGHT, and M. D. DECKER. 1992. Psychoactive drugs and the risk of injurious motor vehicle crashes in elderly drivers. *American Journal of Epidemiology* 136(7): 873–883.

RAY, W. A., W. SCHAFFNER, and C. F. FEDERSPIEL. 1985. Persistence of improvement in antibiotic prescribing in office practice. *Journal of the American Medical Association* 253(12): 1774–1776.

RAY, W. A., D. G. BLAZER, II, W. SCHAFFNER, C. F. FEDERSPIEL, and R. FINK. 1986. Reducing long-term diazepam prescribing in office practice: A controlled trial of educational visits. *Journal of the American Medical Association* 256: 2536–2539.

RAYNES, N. V. 1979. Factors affecting the prescribing of psychotropic drugs in general practice consultations. *Psychological Medicine* 9: 671–679.

RAYNOR, D. K., T. G. BOOTH, and A. BLENKINSOPP. 1993. Effects of computer-generated reminder charts on patients' compliance with drug regimens. *British Medical Journal* 306: 1158–1161.

REEDER, B. A., L. HORLICK, and O. E. LAXDAL. 1991. Physician management of hyperlipidemia in Saskatchewan: Temporal trends and the effect of a CME program. *Canadian Journal of Cardiology* 7(9): 385–390.

REEDER, C. E., and A. A. NELSON. 1985. The differential impact of co-payment on drug use in a medicaid population. *Inquiry* 22: 396–403.

RENAUD, M., J. BEAUCHEMIN, C. LALONDE, H. POIRIER, and S. BERTHIAUME. 1980. Practice settings and prescribing profiles: The simulation of tension headaches to general practitioners working in different practice settings in the Montréal area. *American Journal of Public Health* 70: 1068–1073.

REVIEW COMMITTEE. Study into the Growth in Use of Health Services. 1989. *Report to the Saskatchewan Minister of Health*. Regina.

RIGTER, H. 1994. Recent public policies in the Netherlands to control pharmaceutical pricing and reimbursement. *Pharmacoeconomics* 6 (Suppl. 1): 15–21.

ROBINSON, A. 1995. After years of steady growth, winds of restraint blowing on prescription drug industry. *Canadian Medical Association Journal* 153(1): 85–88.

ROCH, D. J., R. G. EVANS, and D. W. PASCOE. 1985. *Manitoba and Medicare: 1971 to the Present.* Winnipeg: Manitoba Health Services Commission.

ROSS-DEGNAN, D., S. B. SOUMERAI, E. E. FORTESS, and J. H. GURWITZ. 1993. Examining product risk in context: Market withdrawal of zomepirac as a case study. *Journal of the American Medical Association* 270(16): 1937–1942.

RYAN, M., B. YULE, C. BOND, and R. J. TAYLOR. 1990. Scottish general practitioners' attitudes and knowledge in respect of prescribing costs. *British Medical Journal* 300: 1318–1320.

SAFAVI, K. T., A. RODNEY, and M. D. HAYWARD. 1992. Choosing between apples and apples: Physicians' choices of prescription drugs that have similar side-effects and efficacies. *Journal of General Internal Medicine* 7: 32–37.

SALZMAN, C. 1985. Geriatric psychopharmacology. *Annual Review of Medicine* 36: 217–228.

SANZ, E. J., U. BERGMAN, and M. DAHLSTROM. 1989. Paediatric drug prescribing. A comparison of Tenerife (Canary Islands, Spain) and Sweden. *European Journal of Clinical Pharmacology* 37: 65–68.

SAUNDERS, C. E. 1987. Patient compliance in filling prescriptions after discharge from the emergency department. *American Journal of Emergency Medicine* 5(4): 283–286.

SCHAFFNER, W., W. A. RAY, C. F. FEDERSPIEL, and W. O. MILLER. 1983. Improving antibiotic prescribing in office practice: A controlled trial of three educational methods. *Journal of the American Medical Association* 250: 1728–1732.

SCHECTMAN, G., J. HIATT, and A. HARTZ. 1994. Telephone contacts do not improve adherence to niacin or bile acid sequestrant therapy. *Annals of Pharmacotherapy* 28: 29–34.

SCHNARCH, B., R. M. TAMBLYN, P. MCLEOD, et al. 1993. Psychotropic drug prescribing in the elderly: Exploration of the patient gender–physician gender relationship. *Canadian Pharmacoepidemiology Forum*, Toronto (abstract).

SCHRIER, R. W. (ed). 1993. *Renal and Electrolyte Disorders.* 4th ed. Little Brown & Co.

SCHWARTZ, M. A. 1976. The role of the pharmacist in the patient–health team relationship. In *Patient Compliance*, ed. L. LASAGNA. Mt. Kisco: Futura Publishing Co. pp. 83–95.

SCLAR, D. A., T. L. SKAER, A. CHIN, M. P. OKAMOTO, R. K. NAKAHIRO, and M. A. GILL. 1991. Effectiveness of the C Cap in promoting prescription refill compliance among patients with glaucoma. *Clinical Therapeutics* 13(3): 396–400.

SEIDL, L. G., G. F. THORNTON, J. W. SMITH, and L. E. CLUFF. 1966. Studies on the epidemiology of adverse drug reactions. III. Reactions in patients on a general medical service. *Bulletin of Johns Hopkins Hospital* 19: 299–315.

SHEIKH, J. I. 1992. Anxiety disorders and their treatment. *Clinics in Geriatric Medicine* 8: 411–23.

SHORR, R. I., S. F. BAUWENS, and C. S. LANDEFELD. 1990. Failure to limit quantities of benzodiazepine hypnotic drugs for outpatients: Placing the elderly at risk. *American Journal of Medicine* 89: 725–732.

SKEGG, D. C. G., R. DOLL, and J. PERRY. 1977. Use of medicines in general practice. *British Medical Journal* 1: 1561–1563.

SLEATOR, D. J. D. 1993. Towards accurate prescribing analysis in general practice: Accounting for the effects of practice demography. *British Journal of General Practice* 43: 102–106.

SLOAN, F. A., G. S. GORDON, and D. L. COCKS. 1993. Hospital drug formularies and use of hospital services. *Medical Care* 31(10): 851–867.

SMIDT, W. A., and E. G. MCQUEEN. 1972. Adverse reactions to drugs: A comprehensive inpatient survey. *New Zealand Medical Journal* 76: 397.

SMITH, P., and J. ANDREWS. 1983. Drug compliance not so bad, knowledge not so good: The elderly after hospital discharge. *Age and Ageing* 12: 336–342.

SOROCK, G. S., and E. E. SHIMKIN. 1988. Benzodiazepine sedatives and the risk of falling in a community-dwelling elderly cohort. *Archives of Internal Medicine* 148: 2441–2444.

SOUMERAI, S. B., and J. AVORN. 1986. Economic and policy analysis of university-based drug "detailing." *Medical Care* 24(4): 313–331.

———. 1987. Predictors of physician prescribing change in an educational experiment to improve medication use. *Medical Care* 25: 210–221.

SOUMERAI, S. B., and D. ROSS-DEGNAN. 1990. Experience of state pharmaceutical benefit programs in improving medication utilization. *Health Affairs* 9: 36–54.

SOUMERAI, S. B., T. J. MCLAUGHLIN, and J. AVORN. 1989. Improving drug prescribing in primary care: A critical analysis of the experimental literature. *Milbank Quarterly* 67: 268–317.

———. 1990. Quality assurance for drug prescribing. *Quality Assurance in Health Care* 2(1): 37–58.

SOUMERAI, S. B., T. J. MCLAUGHLIN, and D. ROSS-DEGNAN. 1994. Effects of limiting medicaid drug reimbursement benefits on the use of psychotropic agents and acute mental health services by patients with schizophrenia. *New England Journal of Medicine* 33(10): 650–655.

SOUMERAI, S. B., J. AVORN, S. GORTMAKER, and S. HAWLEY. 1987. Effect of government and commercial warnings on reducing prescription misuse: The case of propoxyphene. *American Journal of Public Health* 77: 1518–1523.

SOUMERAI, S. B., J. AVORN, D. ROSS-DEGNAN, and S. GORTMAKER. 1987. Payment restrictions for prescription drugs under medicaid: Effects on therapy, cost, and equity. *New England Journal of Medicine* 317: 550–556.

SOUMERAI, S. B., D. ROSS-DEGNAN, J. AVORN, T. J. MCLAUGHLIN, and I. CHOODNOVSKKIY. 1991. Effects of medicaid drug payment limits on admission to hospitals and nursing homes. *New England Journal of Medicine* 325: 1072–1077.

SOVA, G. 1989. *1989 Corpus Almanac and Canadian Sourcebook*. Vol. 1. Don Mills (ON): Corpus Information Services.

STEELE, M. A., D. T. BESS, V. L. FRANSE, and S. E. GRABER. 1989. Cost-effectiveness of two interventions for reducing outpatient prescribing costs. *DICP, The Annals of Pharmacotherapy* 23: 497–500.

STEWART, R. B., and G. J. CARANASOS. 1989. Medication compliance in the elderly. *Medical Clinics of North America* 73(6): 1551–1563.

STOLLEY, P. D., and L. LASAGNA. 1969. Prescribing patterns of physicians. *Journal of Chronic Diseases* 22: 395–405.

STRANDBERG, L. R., G. W. DAWSON, D. MATHLESON, J. RAWLINGS, and B. G. CLARK. 1980. Effect of comprehensive pharmaceutical services on drug use in long-term care facilities. *American Journal of Hospital Pharmacy* 37: 92–94.

STROSS, J. K., and G. G. BOLE. 1980. Evaluation of a continuing education program in rheumatoid arthritis. *Arthritis and Rheumatism* 23(7): 846–849.

SVARSTAD, B. L., and J. K. MOUNT. 1991. Nursing home resources and tranquilizer use among the institutionalized elderly. *Journal of the American Geriatrics Society* 39: 869–875.

TAMBLYN, R. M. 1996. *The Prediction of Practice Profile by Licensure Examination* (2-year grant). National Health Research and Development Program Project (NHRDP) Reference No. 6605–4101–57E.

———. 1996. Medication use in seniors: Challenges and solutions. *Thérapie* 51: 269–282.

TAMBLYN, R. M., and R. N. BATTISTA. 1993. Changing clinical practice: Which interventions work? *Journal of Continuing Education in the Health Professions* 13(4): 273–288.

TAMBLYN, R. M., M. ABRAHAMOWICZ, L. BERKSON, et al. 1993. *The Feasibility of Using Standardized Patients to Measure the Medical Management of High-Risk Prescribing Situations in the Elderly.* Final Report, NHRDP Project Reference No. 6605-3752-57P.

TAMBLYN, R. M., G. LAVOIE, M. ABRAHAMOWICZ, et al. 1994. *Variation in Specialty Referral Rates in a Universal Health Care System: Can It Be Predicted by Physician Characteristics?* Research in Medical Education. 33rd Annual Research in Medical Education Conference, Boston (MA).

TAMBLYN, R. M., P. MCLEOD, M. ABRAHAMOWICZ, et al. 1994. Questionable prescribing for elderly patients in Québec. *Canadian Medical Association Journal* 150(11): 1801–1809.

TAMBLYN, R. M., G. LAVOIE, L. PETRELLA, and J. MONETTE. 1995. The use of prescription claims databases in pharmacoepidemiological research: The accuracy and comprehensiveness of the prescription claims database in Québec. *Journal of Clinical Epidemiology* 48(8): 999–1009.

TAMBLYN, R. M., P. J. MCLEOD, M. ABRAHAMOWICZ, and R. LAPRISE. 1996. Do too many cooks spoil the broth? Multiple physician involvement in medical management and inappropriate prescribing in the elderly. *Canadian Medical Association Journal* 154(8): 1177–1184.

TAMBLYN, R. M., R. LAPRISE, B. Schnarch, J. Monette, P. McLeod. 1996. Caractéristiques des médecins prescrivant des psychotropes davantage aux femmes qu'aux hommes. *Santé mentale au Québec* 22:239-262.

TAMBLYN, R. M., M. ABRAHAMOWICZ, B. SCHNARCH, J. COLLIVER, S. BENAROYA, and L. SNELL. 1994. Can standardized patients predict real patient satisfaction with the doctor-patient relationship? *Teaching and Learning in Medicine* 6(1): 36–44.

TATRO, David S. 1995. *Drug Facts and Comparisons.* St. Louis: Facts and Comparisons Inc.

TIERNEY, W. M., S. L. HUI, and C. J. MCDONALD. 1986. Delayed feedback of physician performance versus immediate reminders to perform preventive care: Effects on physician compliance. *Medical Care* 24(8): 659–666.

TINETTI, M. E., M. SPEECHLEY, and S. F. GINTER. 1988. Risk factors for falls among elderly persons living in the community. *New England Journal of Medicine* 319: 1701–1707.

UNITED STATES PHARMACOPEIAL DRUG INFORMATION. 1996. *Drug Information for the Health Care Professional by Authority of the United States Pharmacopeial Convention, Inc.* Vol 1.

VAN DER WAALS, F. W., J. MOHRS, and M. FOETS. 1993. Sex differences among recipients of benzodiazepines in Dutch general practice. *British Medical Journal* 307: 363–366.

VAN NOSTRAND, J. F., S. E. FURNER, and R. SUZMAN. 1993. Health data on older Americans: United States, 1992. *Vital and Health Statistics* 3(27): 9–21.

VERBRUGGE, L. M. 1984. How physicians treat mentally distressed men and women. *Social Science and Medicine* 18: 1–9.

VERBRUGGE, L. M., J. LEPKOWSKI, and Y. IMANAKA. 1989. Comorbidity and its impact on disability. *Milbank Quarterly* 67(3–4): 451–484.

VERBRUGGE, L. M., and R. P. STEINER. 1981. Physician treatment of men and women patients: Sex bias or appropriate care? *Medical Care* 19: 609–632.

WADE, O. L., and H. HOOD. 1972. Prescribing of drugs reported to cause adverse reactions. *British Journal of Preventive and Social Medicine* 26: 205–211.

WALLEN, J., H. WAITZKIN, and J. D. STOECKLE. 1979. Physician stereotypes about female health and illness: A study of patient's sex and the informative process during medical interviews. *Women and Health* 4: 135–146.

WANDLESS, I., and J. W. DAVIE. 1977. Can drug compliance in the elderly be improved? *British Medical Journal* 1: 359–361.

WARE, G. J., and R. G. HARRIS. 1991. Unit dose calendar packaging and elderly patient compliance. *New Zealand Medical Journal* 104: 495–497.

WEBSTER, G. 1989. *American Board of Internal Medicine Final Report on the Patient Satisfaction Questionnaire Project.* Philadelphia (PA): American Board of Internal Medicine.

WEINGARTEN, M. A., and B. S. CANNON. 1988. Age as a major factor affecting adherence to medication for hypertension in a general practice population. *Family Practice* 5(4): 294–296.

WEISS, O. F., K. SRIWATANAKUL, J. L. ALLOZA, M. WEINTRAUB, and L. LASAGNA. 1983. Attitudes of patients, housestaff, and nurses toward postoperative analgesic care. *Anesthesia and Analgesia* (Cleveland) 62: 70–74.

WELLS, K. B., C. KAMBERG, R. BROOK, P. CAMP, and W. ROGERS. 1985. Health status, socio-demographic factors, and the use of prescribed psychotropic drugs. *Medical Care* 23: 1295–1306.

WENNBERG, J. E. 1985. On patient need, supplier-induced demand, and the need to assess the outcome of common medical problems. *Medical Care* 23(5): 512–520.

WESSLING, A., G. BOETHIUS, and F. SJOQVIST. 1990. Prescription monitoring of drug dosages in the County of Jamtland and Sweden as a whole in 1976, 1982, 1985. *European Journal of Clinical Pharmacology* 38: 329–334.

WESTERLING, R. 1988. Diagnoses associated with the prescription of psychotropic drugs at a Swedish health centre. *Scandinavian Journal of Primary Health Care* 6: 93–98.

WEYERER, S., and H. DILLING. 1991. Psychiatric and physical illness, sociodemographic characteristics, and the use of psychotropic drugs in the community: Results from the Upper Bavarian Study. *Journal of Clinical Epidemiology* 44: 303–311.

WILCHER, D. E., and J. W. COOPER. 1981. The consultant pharmacist and analgesic/anti-inflammatory drug usage in a geriatric long-term facility. *Journal of the American Geriatrics Society* 29(9): 429–432.

WILCOX, S. M., D. U. HIMMELSTEIN, and S. WOOLHANDLER. 1994. Inappropriate drug prescribing for the community-dwelling elderly. *Journal of the American Medical Association* 272: 292–296.

WILLIAMS, A. P., and R. COCKERILL. 1990. *Report of the 1989 Survey of the Prescribing Experiences and Attitudes Toward Prescription Drugs of Ontario Physicians.* Toronto (ON): Ontario Ministry of Health.

WILLIAMS, P., and D. R. RUSH. 1986. Geriatric polypharmacy. *Hospital Practice* 21: 109–120.

WILLIAMSON, D. H., J. W. COOPER, J. A. KOTZAN, and A. O. GELBART. 1984. Consultant pharmacist impact on antihypertensive therapy in a geriatric long-term care facility. *Hospital Formulary* 19: 123–128.

WONG, B. S. M., and D. C. Normal. 1987. Evaluation of a novel medication aid, the calendar blister-pack, and its effect on drug compliance in a geriatric outpatient clinic. *Journal of the American Geriatrics Society* 35: 21–26.

WOODHOUSE, K. W. 1994. Drug formularies—good or evil? The clinical perspective. *Cardiology* 85(Suppl. 1): 36–40.

WYSOWSKI, D. K., and C. BAUM. 1991. Outpatient use of prescription sedative-hypnotic drugs in the United States. *Archives of Internal Medicine* 151: 1779–1783.

WYSOWSKI, D. K., D. L. KENNEDY, and T. P. GROSS. 1990. Prescribed use of cholesterol-lowering drugs in the United States, 1978 through 1988. *Journal of the American Medical Association* 263: 2185–2188.

YOUNG, F. E. 1987. Questions about your medicine? Go ahead—ask. *FDA Consumer* 21: 2.

YOUNG, L. Y., B. D. LEACH, D. A. ANDERSON, and R. T. RICE. 1981. Decreased medication costs in a skilled nursing facility by clinical pharmacy services. *Contemporary Pharmacy Practice* 4(4): 233–237.

ZAMMIT-LUCIA, J., and R. DASGUPTA. 1995. *Reference Pricing, the European Experience.* Health Policy Review Paper No. 10, St. Mary's Hospital Medical School, London (U.K.).

ZIEVE, F. J., and E. CIESCO. 1993. *Computer-Focused Modification of Physician Prescribing Behavior.* Richmond: AMIA, Inc.

Preventing, Reducing and Stopping the Abuse and Neglect of Older Canadian Adults in Canadian Communities

DAPHNE NAHMIASH

Ph.D. Candidate, Laval University
Adjunct Professor, School of Social Work, McGill University
Adjunct Professor, McGill Centre for Studies in Aging

SUMMARY

This paper surveys American and Canadian literature on abuse and neglect of community-based older Canadian adults by a person in a position of trust. The studies are reviewed through a discussion on health and social indicators that have been observed in abused and neglected older adults, their abusers and the social and cultural context. While no incidence studies have been conducted yet, one empirically rigorous study estimates the prevalence of abuse and neglect of older adults to be 4 percent of the population over the age of 65 years. Although this is not a high percentage, it nevertheless represents a large number of individuals in the population who are subjected to unacceptable behaviour, according to Canadian values. As well, the percentage of abused and neglected older adults is probably underestimated, due to the sensitivity of reporting such facts over the telephone and overall reluctance to report such abuse.

This paper also underscores the fact that there is still little consensus among researchers and intervenors regarding definitions pertaining to elder abuse. This makes it impossible to compare data flowing from research. One simple definition of abuse proposed is "a misdemeanor against acknowledged standards by someone a senior has reason to trust" (Stones 1994). Research methodologies are also diverse, and are based on a variety of theoretical assumptions, caregiver stress theories and family violence theories being the most popular. Neither of these theories appears to be empirically based, since there is no evidence that caregiver abusers are more stressed than caregivers who are not abusers. Further, family violence theories have not been observed to fit all the different types of abuse. However, most practitioners use empowerment concepts which may merit further research.

Many possible indicators of abuse and neglect have been associated with older adults, their abusers and the social and cultural context. Each of these is presented in this paper. Unfortunately, at this time no single risk factor has been singled out as a determinant of abuse and neglect, and to date only two case-control studies have been conducted on the topic of risk factors. This points to the need for more targeted research in this area. Areas for future research include: dependence (though we still do not know who depends on whom, and dependence needs to be better defined); social isolation, depression and substance abuse of the caregiver; lack of family support; and gender. Difficulties in singling out risk indicators may be due to the interaction of other factors from the social and cultural context; these must be taken into account in the studies. Some of these factors may stem from the context in which care is given, such as inadequacy of resources to support family caregivers and care receivers.

Five case studies are presented in this paper. Selection criteria included: innovativeness; origins in both eastern and western parts of Canada; diversity of intervention strategies in the problem of abuse and neglect of older adults; being community-based and housed in different sites; and the presence of an evaluation process. Successful features of these case studies include collaborative links and partnerships with other programs, organizations and universities, and innovative funding strategies, sometimes including partners from federal, provincial, municipal and private agencies, as well as their own fundraising campaigns. As well, the projects studied are based mainly on existing rather than newly added resources.

The programs highlighted in the case studies include a variety of strategies, based on a multidisciplinary and sometimes an intersectoral approach that creates alliances among health and social service agencies, the criminal justice system, community organizations and others. Innovative approaches such as volunteer advocates, peer counselling strategies and support groups for abused older women are used, though individual counselling tends to be the strategy of choice for abused seniors and abused caregivers.

The projects evaluated place emphasis on the involvement of seniors in all aspects of the projects. However, the location of each project influences how senior involvement takes place and whether seniors, not just participants or volunteers, are involved in the design and planning of services. One program housed in a senior centre shows that seniors are more likely to become involved in this type of program rather than in programs that are professionally led.

The recommendations made in this paper focus on continued funding of more evidence-based research and program outcome evaluations. Future studies should focus on: determining the extent of abuse and neglect and the number of new cases; the definition of terms for use in future studies; and risk-controlled studies that will predict who is at risk for abuse and neglect, who is at risk of being an abuser, and in what circumstances and contexts abuse occurs.

The recommendations include:

- *That senior organizations play a leadership role in disseminating existing knowledge, program models and approaches, including to multicultural and Aboriginal communities;*
- *That validated tools and protocols be used;*
- *That provincial and municipal governments ensure that validated screening tools and measures such as the EAST (Stones 1995) are widely known and made accessible to the organizations within their jurisdiction. In addition, each area should have access to trained teams and resources to respond to the abuse and neglect of older Canadians; and*
- *That technical support and resources for rigorous program evaluation studies come from partnerships between community-based agencies, universities, researchers and policymakers. These evaluation studies would be based on outcome measures that can determine which interventions are successful and which are not.*

TABLE OF CONTENTS

TABLE

He who nurtures the teeth to grow will be nurtured when the teeth are falling out.

– African saying

INTRODUCTION

Child abuse came to the forefront of public awareness in the '60s, and spouse abuse became more visible in the '70s. The '80s and '90s have seen increasing attention to other forms of violence, such as dating and school violence, as well as the abuse and neglect of older adults. However, such abuse is not a new phenomenon. It represents a form of societal violence that has always existed, but which only recently has been a focus of public awareness. During the past few decades, the number of persons over the age of 65 has increased significantly, and therefore the presence of this type of abuse and neglect has become more visible.

Multiple studies were first produced in the United States, a few in Great Britain and, as awareness developed in Canada, the first extensive national empirical study by Podnieks et al. was produced in 1990. Other countries are just beginning to become aware of abuse and neglect of older adults as a social problem (Kosberg and Garcia 1995). This paper will focus on the studies from the U.S. and Canada, since they are both more numerous and more applicable to the Canadian context.

In this paper, elder abuse and neglect will be generally defined as *adverse acts of omission or commission against an older person.* Abuse and neglect can be perpetrated in the home or in an institution, by unpaid or paid caregivers, or on the street by a stranger. The paper will describe the current knowledge about abuse and neglect of older Canadian adults living in the community, in terms of the impact upon their health and social well-being. Specifically, the paper will refer to abuse and neglect perpetrated by unpaid, informal caregivers (mainly family members) who are in a position of trust to the care receiver. This emphasis on abuse and neglect by unpaid caregivers stems from the fact that it is both the most common form of abuse (Podnieks et al. 1990), and the most difficult to detect (Thériault 1994).

The extent and nature of the problem will be explored, and the literature will be reviewed for indicators related to the abused, the abusers and the social, cultural and economic environment in which abuse occurs. Issues of the formal and informal care context and older abused persons and their abusers will be described, highlighting specific issues related to gender, poverty and resources.

It will be argued that factors from the care environment and the health and social service system interact with personality or relationship indicators of abused and abuser to produce situations of abuse and neglect. It is therefore not enough merely to look at indicators relative to the individual abused or abuser, as has often been done in past studies. Five specific Canadian case studies of programs to prevent, reduce and eliminate abuse and neglect will be reviewed briefly to highlight their relevance for replicability in other parts of Canada. Specific research planning and program strategies for future directions in this area will be proposed, based on the literature and on the case studies.

It is to be hoped that this paper will provoke more discussion about the problem of abuse and neglect of older adults in Canada. In addition, program interventions to stimulate more research and produce a more responsive, caring social context for older adults and their caregivers should be initiated.

THE NATURE AND THE EXTENT OF THE PROBLEM

Prevalence of Abuse and Neglect

In Canada, it has been estimated that approximately one out of every 25 Canadians is a victim of abuse and neglect every year (Podnieks et al. 1990). As well, in the U.S., the Select Committee on Aging (1981) has estimated that one out of 35, or roughly one million older Americans may be victims of such abuse each year. Thus, according to these estimates, a serious problem exists for older North American adults. Therefore, we will analyze further what research studies say about the prevalence of this phenomenon.

The extent of the problem has been often described but accounts differ significantly according to the methodologies and definitions used. For example, a major problem in the literature is the difficulty in discerning true prevalence and incidence, as studies and research designs tend to confuse such projections (Kozack, Elmslie, and Verdon 1995). Prevalence studies are useful for planning health and social service interventions, whereas incidence studies are better suited to exploring causal models of abuse and neglect, and for evaluating the effectiveness of primary intervention programs (Kozack, Elmslie, and Verdon 1995). The same authors' analysis of prevalence and incidence rates in Canada found that no incidence study has been conducted to date. Their document highlights conclusions from reported Canadian studies.

The first report was the Quebec study of Bélanger et al. (1981). This study, based on a low return rate of 32 percent, reported physical abuse at 21 percent, psychological abuse at 55 percent, material abuse at 24 percent and rights violations at 25 percent among the aged clients of social service workers. Similar results were obtained by Shell (1982) who interviewed 105 professionals in Manitoban health care agencies. These studies were followed by Stevenson's Albertan study (1985), an Ontario study by the Ministry of Community and Social Services (1985), chart reviews by Grand

Maison (1988), hospital visits in Winnipeg by King (1984) and a case recall study by professionals (Lamont 1985).

Only the Podnieks national study (1989) was experimentally rigorous enough to estimate the prevalence of abuse and neglect among community-dwelling seniors in Canada. This study indicated the rate at 4 percent, with slight variations across the country. Material abuse (2.5 percent) which includes financial or property abuse, and chronic verbal aggression (1.4 percent) accounted for most of the self-reported cases.

The Project CARE study from Montreal (Reis and Nahmiash 1995a) found a higher rate of abuse frequency among health and social service care recipients (8–13 percent) than in the general population (3–5 percent). This increase is most likely due to the fact that this was a frailer population group of elderly persons, and that intensive sensitization campaigns were conducted in this community. From these studies, one can conclude that abuse and neglect of seniors exists throughout Canada with some regional variation. Still, more information needs to be gathered as to the extent of the problem and the number of new cases (Kozack, Elmslie, and Verdon 1995). The Podnieks et al. (1990) study results probably underestimate the number of neglected older adults. Many people may not wish to report over the telephone that they are being abused or neglected, partly because of possible repercussions from the abuser, and partly because of reluctance to report such highly personal, sensitive and taboo information. Project CARE estimates may confirm U.S. studies that higher rates may be found in a frailer study population. Studies also need to recognize cohort, language and cultural differences within groups, and assist cultural leaders in identifying abuse issues within cultural groups. Thirty-six different ethnocultural groups were identified in one Canadian study (Pittaway et al. 1995).

Definitions

Definitions and terminology of elder abuse are equally problematic. There is no accepted intrinsic or extrinsic definition or conceptualization of the phenomenon of abuse yet. Several authors have attempted this, including Hudson and Johnson (1986) from the U.S., and Stones (1991) from Canada. While no consensus has yet been reached, the most common forms of mistreatment have been generally defined (Podnieks et al. 1989; Pillemer and Finkelhor 1988; Pillemer and Wolf 1986; Kosberg 1988) as follows:
- *Physical abuse* includes sexual abuse and the infliction of physical pain, burns, rough handling, etc.;
- *Psychological or emotional abuse* includes verbal assault, threats, infantilization, humiliation and isolation or withholding of affection. Psychological abuse entails the violation of rights, and involves acts

that prevent elderly people from making their own decisions, such as forcing them to go into a nursing home;

- *Financial or material abuse* includes misuse of funds or property, exploitation and fraud;
- *Passive and active neglect* involves the withholding of items or care necessary for daily living and can be either intentional or unintentional.

Though not used in most studies, two additional forms of abuse should be drawn to the reader's attention:

- *Social or collective abuse* is any societal abuse which includes ageism and other forms of treating elderly persons at a societal level, in a manner that affects their personal dignity and identity (Gouvernement du Québec 1990). Ageism, as defined by Robert Butler (1969), reflects a deep-seated uneasiness on the part of the young and the middle-aged. It represents a personal revulsion to and distaste for aging, disease and disability, and a fear of powerlessness, uselessness and death. This definition points out that old age in this culture is equated with powerlessness as a result of disease, disability and uselessness;
- *Self-neglect* (Breckman and Adelman 1988) has also been defined as a form of abuse. It consists of an older person's failure to provide an adequate degree of care for himself. This form of abuse differs from the others in that no perpetrator is involved in the mistreatment, but sometimes relatives or others may be aware of it and fail to help. Since no perpetrator is involved in self-neglect, this form of abuse will not be further discussed in this paper.

Stones (1991) points out that the main reason elder mistreatment has been so difficult to define is that its meaning differs depending on who is doing the defining and for what purpose. The multiple meanings depend on the source of the definition and the context in which it is used. Stones (1991) also mentions that the types of mistreatment can be categorized according to legislative reference standards, or those based on vocational, organizational or normative ethics. Violations of normative community mistreatment standards are most difficult to define, as they differ according to the person's cultural background and are indicative of cultural attitudes toward abuse in general. Stones (1991) further notes the following other forms of classifying abuse:

- *Connotative definitions* emphasize the consequences of abuse for the recipient;
- *Definitions based on structural criteria* cite the multiple meanings of abuse;
- *Denotative definitions* elaborate on the behaviour of the instigator.

Stones (1995) concludes that connotative definitions have proved unsuccessful and that structural definitions convey the general meaning of abuse and neglect by acknowledging the diversity of the criteria against which abuse and neglect are evaluated. Stones (1994) offers the following simple structural definition of abuse: "A misdemeanor against acknowledged standards by someone a senior has reason to trust".

The most systematically developed Canadian framework for abuse and neglect consists of the denotative definitions in the EAST tool. This contains 71 items grouped into the following nine categories (Stones 1995): physical assault; excessive restraint; putting health at risk; failure to give care by someone acting as a paid or unpaid caretaker under pressure; humiliating behaviour; abuse in an institution; and material exploitation and verbal humiliation. Stones (1991) found high agreement among seniors and professionals on items indicating greater or lesser abuse. The items rated as most abusive were mainly examples of physical abuse.

Little has been published specifically related to how older, Aboriginal or multicultural groups define abuse and neglect (Pittaway et al. 1995). Most of the abuse studies ignore cultural aspects, and seem to assume that all older adults are similar in their attitudes and perceptions. However, a recent Canadian study (Bergin 1995) explored abuse of older adults in ethno-cultural communities, though Aboriginal communities were excluded. This study found that language barriers and sociocultural factors, such as difficulties in adapting to life in Canada and intergenerational differences in expectations, values and beliefs, affected the abused persons' definitions of abuse and their reluctance to disclose their situations. The Pittaway et al. (1995) study also found particular issues related to First Nations communities, such as the reluctance of abused seniors to leave their home or land, or difficulties in separation from extended families in spite of abuse.

Thériault (1994), from Quebec, similarly found that seniors said that even though "abuse and violence is part of our relationships, interpersonal exchanges and our organizations... the problem is so taboo that intervenors must decode their language, name the unnamable and especially offer places and moments in which such situations can be exchanged in a clear and transparent language for them" (96).

One can conclude from this that no general measures of abuse and neglect can be possible without developing clear operational definitions. In addition, there are still no commonly accepted or used definitions of abuse and neglect of older Canadians. Although the work of Stones presents a good starting point, definitions must refer to intent and nonintent to do harm, as well as to behaviour. Finally, definitions must take into account cultural differences and nuances, and approaches must be discovered to enable and facilitate those who are abused and neglected to express and report the abusive behaviour.

The next section will review the U.S. and Canadian literature to discuss which health and social indicators have been reported as most likely to be present in elders who are abused and absent in those who are not abused, as well as those present in caregivers who abuse versus those caregivers who do not abuse. As well, social, cultural and economic indicators that have been noted in the literature as present in abusive circumstances will be examined, since they may interact with the individual indicators to produce abuse and neglect.

It is interesting to note that most studies have focused on the individual characteristics of either abused seniors or of their abusers, rather than on the interaction of indicators of abuse relating to abused seniors, their abusers, and the environment. This seems surprising in light of the wealth of recent literature focusing on the interacting relationships between health and the social environment (Renaud 1993; Wilkinson 1993).

REVIEW OF THE LITERATURE

Relationships of Health Determinants to Abuse and Neglect of Older Adults

The relationships between health, wealth and well-being have been already well noted in the literature. To summarize some of these relationships, we know that mortality rates are linked to the scale of income inequality in each society (Wilkinson 1993). This demonstrates the close relationships between material and social constraints to the quality of human life. Health within developed countries is clearly linked to socioeconomic status. This is not only based on income but also on interacting psychosocial factors, such as social conditions and how people feel about and attach meanings to their circumstances and themselves (Wilkinson 1993). Since abuse and neglect of older adults would obviously impact upon their quality of life, these links to abuse and neglect are relevant. The World Health Organization defines health broadly as "a state of complete physical, mental and social well-being and not merely the absence of disease". Thus, it can be assumed that physical, psychological or material/financial abuse or neglect of an older adult would constitute a risk to that person's health. As well, since ageism and collective abuse affect a person's sense of identity, status and dignity, these factors would also have an impact on the quality of life of older adults.

Several specific health determinants have evolved from the fundamental prerequisites for the "Achieving Health for All" strategy developed in Canada in the late 1980s. Some of these health determinants are: social and economic environment; physical environment; personal health practices and coping skills; gender and culture characteristics; health services; and community involvement. This paper assumes that these health determinants affect the sense of control that seniors and their caregivers have over their lives. This sense of control may protect them from abusive and neglectful situations. The social and economic environment, and personal income, education level and social status all contribute to the sense of control that people, in general, have over their lives and their capacity to take action or to cope in stressful life situations. The physical environment of older adults may be restricted because of individual health and social conditions. Thus, the sense of control seniors have over their lives can be enhanced or inhibited, depending on their physical and social environments. As well, personal health practices and coping skills affect how older people are able to deal with difficult situations in a positive way. Gender and cultural characteristics affect how seniors maintain their personal and group identity, status and traditions, and contribute to their sense of control. Health services and resources play an important role in an older person's ability to participate in activities of daily living and community involvement. Involvement of the community with the older individual, too, can influence the senior's quality of life. The next section will examine further the main theoretical perspectives on the causes of abuse and neglect of older Canadians, and how these relate to the control seniors have over their health and well-being.

Theoretical Perspectives on Abuse and Neglect of Older Adults

The causes of abuse and neglect by informal caregivers are complex and varied, and depend on the theoretical perspective of the researcher. The major explanatory frameworks in the research literature fall into the following large categories: the Situational Model, Social Exchange Theory and the Symbolic Interaction Approach (MacDonald et al. 1991, 24–25). MacDonald et al. explain the approaches as follows:

- *The Situational Model* posits that mistreatment is an irrational response to environmental conditions and situational life crises. The situational variables include: (1) caregiver-related factors; (2) elder-related factors; (3) sociostructural factors. The three factors are not necessarily mutually exclusive. Caregiver-related factors may result from transgenerational or learned violence, personality traits, web of dependencies, filial crisis and internal stress. Elder-related factors tend to stem primarily from a web of dependencies, although they may also result from trans-generational violence or internal stress. Sociostructural factors may include external stressors and societal attitudes towards the elderly. This model appears to be the most widely used perspective, both by researchers and intervenors. It places emphasis on current social conditions rather than on past problems.

- *Social Exchange Theory*, according to the same authors, posits that as older people age they have less access to power, fewer resources and are progressively less able to perform instrumental tasks. As aging progresses, the imbalance grows and the elderly generally become more powerless, dependent and vulnerable than their caregivers. This theory is much less used than the first theory. The important U.S. studies by Pillemer (1986) found that the problem with this approach is that dependency sometimes operates in a direction opposite to that suggested in the theory. In other words, Pillemer found that the abuser felt powerless and dependent on the abused.

- *Symbolic Interaction* is a process which involves at least two individuals. The process occurs over time, consists of identifiable phases that are recurring and interrelated and requires constant negotiation and re-negotiation. In this approach, which is tied to social learning and modelling, mistreatment is viewed as a recurring phenomenon in the family, a phenomenon that is cyclic in nature and is related to the family's history of violent relationships (Shell 1982). (This theory is also less used than the first theory. Recently the theories on inter-generational transmission of violence have been challenged, since they do not fit with all types of abuse and neglect.)

Less known and used concepts are based on *empowerment*. Empowerment has been defined (Health Canada 1993) as "the process of helping individuals to maximize their confidence, skills and abilities in order to take control of their lives and to make informed decisions that are in their best interests. Empowerment also involves the element of choice and available, accessible options". A recent analysis by this author of the empowerment literature reveals an absence of powerlessness and dependence as characteristics of an empowered person (Lord and McKillop 1990). An inherent cause of powerlessness has been identified as social breakdown (Myers 1993). Myers summarizes this process as occurring in four stages and resulting in "discouraged persons who do not believe they have a chance to win a battle or solve a problem".

The process of becoming empowered involves a struggle and is often provoked by a crisis, unpleasant event or an unattainable objective (Lord and McKillop 1990). A process of powerlessness is observed in the individual, and a helper plays the important role of link between the person and their peers or group (Lord and McKillop 1990). Moving from powerlessness to empowerment implies helping people express themselves and listening to them. It also involves encouraging and facilitating empowerment; recognizing and fostering strengths and competencies; acknowledging and utilizing the wisdom of everyday experience; promoting diversity of ideas and approaches; and strengthening social networks and institutions (Hughes 1987). The process involves the interaction of the person with their environment in a way that influences their sense of control over their life. The variables often used in the empowerment approach studies are self-esteem, social support and control (Geston and Jason 1987).

The empowerment approach has been used widely in research in many different areas, particularly in the areas of social work, family violence, community psychology and health promotion. The approach has been used in both quantitative and qualitative studies, especially as a method to evaluate program interventions (Fetterman, Kaftarian, and Wandersman 1996). Empowerment researchers use the approach to target oppressed persons, groups and communities and focus on a process of helping people who have little control over their lives regain that control.

In reviewing each of these theoretical perspectives, no one theoretical model seems to provide a comprehensive, all-inclusive explanation of elder abuse (Phillips 1986). In fact, MacDonald et al. (1991, 36) suggest that "the scope of theory generation must be broadened beyond the family violence and caregiver stress hypotheses." For this reason, and since most practitioners and theorists who adhere to either the family violence perspective or the caregiver stress theories also seem to embrace empowerment concepts in their approaches, empowerment will be used as the perspective for this paper. Empowerment will be related to abuse and neglect as a process and an outcome of interventions that, according to Lee (1996, 13), entail:
- the development of a more potent sense of self;
- the construction of knowledge and capacity for a more critical comprehension of the web of social and political realities of one's environment;
- the cultivation of resources and strategies, or more functional competence, for attainment of personal or collective goals.

Values and Principles in the Empowerment Perspective

Values and principles are an extremely important part of the empowerment perspective. Since abuse and neglect are value-laden concepts, values represent an important factor in work related to this area. Identified values which must be respected in intervention and research are as follows (Cox and Parsons 1994, 41):
- fulfillment of human needs;
- promotion of social justice;
- more equal distribution of resources;
- concern for environmental protection;
- elimination of racism, sexism, ageism and homophobia;
- self-determination (the fullest possible participation in decisions that have an impact on one's life, both personal and political); and
- self-actualization.

Policies and interventions express values, whether explicitly or implicitly. These form guidelines for worker-client relationships, problem definition and assessment, goal setting and the choice of intervention strategies and techniques. The empowerment perspective expresses the values stated above in policies, intervention and research. Values must be considered when assessing or observing, or making policy about care receiver–caregiver relationships and contexts, since societal, family and individual values play an important role in the diverse motivations for giving care, asking for or receiving help, or creating modalities and conditions in which care is to be provided.

Some of the basic notions about how research is planned and conducted (Holmes, 1992) must also be considered. The empowerment perspective generally assumes a partnership between researchers, practitioners and research subjects, and assumes the following principles for conducting research:

- Empowerment research contributes to knowledge while empowering people, helping to give them a voice and tools to pursue and develop their agendas (Rappaport 1990);
- Methods and designs should never subvert the empowerment of people;
- The problems, solutions, needs and aspirations of research should be formed in terms defined by the group;
- Research questions and designs should be proactive so that information will be of positive use and will benefit the group under study as well as that of the workers and clients.

Lee (1994, 23) emphasizes that "the relationship between the researcher and the interviewees is clearly described in the empowerment perspective as a '1 and 1' (meaning equal) relationship". These values and perspectives are idealistic but can be seen as an attempt to involve seniors and caregivers in the design, planning and provision of their services and care, as well as in evaluations of programs and strategies. One Voice (1994) has offered to take a leadership role to help seniors and senior groups become more involved in attempts to prevent and reduce elder abuse and neglect.

Abuse and neglect clearly have a negative impact on the physical, psychological and social health and well-being of older adults, through the process of rendering people powerless and therefore not in control of their lives. It is important to examine specific individual, family, social, cultural and economic indicators associated with older abused and neglected adults and their abusers.

Indicators of Abuse

The aim of this paper is not to analyze, once again, all studies that have been reviewed on abuse and neglect in the U.S. and Canada by numerous authors (such as Pedrick, Cornell, and Gelles 1982; Pillemer and Wolf 1986; McDonald et al. 1991; and Kozack, Elmslie, and Verdon 1995). Rather, the purpose is to summarize the main conclusions about relationships between health determinants and the abuse and neglect of older adults.

Risk factors have been identified as important in predicting who will become abused or neglected, identifying causes, and detecting the presence of abuse and neglect (Kozack, Elmslie, and Verdon 1995). Kozack, Elmslie, and Verdon (1995) reviewed risk factors correlated with an increased risk of becoming abused or neglected. According to these authors, no single risk factor is a good predictor of abuse and neglect. The difficulties stem from the interactions of any single risk factor with other variables, such as family dynamics, caregiver stress and social isolation.

A second problem is the paucity of research related to risk factors. An ever increasing body of literature exists on factors that appear to place elderly people or their caregivers at risk for abuse and neglect (Pillemer and Finkelhor 1988). However, only two appropriate case-control studies have been conducted on the topic of risk factors in elder abuse (Pillemer and Suitor 1992; Godkin, Wolf, and Pillemer 1989). The results indicate that risk factors are not static dimensions whose presence or absence dictates the incident. Rather, they interact in a dynamic manner. Godkin et al. (1989) reported that abused seniors were not more functionally dependent upon their caregivers than age-matched seniors. Abusive incidents resulted when the caregiver and care receiver were in an interdependent relationship following the loss of a family member's support, increased social isolation and increased financial dependence of the abuser.

The risk factors that have been summarized from diverse studies all involve a complex interaction between socioeconomic, psychological and environmental conditions. All of these may interact to have an impact on the abused or the abuser. Before listing each risk factor, it is important to examine some salient points from the studies:

- Some differences between the risk profiles for abuse and neglect were demonstrated in the Podnieks et al. study (1990). These showed that chronic verbal aggression was more common among spouses, both male and female. Physical abuse, though affecting more males than females, was more violent toward females. This concurred with other findings in the spousal abuse literature (Sonkin, Martin, and Walker 1985).
- The impact of interacting factors has been noted on specific population groups. For example, the risk of abuse for seniors with Alzheimer's disease increased with the caregiver's depression, poor self-esteem, living arrangement and the presence of spousal violence (Paveza et al. 1992); Pillemer and Suitor 1992). Another identified population group is the mentally ill living in rural areas (Weiler and Buckwalter 1992); a third group consists of those abused within a relationship of spousal violence (Giordano and Giordano 1983). In qualitative studies of spousal violence, factors such as fear of reporting and professional reluctance to become involved in perceived family issues were common to young and older battered women (Gesino, Smith, and Keckich 1982).
- Overall, the paucity of research has limited the understanding of risk factors for elder mistreatment, and has stunted the development of effective screening tools; it is not clear which markers must be screened. As well, elder abuse encompasses multiple, often overlapping forms of mistreatment that can be difficult to distinguish from common problems associated with aging (Rosenblatt 1996).
- Research in the area of elder abuse indicators also depends on the researchers' theoretical perspective. Thus caregiver stress factors, family violence, personality or psychopathology of the abuser and/or lack of

community and family support may all be factors guiding the research study. The multiplicity of possible factors presented in the next section, as well as lack of evidence pointing to specific factors as indicative of risk of abuse and neglect make it difficult to point to any one guiding principle.

• Despite the lack of evidence, some indicators have appeared more prominently or more often than others in research studies. It seems that dependency is a key factor, sometimes involving the dependency of the care receiver and, at other times, that of the caregiver. However, as will be explained later, dependency is defined in different ways. As well, the literature points to social isolation and lack of social or family support as factors influencing whether an elder is abused or not, and whether a caregiver is abusive.

Substance abuse has been identified as the single best predictor of a caregiver being an abuser. As well, depression has been observed as a possible variable discriminating abusive caregivers from nonabusive, especially in cases where the dependant suffers from Alzheimer's disease.

Finally, gender issues have often been noted, though there is not enough evidence to draw clear conclusions. One can say that in cases of spouse abuse and physical violence, the violence has greater consequences for women than for men.

A recent review of the literature from the U.S. and Canada (Kosberg and Nahmiash 1996) summarized the main studies of indicators of abused and neglected older adults, their abusers, and the social and cultural environment within which abuse occurs.

Each of these indicators will be briefly discussed next.

The Abused

Ten areas indicating abuse and neglect in older adults have been defined as gender, marital status, health, age, substance abuse, living arrangements, psychological factors, the presence of problem behaviour, dependency and isolation.

Gender – Most studies have found that older women are most likely to be victims of elder abuse (Pillemer and Finkelhor 1988; Wolf et al. 1982). However, it has recently been suggested in the U.S. that the majority of victims might be men (Tatara 1993). In two Canadian studies, most abused older adults were women (Reis and Nahmiash 1995a; Pittaway et al. 1995). As well, gender influences may differ according to the type of abuse. For example, Podnieks et al. (1990) found that material abuse is equally common among males and females living alone, and that although males were more likely to be physically abused, physical abuse by males toward females tended to be more violent.

Marital status – Many studies have found that abused seniors are mainly widows (Pittaway et al. 1995). This is not surprising as most elderly persons are women, the majority of whom are widowed. However, some studies have identified older spouses as abused (Giordano and Giordano 1983; Pillemer and Suitor 1992). Case studies have also indicated similarities between younger and older-aged battered women (Gesino, Smith, and Keckich 1982).

Health – From numerous studies one can conclude that most abused older adults are in poor physical or mental health. However, studies note that impairment is not necessarily a specific indicator of abuse, since those who are not abused may be as impaired as those who are (Pillemer and Suitor 1992; Godkin, Wolf, and Pillemer 1989; Reis and Nahmiash 1995). It does seem likely that abuse would have a negative influence on health, and neglect has been associated with severely impaired health (Paveza et al. 1992).

Chronological age – Advanced age has been associated with abuse of older adults (Kosberg 1980; O'Malley 1987). However, researchers have found that abuse does occur among the young old (Hudson 1994). In general, though, those between the ages of 60–69 years are less likely to be abused (Tatara 1993).

Substance abusers – Older substance abusers have been found to be susceptible to abusive behaviour by others (Kosberg 1988). However, not many studies have observed this.

Living arrangements – Most abused older adults live with a relative rather than living alone (Pillemer 1986; Floyd 1983). In urban areas where elders are often isolated, lonely, easily identifiable, and living alone, elders may be exploited in financial scams, larceny and embezzlement. Shared living arrangements have been particularly related to cases of spousal, physical and psychological abuse, but not to cases of financial abuse.

Psychological factors – Older persons who are depressed or resigned to un-satisfactory situations are prone to abuse (Phillips 1983). Other individuals, who internalize blame, engage in excessive loyalty to family members or display stoicism, are also susceptible to mistreatment (Kosberg 1988).

Presence of problem behaviour – Problem behaviour has been noted in some abused older adults (Paveza et al. 1992). For example, when the care receiver is suffering from advanced Alzheimer's disease and/or engages in aggressive behaviour toward the caregiver, this can result in abuse of the impaired individual.

Dependence – A debate rages about whether dependency of the care receiver is likely to increase the chances of abuse (Quinn and Tomita 1986), or whether the abuser is more likely to be dependent on the abused older adult (Pillemer 1985; Fulmer 1990). Other studies have found that abusive incidents occur when the abused person and the caregiver become increasingly interdependent upon one another due to loss of a family member, decreased support, increased isolation and/or increased financial dependency of the abuser (Godkin et al. 1989; Pillemer and Suitor 1992). Abused and neglected older adults have been described as powerless (Blunt 1993), unwilling to disclose their problems, having low self-esteem, wishing to save face and unwilling to betray family secrets. However, such characteristics may emerge as consequences of long-term abuse rather than as etiologic factors.

Isolation – Social isolation and a lack of social support have been portrayed as indicators of abuse (Pillemer 1984). Isolation from others permits the abuse to continue without detection and intervention.

The Abuser

Studies have generally found that a typical abuser of older adults is a son or daughter caregiver, under 60 years of age and living with (or in close proximity to) the abused older adult (Wolf, Strugnell, and Godkin 1982; Quinn and Tomita 1986). Project CARE found that more abusers were males than females (Reis and Nahmiash 1995a) as did the Pittaway et al. (1995) study. However, one should be cautious in generalizing from these studies. Even though this paper will not deal with institutional abuse, it should be noted that abusers in institutions are usually female (Gnaedinger 1989) and predominantly in low-paid, high-stress jobs.

Ten indicators of abusers of older adults have been defined, as follows: substance abuse; mental/emotional illness; caregiving inexperience; caregiving reluctance; history of receiving abuse; dependency on the care recipient; confusion and dementia; burden and stress of caregiving; personality traits (related to control, depression, blame, being overly critical and unsympathetic) and lack of social support. Each indicator will be summarized below:

Substance abuse – This seems to be the single best predictor of a caregiver being an abuser (Floyd 1983; Pillemer and Wolf 1986; Reis and Nahmiash 1995b).

Mental and emotional illness – Some caregivers with emotional problems appear to be unable to curb their behaviour, which interferes with their ability to meet the needs of care receivers (Kosberg 1988; Reis and Nahmiash 1995b).

Lack of experience – It cannot be assumed that a person who has never undertaken the task of caregiving will automatically know how to do the job appropriately (Kosberg 1988).

Reluctance – Some caregivers are reluctant to take on the helping role for an older relative (Cairl, Kelner, and Kosberg 1984). These caregivers may be influenced by professionals to take on the role, with possible adverse consequences for the care receiver.

History of abuse – Violence appears most likely in families with lifelong patterns of violent behaviour, especially cases such as spousal or child abuse (Gelles 1974; Sengstock and Hwalek 1987). The behaviour may have been learned in the family, or may result from an unconscious need for retribution. One study noted the relationship between Aboriginal abused seniors and their early experiences in residential schools (Pittaway et al. 1995).

Stress and burden – Feelings of stress and being overburdened have frequently been associated with abuse of older relatives (Hudson 1986; Block and Sinnott 1979, Hickey and Douglass 1981; Galbraith and Davison 1985). Yet the actual stress may be a less important predictor of abuse than the caregiver's perception of the stress (Steinmetz and Amsden 1983; Zarit, Reever, and Bach-Peterson 1990). As well, burden and stress have been associated with nonabusive caregivers.

Dependency – As noted above, some studies (Pillemer 1985) suggest that the caregiver is frequently dependent on the older person for financial, emotional or social support.

Confusion and dementia – Abuse of older persons with confusion and dementia has been observed (Steinmetz 1988; Hamel et al. 1990). Further, as the population ages, there is an increasing possibility that the caregivers themselves may be elderly and suffering from cognitive impairments (Giordano and Giordano 1983).

Personality traits – People who display hypercritical or unsympathetic attitudes toward the needs of others are more likely to become abusers (Sengstock and Hwalek 1987; Reis and Nahmiash 1995). In addition, abusers include people who blame the older person for problems, those with unrealistic caregiving expectations, and those who lack understanding of the care receiver's condition (Quinn and Tomita 1986; Reis and Nahmiash, 1995).

Other indicators include *depression* (Paveza et al. 1992; Reis and Nahmiash 1995) and *loss of self control* (Bendik 1992; Reis and Nahmiash 1995) which can result from the caregiver's feeling a loss of personal control or freedom (Pillemer 1986; Gottlieb 1991).

The Social Context

Six additional indicators relating to the social context of the caregiving situation have been identified in the literature. These indicators, including financial problems, family violence, lack of social support, family disharmony, living arrangements and intergenerational transmission of violence, may interact with one another in abusive situations. Some of these may overlap with the aforementioned indicators.

Financial problems – Difficulties resulting from unemployment have been noted to cause resentment in a caregiving situation (Lau and Kosberg 1979). However, few other studies support this.

Family violence – In situations where family members are in conflict with one another, abuse is often hidden, and elderly members are fearful of revealing their problems (Steinmetz 1988). Such patterns of intrafamily violence might be so long term as to be viewed as normative (Myers and Shelton 1987; Griffin 1994). Family violence has been especially explored in smaller case studies of abused women (Gesino, Smith, and Keckich 1982).

Lack of social support – This has been linked to abusive behaviour (Pillemer 1984). Abused older adults have been found to be more socially isolated and to have fewer social contacts than nonabused older adults (Pillemer 1984). As well, when families are isolated from the support of their relatives, older members are at greater risk and abusive behaviour may go undetected (Pillemer and Finkelhor 1988).

Family disharmony – Problems such as marital disputes may increase the vulnerability of older adults to family violence (Douglass, Hickey, and Noel 1980). Parent-child conflicts have been noted (Cicirelli 1981), as have mother-daughter and husband-child rivalry. Conflicts regarding household management or the sharing of responsibilities can be additional factors (Steinmetz and Amsden 1983).

Living arrangements – Most people in North America would prefer not to share a household with adult children and their families, even when they are ill (Anetzberger 1987). Overcrowding and lack of privacy have been associated with intrafamilial conflict and can result in anger toward the older adult (Kosberg 1988). As well, shared living arrangements have been associated with spousal abuse and physical and psychological violence (Giordano and Giordano 1983). Environmental barriers, such as high crime in neighbourhoods, inaccessible areas for wheel chairs and lack of telephones (Harshbarger 1993) have been noted as barriers to abused seniors seeking help. Housing issues can also interact with abuse problems of older clients. Substandard housing conditions can include structurally unsound buildings with safety problems (Pittaway et al. 1995); minimal standards of cleanliness; and deterioration of homes. Health violations, such as pests or insect infestation and trash and garbage that is not disposed of (Pittaway et al. 1995) can be part of this problem.

Intergenerational transmission of violence – It has been stated that problems between parent and child do not decrease with time and may even intensify as the parent becomes dependent on the child (Blenkner 1965). Although this is a popular theory, there seems to be very little evidence to support it.

The Cultural Norms

Another dimension in the area of abuse and neglect of older adults is the cultural milieu within which abuser and abused find themselves. Attitudes and values can influence individuals to engage in, or deter them from engaging in the mistreatment of elderly persons. Six such considerations are: ageism, sexism, cultural attitudes towards violence, reactions to abusive behaviour, attitudes towards disabled persons and the culturally-produced imperative of family caregiving.

Ageism – This has been previously defined in this paper. Negative societal attitudes about older adults can result in a climate favourable to abuse and neglect (Gouvernement du Québec 1990). Unfortunately most studies have not really addressed this type of abuse.

Sexism – Some authors have pointed out that older women are the primary victims of violence (Canadian Panel on Violence against Women 1994) and that the unequal status of women, in general, and older women in particular can contribute to the existence of abuse and neglect. Currently, only two recent studies note that more female victims are abused and that the consequence of physical violence to women is more severe than to men.

Cultural attitudes towards violence – These attitudes may influence the use of violence against dependent family members. Some ethnic groups rely extensively on the family and are reluctant to report cases of intrafamily violence (Nahmiash 1994a), making identification particularly difficult. Within some ethnic or minority groups, abuse is often perceived as a "family affair". Poverty, resistance to formal assistance, and religious beliefs (Pittaway et al. 1995) can exacerbate this situation.

Reactions to abuse – Personal beliefs of abused seniors or abusers may emanate from religious convictions and family or cultural backgrounds. Whether a situation is perceived as abusive or not has been found to influence help-seeking patterns (Moon and Williams 1993) for both the abused and the abuser.

Attitudes towards people living with disabilities – In cultures that deem people living with disabilities to be unworthy, abuse can be condoned or tolerated (Heisler 1991). In such cultures, abusive treatment may not be perceived as wrong.

Imperatives for family caregiving – Social beliefs about the duty of family members can influence behaviour and perceptions regarding abusive behaviour (Pepin 1992). In such cases, cultural expectations of family caregiving, coupled with a lack of formal service assistance and alternatives may place the care recipient in a potentially dangerous situation. However, studies have not really explored these issues in sufficient depth to draw conclusions.

The above indicators relate to societal attitudes that can produce an environment where violence is learned, condoned and allowed to continue. Such attitudes are obviously difficult to change, and require a more pervasive educational approach to promote new social and community values. Most studies have not yet explored the impact of these indicators on abuse and neglect of older adults.

The Economic Context

A final dimension of abuse and neglect is the economic context in which it takes place. There is some indication that poverty and limited finances are related to situations of abuse and neglect (Pittaway et al. 1995). Poverty can be a characteristic of abused seniors, as well as a barrier to seeking help. Similarly, lack of formal and informal resources has been linked to abusive situations (Pittaway et al. 1995). These factors will be detailed later in this paper.

Table 1 illustrates the interacting risk indicators of abused seniors, their abusers and the context. The asterisks note the indicators which probably merit further exploration.

Table 1
Interacting indicators of victims, abusers and the context

Social context	Economic context
Financial problems, family violence, * **Lack of social support,** **Family disharmony,** * **Shared living arrangements,** Intergenerational transmission of violence	Poverty, limited finances, Lack of informal and formal resources
Abused	**Abuser**
* **Gender** (women) Marital status (widows) Health (poor) Advanced age Substance abuse problems Living arrangements Psychological factors (depression) Problem behaviours * **Dependency** * **Lack of social support** * **Social isolation** Unrealistic expectations	* **Substance abuse** Mental/emotional illness Caregiving inexperience Caregiving reluctance History of abuse * **Dependency on the care** **recipient** Confusion/dementia Stress and burden * **Personality factors** * **Lack of social support**

*Cultural norms
Ageism, sexism, cultural attitudes toward violence,
reactions to abusive behaviour,
attitudes towards disabled,
context of family caregiving.

Conclusions from the Studies

The phenomenon of abuse and neglect affects approximately 4 percent of the population over the age of 65 years, but this may be an underestimate.

Definitions of abuse and neglect are diverse and not comparable. Researchers need to arrive at a consensus based on empirical studies of definitions, although the work of Stones provides a good starting point.

Methodologies are varied and samples are often small. There are often no control or contrast groups. Studies are mainly quantitative, not qualitative, and data is mainly from client records, health and social service personnel and not from clients, a more reliable source of data.

There are not yet enough evidence-based studies of indicators of abuse or risk factors to draw clear conclusions. Only two U.S. studies (Pillemer and Finkelhor 1988; Gioglio and Blakemore 1983) and one Canadian study (Podnieks et al. 1990) were considered rigorous enough to justify an in-depth analysis of risk factors.

Most researchers focus on individual indicators related to either the abused or the abuser. Recently, the focus has turned to caregiver rather than care receiver indicators, discriminating abusers from nonabusers rather than abused from nonabused elders.

Many of the indicators may overlap. As well, they probably interact in combination with indicators from the social, cultural and economic environments of both abused and abusers, and they may vary according to the theoretical perspective of the researcher. The current social context of care within which abuse occurs creates a particularly vulnerable environment: abusive circumstances may not only occur but may be provoked in situations where family support is lacking and shared living arrangements are necessary.

Six indicators related to abuse and neglect are described most often. These are dependency, social support/isolation, substance abuse, depression gender, and living arrangements. However, the terms used, such as dependency, may have different meanings in different studies. For example, dependency may refer to functional inability to perform activities of daily living, or it may refer to affective relationships between care receivers and caregivers. In some studies, dependency is described as an indicator that discriminates the abused from the nonabused, while in others it discriminates the abuser from the nonabuser. Dependency does seem to be an important variable, but we do not know yet who is dependent upon whom. Similarly, social support has been variously defined, according to researchers' different perspectives (Gottlieb 1991). However, there seem to be links between social isolation and lack of support, and cases of abuse and neglect. Substance abuse, particularly alcohol abuse, has been flagged as the best single predictor of a caregiver abuser versus a caregiver nonabuser. As well, caregiver depression has been noted as an indicator, particularly where severely dependent persons with Alzheimer's disease have been abused or neglected.

It must be noted that a primary reason that clear indicators have not yet been identified is that elder abuse and neglect covers a broad area. Therefore, indicators may relate to one type of abuse but not others. For example, spouse abuse may be specifically linked to physical and psychological abuse, but not to financial/material abuse and neglect. Rather, these may be common to elders living alone.

In the case of gender, there are conflicting and mixed reports. In some studies there is evidence that more males are abused (Pillemer and Finkelhor 1988), while in others, females are said to be more frequently abused (Gioglio and Blakemore 1983). One can conclude that gender is a variable affecting both the abused and the abuser. Still, there is not yet any clear evidence about how and whom, nor in what context, gender affects abuse. It does seem that in cases of spouse abuse, the consequences of violence, both physical and psychological, are more severe for women than for men. Shared living arrangements are also an indicator in this type of violence, but not in cases of financial abuse.

Causes of abuse and neglect have not yet been determined. In general, though, being abused and neglected results in a state of powerlessness and a loss of control over one's life, health and environment, especially in a context of dependency and a conflictual caregiver–care receiver relationship. An empowerment perspective implies a supply of adequate resources, a values-based approach to practice, policy and research, and involvement by seniors and caregivers in the planning of programs, resources and evaluations of intervention strategies.

SOCIAL POLICY ISSUES

This section will explore the social context within which care is given, to discover the tasks and pressures involved in caring for a dependent relative. Family support is characterized by diversity (Garant and Bolduc 1990). It consists of emotional support, financial help, mediation between the formal service system and the senior, multiple concrete services and the assurance of a continuous presence. The objective burden of care has been described as heavy, and the length of the helping situation as long. Caregiving has often been described as a constant source of stress and emotional tension, as well as financial strain. Support for people suffering from dementia is particularly difficult and stressful (Garant and Bolduc 1990). However, it must be noted that most family caregivers are not abusive. Caregiver depression, substance abuse and lack of family or social support may be more indicative than stress in determining whether caregivers become abusive or not.

Adequacy of Resources

Little research, other than the Victoria study (Pittaway et al. 1995), has been carried out on whether adequacy of formal resources plays a role in influencing whether caregivers become abusive. However, some information about the importance of resources to family caregivers does exist. This is relevant in our current Canadian economic context of increasingly scarce resources.

Families do count on the state to play an essential assisting role, over which families can exercise control (Lesemann and Chaume 1989). However, public policy is not necessarily responding to the need for adequate resources and supports for family caregivers. There have been budgetary cutbacks in the public sector, and there has been a push toward privatization and growing reliance on the family (Stryckman and Nahmiash 1994). Chappel's study (1989) adds that even when resources do exist, caregivers only use formal services as a last resort, after all informal supports have been used. When they ask for help, they are usually at the end of their rope: their dependant's health is severely impaired, in the terminal stage of illness.

Other authors (Vezina and Roy, in press) note that research exploring dynamics such as those in caregiving relationships, the ambience of care settings, or ease of access to service settings, will be irrelevant without adequate resources to provide services and supports to caregivers. It can be concluded that caring requires a set of specific conditions and a complex organization of resources and supports (Maheu and Guberman 1992). In other words, in situations where family members need more help in caring for a dependant, for example in cases where caregivers are depressed, are substance abusers or lack family support, resources must be adequate, accessible and appropriate. The community, not just individual family members, must assume responsibility for care.

The adequacy of the public service sector and its engagement or disengagement from providing resources and supports to families giving care is relevant in preventing abuse and neglect of older adults. This is particularly true where caregivers are depressed, are substance abusers and lack social support. The state and market sectors can assist family members in their social obligations of caring (Godbout and Caillé 1992), thus protecting social bonds and relationships in society. If the state's ability to provide such services and supports continues to decline, as seems likely in the predictable future, and if pressures and stresses on caregivers increase due to demographic and social policy factors, it seems possible, even likely, that abusive behaviour, situations and conditions will also increase.

Recently, Canadian policies and discourses have emphasized the social obligation of families in providing care, and the responsibility of individuals to provide their own care. Program evaluations have shown that less assistance is given when a family member is present (Gouvernement du Québec 1994).

In contrast, some European countries, such as Sweden, have developed a state model of welfare in which the state pays for all care, including informal care. Thus, to provide or not to provide adequate, paid care is a political choice based on political philosophy and strategy. Unfortunately, statistics are not yet available from Sweden to determine whether this form of social welfare reduces abuse of older adults.

Finally, it is important to note that when the state provides more services, the substitution effect does not happen. Families continue to give as much care as before, rather than decreasing their obligations (Vézina and Roy, in press).

In conclusion, although most caregivers are not abusive, this situation is at best precarious and could lead to the social breakdown described by Myers (1993) and Myers and Shelton (1987). Particularly in the presence of indicators such as depression, substance abuse and lack of family support, abuse and neglect of older adults by caregivers can result in the powerlessness of care recipients. These indicators, which probably interact, need to be explored in future research studies to determine their relationship to abuse and neglect.

Gender and poverty may also relate to the current social context of care, and the abuse and neglect of older adults.

Gender Issues

According to Neysmith (1995, 44), "abuse reflects the gender nature of attitudes, behaviour and expectations in Canadian society. Thus we would expect to find differences between the experiences of older men and women, despite the gender neutrality of the term 'elder abuse'." In the Podnieks et al. (1990) study, both men and women were equally subject to all types of abuse. However, in two other recent studies, though not representative samples, (Pittaway et al. 1995; Reis and Nahmiash 1995), women out-numbered men as abused older adults, and males outnumbered females as abusers, in spite of most caregivers being female. Referring to the Podnieks study, Neysmith (1995) points out that women have been found to have a higher tolerance threshold before considering behaviour abusive. As well, abuse must be named and legitimated before one can speak of it. It is very possible that financial abuse, most prevalent in the Podnieks study, is the least stigmatizing type of abuse to acknowledge, particularly when questions are asked over the telephone. Unfortunately, while these results are not clear enough to draw conclusions nor to generalize from, they indicate directions for future research.

Not enough Canadian research has been done to determine the etiology of abusive situations among older adults. Nor have studies generally separated conjugal types of abusive behaviour from other types of abuse, such as financial, to determine if the dynamics are different. However, we do know that verbal aggression is usually perpetrated by men and that physical violence is seldom initiated by women (Saunders 1988). Physical abuse by males toward females tends to be more violent. Neysmith (1995) poses a question in relation to the Podnieks study for further exploration: "Does the dynamic of a relationship change when a formerly abusive spouse becomes incapacitated?" (49). The other issue is that sustained injuries are reported to be much higher for women than for men where physical force is used (Pillemer and Finkelhor 1988). These findings suggest that the family violence perspective may be relevant at least in cases of physical and spouse abuse, although there is not yet enough evidence to confirm this. However, it is known that kin-based abuse is more likely to occur when one person wields power over another, whether spouse, parent, child or other individual is placed in a dependent position (Lee 1992). Since abuse usually happens in a relationship of trust, it follows that if one person depends on another for material or other essential resources, this may create a precarious and vulnerable situation.

Finally, in the Pittaway et al. (1995) study, not only were most of the abused people females (74 percent), but most were also widows with limited support and advocacy from families, friends or volunteers. In the Project CARE study (Reis and Nahmiash 1995a) the difference between the sampled abused seniors from the health and social service agency and the community nonabused seniors, was the lack of support. Thus, it seems that gender issues may become even more prominent for people such as widows, who have less social support and depend on health and social service agencies for assistance. Support services and advocacy seem to be extremely significant for this high risk group.

Poverty and Socioeconomic Issues

At the macro level, abusive behaviour has been linked with poverty. For example, unemployment has been linked with abusive behaviour (Lau and Kosberg 1979), though there is little evidence to support this. Nevertheless, this may be significant at a time when unemployment in Canada is high, since links have been observed between poverty and crime or violence, as well as poverty and poor health, in areas other than elder abuse.

In studies of abuse and neglect of older adults, there is not much evidence of a link between poverty and social class or education with abusive behaviour. However, given the fact that there are few empirical studies in Canada, these may be areas to examine further. There are indications in some studies that poverty may be related more to certain types of abuse, such as financial. For example, in the Pittaway et al. (1995) study, the only project to explore abuse and neglect among Aboriginal communities, there emerged a clear relationship between the historical conditions of Aboriginal peoples and the current abusive situation. Examples were racist attitudes reinforced through residential school experiences, and the internalization of oppressive stereotypes of Aboriginal peoples. In addition, the displacement of Aboriginal peoples from reserves to urban centres highlighted economic situations.

In the Pittaway study (1995), more than half of the abused adults' revenue was from old age security pensions, and approximately one-third received the guaranteed income supplement. Limited finances played a role in some abusive situations. For example, one woman felt trapped in her abusive daughter's home as she did not have the funds to move out. Another woman shared a story of how her mother was using money as a means of control and power to keep her being dependent. Unfortunately, results from this study cannot be generalized due to the sampling techniques, but they point to areas for further exploration.

As already mentioned, living arrangements, such as overcrowding and lack of privacy can interact with limited finances and abusive situations (Kosberg 1988) on the micro level. In the Pittaway study almost one-third of abused and abusers lived together. It has already been mentioned that financial dependence, whether on the caregiver (Quinn and Tomita 1986) or on the care receiver (Pillemer and Suitor 1992) has been cited as a risk factor for abusive behaviour.

In the above sections it is noted that adequacy of formal resources in the caregiving setting might influence whether or not abuse and neglect occurs. Direct links from which generalizations can be drawn have not yet been made in this area. Gender issues must also be taken into account, particularly in the areas of spousal and physical violence. Some suggestions have also been made in research studies about the links between elder abuse and neglect, and poverty and lack of finances. This has been noted particularly in relation to Aboriginal communities. These results cannot be generalized, but suggest that future study in this area might be worthwhile.

CANADIAN CASE STUDIES OF ABUSE

The next section will assess five case studies of programs and strategies to help abused and neglected adults. This proved a difficult task because, while there are many innovative and extensive programs for combating and intervening in elder abuse and neglect, few have been submitted to rigorous outcome evaluation testing.

Review of Programs and Strategies

Many authors have noted (McKenzie, Tod, and Yellen 1995; MacDonald et al. 1991) that most intervention models fall into one of four categories: domestic violence/family therapy; advocacy and information; adult protection; and multidisciplinary programs. For this reason, case studies

from each intervention model category were selected. Other selection criteria included:
- programs from eastern and western parts of the country;
- diversity of strategies to intervene in abuse cases;
- programs serving abused seniors living in the community;
- programs which have been submitted to an evaluation;
- innovative models; and
- programs housed in diverse sites.

Because of time constraints and lack of information about program costs and funding of all programs, a cost-effectiveness analysis was not possible.

Each program was assessed as to its program orientations and assumptions, evaluation outcomes, the types of actors, and the funding agencies and strategies. Assessments were based on the extent and type of senior involvement in the program, the variety of program strategies and their effectiveness, as well as the links to resources and the program's capacity to continue with few added costs.

Domestic Violence/Family Therapy Model

Domestic violence/family therapy programs can be illustrated by *case study number 1*, the *Elder Abused Woman Project* (Dale 1995) in Toronto. The centre focuses on identifying the predominant barriers to older abused women seeking help. It is assumed that many women are subjected to a lifetime of abuse that begins with physical and sexual abuse in childhood. Then they marry and find they are victims of spouse abuse, and as they grow older, they become victims of elder abuse. Clients in this project were over 55 years old, and the project consisted of building a scrapbook as a tangible way for abused women to tell their stories (many for the first time), express their emotions through art, collect, recollect and recreate lost artifacts and express hidden aspects of self. Group work was the modality chosen because the women overwhelmingly requested it. The small groups aimed to break the women's social isolation, help them develop social networks, destigmatize their individual difficulties, and provide a "minisociety" in which to establish formative relations and try out new behaviours, pool resources and share information. The program is housed in a women's health centre.

Evaluation of the Elder Abused Woman Project

Client empowerment was the overall goal of the group, with elements of popular education approaches, feminist counselling and social work with group strategies. Groups were co-led by a full-time project coordinator and a part-time cofacilitator with expertise in the arts. The project lasted approximately one year, and two groups were run over a six-month period of two sessions. A total of 13 women attended the first-cycle sessions, 11 attended the second, and overall attendance was high, with 70 percent attending after the end of the first session. The average age was 63 years, and women came from a diversity of ethnocultural backgrounds, including First Nations communities. The groups were flexible, to allow those women who wished to continue to attend the second cycle of groups.

The analysis of the groups was a qualitative process evaluation, including completion of group evaluation forms. All participants agreed that attending the groups had been a positive experience. The evaluation identified what worked and what could be improved. This type of evaluation is often used in small family violence projects. However, the women could have been encouraged to make negative, as well as positive comments.

Outcomes noted were that the women made friends, felt less lonely, obtained more daily structure, dealt with past hurts, dealt with emotional upsets and stress, were able to experience being good to themselves, saw how old messages affected them in the present, began to express some emotions through art, learned what they needed to feel safe/secure, and learned more about woman abuse. Other program strengths were the links made with other community and health programs, development of training programs, and an innovative pilot project of programming for older abused women at a homeless women's shelter.

Conclusions from the project were that services for abused women are frequently geared to younger rather than older women, who have a different historical understanding of the roles of women. The program strengths included:

- its nonmedical approach to mental health;
- its multiethnic approach;
- the participation of Aboriginal women;
- the use of a community advisory panel;
- the use of individual as well as group counselling strategies;
- the development of an inventory of resources for the use of abused women;
- the group process, which enhanced the victim-to-survivor understanding of trauma;
- the low cost of the project (it was funded by Health Canada), and the few resources required; and
- that it provided an interesting, detailed model that can be used by other workers in this area.

The weaknesses of the project included:

• The quality of the outcome evaluation: for example, the project included no criticisms from the women;
• The limited number of women who are able to participate in the small group process, and the fact that the small groups targeted a particular small group of abused seniors;

- The limited outreach to other isolated, eligible women (a program that targets such women was, however, recommended for the future);
- That no specific mention was made in the final report to the effect that the project would continue in the future (the project was affiliated with an existing women's health centre whose staff could presumably continue the project);
- That although seniors were involved in this project, the project was not driven by seniors.

It is to be hoped that in the future, the women would be trained to lead other such support groups.

Advocacy and Information Models

An example of an advocacy and information service approach is *case study number 2, Project Synergy II* from Kerby Centre, Calgary, which has a "one-stop shopping" approach to intervention services. This project, located in a centre for seniors, represents an example of senior involvement and participation in all aspects of the phases of detection, prevention and intervention in cases of abuse and neglect of older adults. *Project Synergy II* had ten objectives:

1. To formally establish a community-based consultation team;
2. To publicize as widely as resources permit the services to be offered;
3. To identify or devise treatment options and strategies to address violence within older families, building on existing resources at Kerby Centre;
4. To provide training and consultation services to front-line professionals;
5. To undertake education programs to sensitize the public to the recognition of, incidence and prevention of abuse;
6. To recruit and train a corps of senior volunteers to be utilized as an integral part of the treatment strategy;
7. To recruit and train a corps of senior volunteers to staff a community 24-hour crisis line, in collaboration with an existing crisis service agency;
8. To collect detailed information about older people and families involved in violent family relationships;
9. To evaluate the effectiveness of intervention strategies used by assessing the changes in the clients, their characteristics and circumstances; and
10. To develop complete documentation covering all aspects of this project.

Program assumptions were not explicit in this study. However, implicitly the research seems to fit the situational model, with its emphasis on caregivers and the societal impacts of ageism on both the abused and the abusers. According to the *Project Synergy II* report, all these study objectives were met.

Evaluation of Project Synergy II

Through *Project Synergy II*, 120 clients were assisted, but were not included in the research study because their intervention required less than six hours of professional expertise. One hundred and thirty clients were included in the study, and were involved in a series of pre- and posttest instruments. Treatment modalities offered included a combination of individual, group and peer counselling strategies. Treatment support was obtained from the community, in the form of volunteer professionals who sat on a consultation team. Twenty standardized outcome measures of the intervention strategies were chosen in collaboration with seniors. These included self-esteem of abused and abuser, physical, psychological, material abuse and violation of rights, neglect, economic, emotional and physical indicators, trust, mobility, cognitive, social, loneliness, happiness, general life experiences, stress assessed by the abused and by the abuser, and ageism.

Three treatment options were available for clients but all the clients were first offered individual counselling. Unfortunately, the two groups choosing peer and group counselling were too small to reach statistical significance. Overall client satisfaction measures demonstrated high satisfaction with the programs. There were overall changes in scores in outcome measures. Levels of abuse decreased significantly in all five areas. Loneliness and isolation decreased following counselling, and client self-esteem increased, as did happiness. However, these measures were only effected on 80 clients following professional counselling. Client functioning showed improvement in seven areas: emotional balance, social support, economic resources, trust, mobility, cognitive status and physical health.

Thirty-three abusers took part in the study. Results showed a decrease in their self-esteem and an increase in their stress levels. However, their levels of abuse and their attitudes of ageism decreased significantly.

Problems noted in this study included:

- That too many instruments and outcomes were used, which became tiring for the study participants. A maximum of five instruments and outcomes was recommended for future studies;
- That community professionals only referred 18 cases to the consultation team over the course of the three-year project;
- That many of the standardized scales were found to be inappropriate for use in the study. These scales were consequently adapted by the research team in collaboration with seniors from the community;
- That only one treatment modality was measured in the project, and factors that might have influenced counselling strategies were not taken into account. A random assignment into the three treatment modalities to equalize numbers in treatment groups would have prevented small numbers in two of the groups. The freedom to choose on the part of the client was considered more important, and is in line with the

empowerment perspectives of freedom of choice of available, accessible options. However, seniors were obliged to accept individual counselling before the other strategies, limiting their freedom of choice;

- That there is inconsistency in the analysis: Abused seniors were offended by the Fabroni Ageism Scale, and it was recommended that this scale not be used in further studies. However, the Ageism Scale was used successfully by the abusers, who did not object to it, the reasons for which are not given in the study report.

Highlights of this project were:

– the high degree of senior involvement;

– the quality of the outcome evaluation study; and

– the offer of services to abusers as well as to the abused.

The study contains useful research information as well as information about training and intervention programs and modalities which are useful for other programs and workers.

Funding modalities were collaborative, and the project was based on principles of little added cost and existing resources. Funding for the project was provided by Health Canada, Alberta Family and Social Services and the Office for the Prevention of Family Violence, from three municipal service agencies and from private sources. These mixed funding sources provided a particularly successful way of undertaking a large collaborative project.

One weakness in the project was that there were relatively few participants in the study, and that 120 abused seniors had to be excluded. In addition, the sample of program participants may not have been representative of the population of abused and neglected older adults in general, as the program was mainly based in a seniors centre and few referrals were made from the community.

A second example of an advocacy organization which is different from *Project Synergy II* and illustrates how the rights of abused elders can be upheld and respected on a province-wide basis is shown through *case study number 3, North Shore Community Services Centre* from Vancouver, British Columbia.

This agency has received funding from Health Canada's Seniors Independence Project from 1990–1995 to:

– measure the awareness of the presence or risk of abuse of older persons, primarily as it relates to legal and financial concerns;

– measure knowledge of the types of abuse suffered by older persons and the services available for older persons experiencing or at risk of abuse;

– determine some of the attitudes, beliefs and opinions of service professionals and the public with regard to abuse and risk factors related to abuse, in the senior population;

– identify in Phase 1 of the survey some of the training and public education needs on the topic of abuse and in the senior population; and

- identify in Phase 2 of the survey the effectiveness of training provided by the North Shore Information and Volunteer Centre in connection with the Seniors Project.

North Shore Community Services Centre offers information on community services to the elderly, legal services and information on government services and benefits, and information on issues and rights, such as low-cost housing. The Centre stresses advocacy and legal rights as an intervention model for the prevention and treatment of abuse and neglect. However, the program itself emphasizes the view of seniors as independent, shifting the emphasis from the service provider's response to the senior, returning autonomy to the senior, and promoting conditions that support equality and autonomy. A major component is the use of language that promotes positive images of seniors, and the identification of seniors as participants, users or consumers rather than as clients, patients or care recipients. North Shore projects are based on a feminist and family violence approach.

North Shore Community Services Centre is a nonprofit society which, in addition to offering advocacy information and referrals to seniors, has been responsible for a community survey to assess attitudes about abuse and neglect of older adults. In addition, it has provided support to 12 diverse communities in British Columbia as they have developed effective Community Response Networks to support, improve and integrate services and responses to abused older adults. As well, a Guide to Legal Issues in Elder Abuse Intervention, with related teaching and educational materials, have been produced.

Evaluation of the North Shore Community Services Centre

The agency has not been rigorously evaluated, but rather submitted an "impact assessment" to Seniors Independence Projects, Health Canada. This evaluation showed that the project reached more than 1,000 seniors through workshop activities, training and educational sessions. The group was involved in lobbying for new legislative policies and acts in British Columbia, which may serve as a model for older abused adults in the rest of Canada. New service delivery modalities for seniors in British Columbia were put in place, and a B.C. Coalition to Eliminate Abuse of Seniors was set up. This coalition continues to function to ensure that all activities are maintained. Each of these will be discussed in more detail.

The evaluation of *North Shore Community Services Centre* was done through a survey using checklists, ranking exercises and some open-ended questions. These were used to assess levels of awareness and knowledge, attitudes and beliefs and opinions of five different subject groups. The groups were solicited from potential users of the Seniors Project, health care workers, representatives from the criminal justice system, financial service workers and social service workers. Each organization was mailed a package of questionnaires to be distributed, completed and returned. Only 54 percent returned the questionnaires, a relatively low response rate.

The community survey, based on a three-month period, produced some interesting results. One hundred and ninety-nine clients were seen individually, 75 percent of whom were female, and 44 percent of whom were asking for brief information and referral services. The case load also showed a 24 percent increase over the previous quarter. Eighty percent of the cases required less than 90 minutes to resolve, the remaining 20 percent slightly less than three hours of a case worker's time. One in four clients was referred by other community agencies, and *North Shore* referred one in six clients to other resources. On the basis of self-reports of material, physical or emotional injury, or interference with decision making, 16 percent of all clients were identified as victims of abuse.

Staff activities included case work, the development of training programs, publicity through the media and educational activities. A video was made and handout materials prepared, and a public lecture series was coordinated as part of the public awareness component. Community awareness and links were promoted through community meetings and consultations. The staff also developed policies and policy manuals for their own use and the use of other organizations.

In the evaluation, the need to disseminate the knowledge gained by the project coordinator, to delegate responsibility for follow-up, and to ensure future efforts did not depend on one individual were noted. A second change in direction was in the role of seniors from service recipients to peer advocates.

One major impact of the project has been an extensive community consultation process, through which standards for all models of service provision have emerged for British Columbia. The standards are based on the following principles:

- All adults have a right to autonomy and self-determination, and to the presumption that they are capable of living and entitled to live in any manner they wish;
- When they need it, all adults are entitled to assistance, support or protection that returns power to them by means of the least restrictive, intrusive or stigmatizing form of intervention possible. This entitlement recognizes that there is no justification for abuse;
- Adults are entitled to the legal presumption that they are capable of making decisions and they shall be supported in making informed decisions;
- Court interventions occur as the last resort; and
- All procedures, protocols and other processes associated with the provision of services shall be accessible to all adults (British Columbia Joint Working Committee 1992).

These principles have led to the development of 12 Community Response Networks throughout British Columbia. In cases of abuse and neglect, the networks will offer the individual a choice between self-advocacy, naming an advocate among friends or relatives or, when an advocacy service is available, having someone assigned from the service. The aim is to spread the work of the *North Shore Community Services Centre* to other parts of British Columbia, to assure a service delivery network through existing health and social service agencies, agencies from the criminal justice system and community organizations. The groups are brought together through periodic meetings of the B.C. Coalition to Eliminate Abuse of Seniors. As well, an extensive six-part guide has been produced for communities wishing to establish similar Community Response Networks.

A third outcome of the work of *North Shore Community Services Centre* has been innovative changes to four new bills being passed by the House of Legislature. For example, British Columbia has recently undertaken new initiatives with the enactment of their Adult Guardianship Act, S.B.C. 1993. This confers extensive powers of investigation on designated agencies, but also provides that the court must choose the most effective, least restrictive way of providing support and assistance. This represents an attempt to balance the need to protect vulnerable adults from abuse and neglect, with the need to respect the rights of these individuals to make their own autonomous decisions.

A fourth highlight relates to multiple funding sources. Funding was obtained from federal Seniors Independence Project grants, provincial grants from the Office of the Public Trustee in British Columbia and from the Office for Seniors, as well as grants from the Notary Foundation.

Weaknesses of this project lie in its lack of response to abusers, as the focus is clearly on the abused. As well, the project evaluation is based on process and not on outcome. The project emphasizes legal and advocacy approaches to abuse rather than long-term counselling strategies. The latter have been effective in other programs, such as *Project Synergy II* and *Project CARE*. Nor does the *North Shore Community Services Centre* offer support groups for survivors and/or abusers, such as in case study number 1.

Multidisciplinary Approaches

Although many projects incorporate multidisciplinary approaches, two models in Quebec, *Project CARE* (Reis and Nahmiash 1995b) of CLSC NDG/Montreal West and the *Elder Abuse Project* of CLSC René-Cassin are both based on a multidisciplinary approach to intervention. *Project CARE* will be used as *case study number 4* to illustrate this approach. The project is based on the use of existing resources in the community, whose personnel are part of a home care team located in a local community service centre

(CLSC). *Project CARE* developed a seven-element abuse intervention model, including:

- a tool package for screening and planning measures;
- a home care team trained in abuse interventions;
- a small professional multidisciplinary team for abuse case consultation from existing home care team members;
- an intersectoral professional team for specialized expert help;
- an empowerment group for abused seniors and support groups for caregivers and abuser-caregivers;
- a team of trained volunteer buddy advocates to assist abused seniors (some of whom were seniors); and
- a community committee (consisting of fourteen organizations, including seniors agencies) to act as advocates and educators to prevent and build public awareness of elder abuse.

Professionals and nonprofessionals from the home care team were trained to incorporate the principles of detection, prevention and intervention of abuse and neglect of older adults, as part of their home care roles. They were trained to use four screening and planning tools as part of the approach (Reis and Nahmiash 1995b). Each team member was trained to use the Brief Abuse Screen for the Elderly (BASE). The BASE was completed three different times to confirm suspicion of abuse and neglect: following the initial request for help; following a 2 1/2-hour assessment in the person's home; and at the multidisciplinary team meeting, when a confirmation of abuse and neglect was made.

The intervention approach was based on empowerment principles. Empowerment support groups for abused seniors, family support groups for abuser-caregivers, and one-on-one matched volunteer buddy advocates, often trained seniors, were the main intervention strategies. Multidisciplinary teams consisted of social workers, nurses, homemakers, physicians, occupational and physical therapists and volunteers. Collaborative links between community organizations, the health and social service agency and a public day centre located in a nursing home were emphasized, to ensure maximization of resources and coordination, and case management of such resources to the abused and the abuser-caregivers.

Project CARE's multidisciplinary team members worked with an interdisciplinary consultant team of professionals from the criminal justice system, financial agencies, psychogeriatric team members (a psychogeriatrician and a psychologist), human rights and public guardianship organizations. During monthly team meetings, and for individual consultations where extra help was required, these consultants provided expertise on a volunteer basis. The teams focused their interventions on both the abused and the abuser-caregivers or potential abusers. A community elder abuse committee consisting of 14 local organizations and volunteers, many of whom are seniors, coordinated elder abuse initiatives, training and education in the community and for the public. This was done mainly through a public speakers' bureau of trained seniors and volunteer professionals. Senior involvement was encouraged, and community seniors were trained through community-based support groups called "Stand Up and Be Counted".

Evaluation of Project CARE

An empowerment perspective was used in the project. The focus was on involvement of seniors in all aspects of the project, including intervention strategies and participation in the research study. Ethical considerations were taken into account and confidentiality procedures clearly respected.

Initially, 965 health and social service agency clients over the age of 60 years were screened for abuse, and 512 were screened for a second and third time. From this pool, abuser and nonabuser group placements were made. From the same community, a group of nonabusive caregiver–care receiver pairs were recruited, to contrast with the first two groups. A questionnaire package was administered to the three groups, containing standardized measures of general health, personality traits, caregiving aspects, happiness and the likelihood of abuse. Univariate and multivariate analyses assessed the changes before and following program interventions to evaluate the outcomes.

Three screening measures (BASE, the CASE and the IOWA) were validated in this project and proved useful, both for detecting and confirming abused and neglected seniors and abusive or potentially abusive caregivers (CASE). The IOWA provided a list of 22 indicators of abuse that discriminated between abusive and nonabusive caregivers and abused and nonabused seniors. Caregiver indicators were found to be the most important discriminators. A fourth tool (AID) is an intervention planning tool that helped identify successful and accepted versus unsuccessful and unaccepted or unavailable intervention strategies.

The results of the outcome evaluation showed an overall 25 percent decrease of the confirmed abuse categories. There was a definite decrease in physical, financial abuse and neglect. However, there was a slight increase (8 percent) in psychosocial abuse after abuse intervention. Improvement in the physical health of care recipients was demonstrated, but not improvement in anxiety levels. An improvement in depression levels for caregivers was shown, and the total number of caring activities of caregivers diminished, while use of services increased.

Overall, the results suggested decreases in abuse cases and types of abuse. While it was not possible to assess the effectiveness of individual elements of the intervention, concrete home care intervention strategies (medical, nursing, homemaking and personal care) were rated most successful and accepted by abused seniors. Education and counselling interventions to assist caregivers on a one-to-one basis were also ranked as highly successful and accepted by abuser-caregivers. Next most successful and accepted were the empowerment interventions, including support groups and volunteer advocates. The use of expert consultants, and referral to specialized treatment programs, such as substance abuse programs, did not prove successful in this program evaluation. It was felt that intervenors ought to encourage abused clients to use financial, legal and other expert services and treatment programs more often.

It can be concluded from this brief overview that *Project CARE's* strengths included:
- its comprehensiveness, in that the model contained seven program elements;
- its cost-effectiveness. The program trained an interdisciplinary team of existing resources. The research study was the only cost of this model, and additional funding for project continuation after three years was not required;
- that funding was provided by the Family Violence Prevention Division of Health Canada, with some additional material and human resources from Concordia University and the CLSC NDG/Montreal West;
- the collaborative partnership between the funders in Health Canada, the university-based researchers, a local health and community service centre, a day centre program and 14 community-based organizations;
- the three-year length of the project which enabled the partners to design, implement and evaluate the program, as well as to disseminate the findings through journal articles and a guidebook;
- the training programs for all team members and volunteers.
  Project CARE's weaknesses included:
- the inability of the project to evaluate each of its specific elements, such as the multidisciplinary team versus the volunteer buddy program;
- the fact that the volunteer buddy program was also too small to yield many findings during the project evaluation;
- that the researchers used existing definitions of abuse and neglect rather than producing new and more complete ones;
- that the tools were only able to be validated in English during this project, and not in French;
- that although seniors were involved in the project, they needed to be continually encouraged, and a specific new program needed to be developed ("Stand Up and Be Counted") to train seniors to initiate more leadership. When a program is centred in a health and social service centre, it tends to be more driven by professionals than by seniors.

Adult Protection Services

Some provinces, such as the Atlantic Provinces, use the protection approach for older adults who are victims of abuse and neglect. This approach is characterized by special powers of investigation and intervention and mandatory reporting. Intervention strategies include the power of removal, and compulsory custody and services. The legal intervention role assigned to practitioners in the enforcement of protection services has been subject to considerable scrutiny (MacDonald et al. 1991), respecting the need to safeguard individual rights, the right to refuse services, and issues around guardianship. The legal intervention approach, as well as mandatory reporting, has also been criticized in the U.S. as treating older adults as children under child welfare legislation (Pillemer 1985).

Rather than taking an example of a provincial program which uses a legal protection approach, *case study number 5, Maison Jeanne Simard,* presents an innovative approach: a shelter which provides protection, on a voluntary basis, for abused elders who cannot stay in their own homes.

Maison Jeanne Simard in Montreal was the first shelter of its kind established in Canada. The shelter receives, on a temporary basis, male and female seniors who are victims of all types of violence. The aim is to provide shelter, and to help the abused regain self-confidence and eventually find satisfactory living conditions. The seniors are self-referred or referred through health and social service agencies. *Maison Jeanne Simard's* staff also provide consultation through an interdisciplinary team to other agencies. The agency does not take a feminist approach to abused women, but rather a geron-tological approach, emphasizing the autonomy and independence of the seniors. In the documents reviewed, the assumptions were not made explicit.

Evaluation of the Project

In a small study of clients during the 12-month period of 1994, the shelter received 81 seniors, 90 percent of whom were women, with an average age of 75 years. The reason for the high percentage of women was not that abused women were more prevalent, but that only one room was available for men. Most of the seniors were widows or married, though 16 percent were separated or divorced. Only 3 percent were single. Most residents (48 percent) stayed for less than one month, while 69 percent stayed for less than two months. The average length of stay was 90 days. 52 percent of the victims had suffered more than one type of abuse or neglect, and the most common types of abuse were psychological and physical, followed by financial. Abusers were mainly children (44 percent) or spouses (42 percent) of the abused seniors.

The evaluation of this project noted that many of the abused seniors chose to renew contact with their families, who were often their abusers, when they left the shelter. There was great resistance to leaving the abuser, and a preference for a bad relationship over no relationship, especially where the abusers were children of the abused. For this reason, the shelter encour-aged continuing relationships between the abused senior and the abuser-child or abuser-spouse, except in cases of what the shelter defined as "gross" abuse. This term was not clearly defined by the shelter.

Diverse funding was obtained for this project, mainly from the Family Violence Prevention Division, Health Canada and private foundations, as well as the shelter's own fundraising campaigns.

Strengths of the model include:

- the useful bilingual guide produced by *Maison Jeanne Simard* (1995) enabling other shelters to replicate the model;
- that the shelter provides an alternative living arrangement on a temporary basis to abused seniors, both men and women, who need to leave their abusive situations;
- that few staff are required;
- the energy, dedication and volunteer work of one family. One downside of this is that it may be difficult to find others who would replicate the project at the same cost;
- the innovative consultation outreach team to the community, which functions on a volunteer basis similar to that described in case study number 4.

Some of the weaknesses of this model include:

- lack of an effective outcome evaluation of the model and the expenses involved in running and maintaining the shelter;
- lack of utilizing existing resources, except in the case of the consultation team of experts;
- little involvement on the part of seniors, since the project favours a more professional gerontological approach to services.
- difficulty in acquiring continued funding for maintenance and operational costs, making continuity problematic. Although some seniors pay for their rooms, it is evident that many find it impossible to pay when they enter the shelter, particularly in cases of financial abuse. Consequently much of the energy of the staff goes into fundraising efforts.

Conclusions from the Case Studies

An overall conclusion is that most of these studies, with the exception of *Project CARE* and *Project Synergy II*, have not been submitted to empirical outcome evaluations, though each has been evaluated. For this reason, care must be taken in interpreting the evaluations; they were drawn from available information that may not lend itself to generalizations. However, some overall similarities and differences between the case studies are useful to note.

First, each study was initiated through grants from Health Canada, but funding was also obtained from additional sources—provincial, sometimes municipal and private. Most projects received funding over at least a three-year period which enabled them to create relatively comprehensive models. Each project takes a different approach, and the approaches themselves are well documented and replicable in other parts of Canada through guidebooks, protocols, training and educational materials. Although it is not possible to establish each project's cost-effectiveness since not all the budget information required is available, all are currently continuing without further funding from Health Canada. Except for *Maison Jeanne Simard*, each project focuses on making use of existing rather than newly added resources, a cost-effective approach that is replicable elsewhere.

As well, each project depended on coordinating with many other health and social service organizations, community groups (who referred clients or consulted with the project staff), and intersectoral groups, mainly from the criminal justice system. In each case study notable partnerships were established between researchers, policymakers and funders, as well as with the community-based organizations. For each case study, research projects were organized and designed by the community-based organizations.

Each project explicitly stressed the empowerment of seniors as a goal. As well, each project observed the involvement of seniors. This was reflected in different ways. For example, *Project Synergy II* was based in a seniors centre, whereas in the *North Shore Community Services Centre* model, seniors were defined as participants, advocates and peer supports as the project evolved. *Project CARE* began in a health and social service agency but developed a model of senior volunteer advocates and a community-based committee with senior organizations as participants. Seniors were encouraged to participate in the research study as research assistants. However, in the cases of *Project CARE* and *Maison Jeanne Simard*, the approach was service-based professionalism, rather than initial senior involvement in the design and planning of projects.

Differences are also evident in the approaches. Each model demonstrates a different approach to the problem of senior abuse. Philosophies and assumptions underlying programs differ, in that *North Shore* and the *Elder Abused Woman Project* are based on a feminist and family violence approach to violence. In contrast, *Maison Jeanne Simard*, although it mainly serves abused women, is based on a more global gerontological approach, emphasizing the autonomy of seniors. *Project CARE* and *Project Synergy II* are based on the assumption that most abuse and neglect is by family caregivers, and that the care situation contributes to abuse and neglect.

There are differences in the staffing of the various projects, though all seem to favour multidisciplinary and interdisciplinary or intersectoral approaches. Staff choices depend on who houses the project. *Project Synergy II* and *North Shore Community Services Centre* are based in community organizations and staffed by the personnel of these organizations. However, *North Shore* puts more emphasis on legal issues and expertise, mostly determined by the project coordinator having such expertise. Thus the collaboration with the criminal justice system and emphasis on changes in the legal system are greater in this project than the others. This may be difficult to maintain when the current project coordinator leaves. *Maison Jeanne Simard* is staffed by a professional social gerontologist and an accountant, and the *Elder Abused Woman Project* by a social group worker. Orientations of both projects are influenced by the background of these staff members. *Project CARE* is staffed by a multidisciplinary team of professionals and volunteers from a home care project, including an interdisciplinary team and community-based organizations. Multicultural approaches, though probably implicit, are not explicit in the reporting of the projects. The exception is the *Elder Abused Woman Project*, which includes Aboriginal women as well as women of other ethnicities.

Programs and services also reflect the composition of the team members and projects. All programs offer information and referral and individual counselling services. Some projects, such as the *Elder Abused Woman Project*, *Project CARE* and *Project Synergy II*, offer specific types of group counselling, though each type seems to fulfill different needs of specific population groups. For example, the group for abused women targets only abused women whereas the *Project CARE* empowerment group targets abused women and men (though mainly women attended). The family support group targets abusive or potentially abusive family caregivers, both male and female. All groups are professionally led, although self-help is an eventual goal. Only *Project Synergy II* offers a telephone help line for abused seniors, but the service is too new to be evaluated. Peer counselling strategies, involving one-to-one matching of an abused senior with a trained volunteer senior, are not the preferred choice of most seniors either in *Project Synergy II* or in *Project CARE*. This treatment modality is noted in the *North Shore Community Services Centre* as well as *Project Synergy II* and *Project CARE*. In all projects except the *Elder Abused Woman Project*, individual counselling is chosen by abused elders as the most popular intervention strategy, although it seems that in *Project Synergy II* individual counselling is not a real choice. Not all projects offer services to abusers, though *Project CARE* and *Project Synergy II* offer specific interventions, and *Maison Jeanne Simard* notes the importance of maintaining relationships with family members.

More outcome data is provided by *Project CARE* and *Project Synergy II* due to the large-scale empirical research studies. Thus data from all groups are not comparable. However, these two projects yield some useful data on which further research and some indications of future interventions can be based. Both projects show a decrease in levels of abuse following interventions. In *Project Synergy II*, being female correlates with physical abuse, and in *Project CARE* most abused seniors were female and most abusers male. However, gender does not correlate with types of abuse in *Project CARE*. Both studies show that abused seniors tend to be isolated. *Project Synergy II* notes that the isolation decreases following interventions. As well, self-esteem and client happiness are observed to increase significantly after participation in the *Project Synergy II*. It also notes an improvement in social support to the client when the perpetrator is not involved in treatment. *Project CARE* cites lack of family support as a discriminating factor between caregivers who are abusive and those who are not. Similar to earlier studies, *Project CARE* assesses that abusive caregivers have poorer premorbid caregiver–care receiver relationships, poorer physical health, more depression, a disposition to more unhappiness and neuroticism, less disposition toward agreeableness, and less control and commitment. *Project CARE* notes an improvement in depression levels of caregivers following intervention.

Finally, *Project Synergy II*, like the *North Shore Community Services Centre*, reports some interesting findings on the relationship of ageism to abused seniors and their abusers. The *North Shore Community Services Centre* notes a change in ageist attitudes following intervention, and *Project Synergy II* notes that the perpetrators' ageism scores drop significantly after intervention. However, *Project Synergy II* abused seniors find the Fabroni Ageism Scale offensive. Ageist attitudes correlate significantly with specific types of abuse, such as violation of rights and neglect, both before and after intervention.

FUTURE DIRECTIONS AND RECOMMENDATIONS

In light of this literature and study review it seems that there is not yet enough empirical evidence upon which to base clear future directions for social policy in the area of abused and neglected older adults. Nevertheless, what is known can be summarized, and suggestions for future research, program planning and prevention of abuse and neglect can be made.

Existing evidence shows that 4 percent of the Canadian population of older adults are likely to be victims of abuse and neglect. These prevalence rates are probably underestimated due to the methodology of collecting sensitive data over the telephone, and in view of reluctance to report abuse and neglect. This suggests that a serious problem of elder abuse and neglect exists, with serious impacts on seniors' health, well-being and quality of life. Even though the percentage is small, it translates into an impressive number of individuals in the population at large. However, program planning is difficult, since operational definitions of the problem are not yet in place. Research has not yet clearly established which factors discriminate abused elders from nonabused and abusers from nonabusers, though there are some indications.

The literature and case studies point to substance abuse as the best single predictor of an abuser-caregiver. Situations of dependence seem to be indicators, though the definition of dependence varies in the studies. It is not clear whether the abused elder is dependent on the abuser-caregiver, whether the abuser-caregiver is dependent on the abused elder, or whether there is an interdependent relationship between the abused and the abuser. Nevertheless we know that most abuse occurs in the community, in a situation where there is a trust relationship between two persons, one of whom is dependent upon the other for care. We also know that social isolation discriminates the abused from the nonabused, and family support seems to discriminate the abusive caregiver from the nonabusive caregiver. Thus program planners should direct their attention to problems of substance abuse, especially since treatment programs in this area are not used effectively in the prevention of abuse, according to the limited available data. As well, those who lack social support and who are socially isolated and severely dependent should be targeted for social and health service delivery, since it is not feasible to wait for empirical evidence to be established to intervene in cases of abuse and neglect.

Evidence from the case studies points to individual counselling as the intervention of choice for most abused seniors and their caregiver abusers. Individual counselling decreases isolation and depression, as well as reducing the level of abuse. There is no evidence, however, that any abuse interventions totally stop abuse. Except in the Podnieks study, physical abuse seems to be correlated with gender, with women as victims. In the case of such abused women, small groups like those presented in case study number 1 may be the intervention of choice, though there is not yet much hard evidence to support this.

Although they have not been empirically demonstrated, all the case studies support the literature in pointing to the usefulness of multi-disciplinary teams and interdisciplinary team interventions. This is particularly important in view of the complexity of cases of elder abuse. We do not know which cases are best handled by which team members, or if and when a multidisciplinary or an interdisciplinary approach is necessary. In the *Project CARE* evaluation, the interdisciplinary team was little used; only 18 cases were referred by the community to *Project Synergy II*, though it was difficult to assess the reasons for this.

There does not seem to be one overarching theoretical approach or cause related to all types and cases of elder abuse, though victims have been described as powerless in most studies and empowerment has been an intervention goal of most case studies. The approach depends on the philosophy of the researcher, and the perspective of researchers and intervenors guides the research and interventions.

It is clear that funding through Health Canada has provided considerable leadership in putting the problem of abuse and neglect of older adults on the public and professional agenda in the past five years. All the above case studies and most of the Canadian research was funded by Health Canada, though some included other provincial, municipal and private funding sources.

These funding efforts have produced some innovative models and well-documented educational initiatives, guides, protocols and research as well as influencing changes to some provincial legislative acts.

Literature and case studies bear out the observation that relatively flexible legislative changes and advocacy approaches appear to be favoured by intervenors. Legal enforcement approaches have been much criticized in the research (McDonald et al. 1991; Robertson 1995). As well, mandatory programs made little impact (Wolf and Pillemer 1989).

Issues around legal approaches to elder abuse have not been addressed here, since this has been done by other authors (Robertson 1995). However, the complete revamping of British Columbia laws relating to the protection of vulnerable adults may serve as a model for other provinces.

In light of the above observations, the following recommendations are suggested:

- More empirical research needs to produce operational definitions and terminology of abuse and neglect of older adults upon which researchers can base studies, so that comparative evidence-based data can be developed in this area. Funding needs to continue to support such research efforts.

- Research needs to focus on pinpointing which health indicators discriminate abused from nonabused elders, and abusive from nonabusive caregivers. Such research should focus on the interaction of several risk factors that seem to relate to abused versus nonabused and abusers versus nonabusers. For example, the indicators which seem to be most related are substance abuse, social isolation, dependency, depression and gender. It would also be important to include interacting factors from the social and family context of care, such as adequacy of resources, living arrangements or lack of family support, which may relate to these variables. Different types of abuse should be explored separately. Qualitative as well as quantitative studies are also suggested, as they may yield additional important information about the complex nature of the phenomenon of abuse and neglect of older adults.

- Health Canada should assist in the dissemination of existing information, facts and models from research and interventions to as many communities in Canada as possible, including multicultural and Aboriginal communities. The information must be disseminated in clear, comprehensible language in order to be useful to consumers and health care professionals. Senior organizations could be encouraged to lead the dissemination process as a means of becoming involved in the public sensitization process. One Voice (1994) has already expressed an interest in assuming leadership in this area.

- Provincial and municipal governments could assume leadership to ensure that existing validated screening measures and protocols (such as the EAST) are widely known. These governments should make the tools accessible to organizations within their jurisdictions. Each area must have access to existing knowledge, training programs and approaches, such as to multicultural or Aboriginal groups, and trained resources to respond to cases of abuse and neglect. The Community Response Network Teams and Guides from British Columbia provide a useful model for other communities. Models such as those in the case studies that rely on existing rather than newly added resources should be promoted. The possible exception could be a shelter for each region to provide temporary placement for abused seniors. Outcome evaluation of programs and interventions should be encouraged and funded. In this area, partnerships between community-based agencies, university researchers and policy-makers must be encouraged, to provide the technical and financial support and expertise required for rigorous evaluation studies. In this way, more information can be collected and shared about which interventions are successful and why others are not.

CONCLUSIONS

This paper has summarized the literature and analyzed five case studies regarding abuse and neglect of older Canadians, living in the community and abused by persons in a position of trust.

Although much leadership has been provided by Health Canada in this area through highlighting problems, creating model interventions, innovative partnerships and providing empirical research in the area, much information is still missing upon which evidence-based policies and programs can be founded.

It is to be hoped that funding will continue, to ensure that research and empirically based evaluations of interventions will not only identify abused and neglected older persons and their abusers, but also tell us more about what interventions and strategies are successful in this area. Indications have been provided. However, if funding, research, education and inter-vention are not continued, it is possible that the problems will increase. The numbers of the elderly in need of care are increasing, and without adequate funding, solutions will neither multiply nor become more effective.

Daphne Nahmiash *is a doctoral candidate at the Laval University School of Social Work in Quebec City. She is also an adjunct professor at the McGill University School of Social Work and at the McGill Centre for Studies in Aging, Montreal. She recently coauthored a book with Myrna Reis entitled* When Seniors are Abused.

BIBLIOGRAPHY

ANETZBERGER, G. J. 1987. *The Etiology of Elder Abuse by Adult Offspring*. Springfield (IL): Charles C. Thomas Publisher.

BAINES, C., P. EVANS, and S. NEYSMITH, eds. 1991. *Women Caring: Feminist Perspectives on Social Welfare*. Toronto (ON): McClelland and Stewart.

BAKER, M. 1988. *Aging in Canadian Society. A Survey*. Toronto: McGraw Hill Ryerson.

BÉLANGER, L., T. D'ARCHE, H. DE RAVINEL, and P. GRENIER. 1981. *L'envers du crime*. Étude criminologique. Montréal: Université de Montréal. Centre international de criminologie comparée. Les cahiers de recherche criminologique.

BENDIK, M. F. 1992. Reaching the breaking point: Dangers of mistreatment in elder caregiving situations. *Journal of Elder Abuse and Neglect* 4(3): 39–59.

BERGIN, B. 1995. *Elder Abuse in Ethnocultural Communities: An Exploratory Study with Suggestions for Intervention and Prevention*. Ottawa: Family Violence Prevention Division, Health Canada.

BLENKNER, M. 1965. Social work and family relationships in later life with some thoughts on filial maturity. In *Social Structure and Family Generational Relations*, eds. E. SHANAS and G. STREIB. Englewood Cliffs (NJ): Prentice Hall. pp. 46–59.

BLOCK, M. R., and J. P. SINNOTT. 1979. *The Battered Elder Syndrome: An Exploratory Study*. Unpublished manuscript. University of Maryland, Center on Aging.

BLUNT, A. P. 1993. Financial exploitation of the incapacitated: Investigation and remedies. *Journal of Elder Abuse and Neglect* 5(1): 19–32.

BOYACK, V. J., L. M. MCKENZIE, and E. K. HANSELL. 1995. *Synergy II: A Demonstration Project to Address the Issues of Violence in Older Families*. Ottawa: Family Violence Prevention Division, Health Canada.

BRECKMAN, R. S. and R. D. ADELMAN. 1988. *Strategies for Helping Victims of Elder Mistreatment*. Newbury Park (CA): Sage.

BRILL, N. I. 1985. *Working with People: The Helping Process*, 3rd ed. White Plains (NY): Longman Inc.

BRITISH COLUMBIA INTERMINISTRY COMMITTEE ON ISSUES AFFECTING DEPENDENT ADULTS/ THE PROJECT TO REVIEW ADULT GUARDIANSHIP. 1992. *How Can We Help? A New Look at Self-Determination, Independence, Substitute Decision Making and Guardianship in Bristish Columbia*. Discussion paper by The Joint Working Committee. Vancouver (BC).

BUTLER, R. N. 1969. Ageism: Another form of bigotry. *The Gerontologist* 9(2): 243–246.

CAIRL, R. E., D. M. KELNER, and J. I. KOSBERG. 1984. Factors associated with the propensity to take on a caregiver role. Paper presented at the Gerontological Society of America, San Antonio (TX).

CANADIAN PANEL ON VIOLENCE AGAINST WOMEN. 1994. Older women report. In *Changing the Landscape: Ending Violence—Achieving Equality*. Ottawa: Ministry of Supply and Services Canada.

CHAPPELL, N. 1989. *Formal Programs for Informal Caregivers of the Elderly in Supporting Elder Care*. Winnipeg: University of Manitoba.

CICIRELLI, V. G. 1981. *Helping Elderly Parents: The Role of Adult Children*. Boston: Auburn House.

COX, E. O., and R. J. PARSONS. 1994. *Empowerment-Oriented Social Work Practice with the Elderly*. Belmont (CA): Brooks/Cole Publishing Co.

DALE, A. 1995. *Elder Abused Woman Project: Final report*. Ottawa: Health Canada.

DESPERITO, A. 1994. *Empowering Older Female Victims of Abuse: A Group Work Process*. Research report for masters degree in social work. Montreal: McGill University.

DOUGLASS, R. L., R. HICKEY, and C. NOEL. 1980. *A Study of Maltreatment of Elderly and Other Vulnerable Adults. Final Report*. Ann Arbor (MI): Institute of Gerontology, University of Michigan.

FETTERMAN, D. M., S. J. KAFTARIAN, and A. WANDERSMAN. EDS. 1996. *Empowerment Evaluation: Knowledge and Tools for Self-Assesment and Accountability.* Thousand Oaks (CA): Sage.

FLOYD, J. 1983. Collecting data on abuse of the elderly. *Journal of Gerontological Nursing* 10(12): 11–15.

FULMER, T. T. 1990. The debate over depenency as a relevant predisposing factor in elder abuse and neglect. *Journal of Elder Abuse and Neglect* 2 (1,2): 51–57.

GALBRAITH, M. W., and D. E. DAVISON. 1985. Stress and elderly abuse. *Focus on Learning* 1 (9): 86–92.

GARANT, L., and M. BOLDUC. 1990. *L'aide par les proches: mythes et réalités.* Gouvernement du Québec: Direction de l'éducation, Ministère de la Santé et des Services Sociaux.

GELLES, R. 1974. Child abuse as psychopathology: A sociological critique and reformulation. In *Violence in the Family,* eds. S. STEINMETZ and M. STRAUS. New York: Dodd, Mead. pp. 190-204.

GESINO, J. P., H. H. SMITH, and W. A. KECKICH. 1982. The battered woman grows old. *Clinical Gerontologist* 1(1): 59–67.

GESTON, E. L., and L. A. JASON. 1987. Social and community interventions, *Annual Review of Psychology* 38: 427–460.

GIOGLIO, G. R., and P. BLAKEMORE. 1983. Elder abuse in New Jersey: The knowledge and experience of abuse among older New Jerseyans. Unpublished manuscript. Trenton (NJ): Department of Human Services.

GIORDANO, N. H., and J. A. GIORDANO. 1983. Family and individual characteristics of five types of elder abuse: Profiles and predictors. Paper presented at the Gerontological Society of America, San Francisco (CA).

GNEADINGER, N. 1989. *Elder Abuse: A Discussion Paper.* Ottawa: Family Violence Prevention Division, Health Canada.

GODBOUT, J. T., and A. CAILLÉ. 1992. *L'esprit du don.* Montréal: Boréal.

GODKIN, M. A., R. S. WOLF, and K. A. PILLEMER. 1989. A case-comparison analysis of elder abuse and neglect. *International Journal of Aging and Human Development* 28(3): 207–225.

GOTTLIEB, B. H. 1991. Social support and family care of the elderly. *Canadian Journal on Aging* 10(4): 359–375.

GOUVERNEMENT DU QUÉBEC. 1990. *Vieillir en toute liberté.* Rapport du Comité sur les abus exercés à l'endroit des aînés. Québec: Bibliothèque Nationale du Québec.

———. 1994. *Services à domicile de première ligne: cadre de référence.* Québec: MSSS.

GRANDMAISON, A. 1988. *Protection des personnes âgées: étude exploratoire de la violence à l'égard de la clientèle des personnes âgées du CSSMM.* Centre des services sociaux du Montréal métropolitain. Direction des services professionnels.

GRIFFIN, L. W. 1994. Elder maltreatment among rural African Americans. *Journal of Elder Abuse and Neglect* 6(1): 1–29.

HAMEL, M., P. D. GOLD, D. ANDRES, M. REIS, D. DASTOOR, H. GRAUER, and H. BERGMAN. 1990. Predictors and consequences of aggressive behaviour by community-based dementia patients. *The Gerontological Society of America* 3(2): 206–211.

HARSHBARGER, S. 1993. From protection to prevention: A proactive approach. *Journal of Elder Abuse and Neglect* 5(1): 41–55.

HEALTH CANADA. 1993. *Older Canadians and the Abuse of Seniors: A Continuum from Participation to Empowerment.* Ottawa: Family Violence Prevention Division, Health Canada.

HEISLER, C. J. 1991. The role of the criminal justice system in elder abuse cases. *Journal of Elder Abuse and Neglect* 3(1): 5–35.

HICKEY, T., and R. L. DOUGLASS. 1981. Mistreatment of the elderly in the domestic setting: An exploratory study. *American Journal of Public Health* 71(5): 500–507.

HOLLAND, S. 1990. *North Shore Information and Volunteer Center: Seniors Project Community Survey. Phase I Report.* Ottawa: Seniors Independence Program, Health Canada.

HOLMES, G. E. 1992. *Social Work Research and the Empowerment Paradigm.* New York: Longman Publishing Group.

HUDSON, M., and T. F. JOHNSON. 1986. Elder neglect and abuse: A review of the literature. *Annual Review of Gerontology and Geriatrics* 6(1): 1–134.

HUDSON, M.F. 1994. Elder abuse: Its meaning to middle-aged and older adults. Part II: Pilot Results. *Journal of Elder Abuse and Neglect* 6(1): 55–83.

KIEFFER, C.H. 1984. *Citizen Empowerment: A Developmental Perspective.* Binghampton (NY): The Haworth Press.

KING, N. R. 1984. Exploitation and abuse of older family members: An overview of the problem. In *Abuse of the Elderly: A Guide to Resources and Services,* ed. J. J. COSTA. Lexington (MA): Lexington Books, Heath.

KOSBERG, J. I. 1980. Family maltreatment: Explanations and interventions. Paper presented at the Meeting of the Gerontological Society of America, San Diego (CA).

_____. 1988. Preventing elder abuse: Identification of high-risk factors prior to placement decisions. *The Gerontologist* 28(1): 43–49.

KOSBERG, J .I., and D. NAHMIASH. 1996. Characteristics of victims and perpetrators and milieus of abuse and neglect. In *Abuse, Neglect and Exploitation of Older Persons: Strategies for Assessment and Intervention,* eds. L. A. BAUMHOVER, and S. C. BEAL, Baltimore (MD): Health Professions Press. pp. 31–50.

KOSBERG, J. I., and J. L. GARCIA. 1995. *Elder Abuse in World-Wide Perspective.* Binghampton (NJ): The Haworth Press Inc.

KOZACK, J., T. ELMSLIE, and J. VERDON. 1995. Epidemiology of the abuse and neglect of seniors in Canada: A review of the national and international research literature. In *Abuse and Neglect of Older Canadians: Strategies for Change,* ed. M. MACLEAN. Toronto: Thompson Educational Publishing Inc. pp. 129–142.

LAMONT, C. 1985. La violence à domicile faite aux femmes âgées. Travail présenté pour le Cour EAN 6670: "Condition feminine et éducation continue." Université de Montréal.

LAU, E. E., and J. I. KOSBERG. 1979. Abuse of the elderly by informal care providers. *Aging* (Sept.-Oct.): 10–15.

LEE, G. R. 1992. Gender differences in family caregiving: A fact in search of a theory. In *Gender, Families and Elder Care,* eds. J. W. DWYER, and R. T. COWARD. Newbury Park (CA): Sage Publishing. pp. 120–131.

LEE, J.A.B. 1994. *The Empowerment Approach to Social Work Practice.* New York: Columbia University Press.

LESEMANN, F., and C. CHAUME. 1989. *Familles providence: la part de l'État.* Montréal: Éditions Saint-Martin.

LORD, J., and F. MCKILLOP. 1990. Une étude sur l'habilitation: répercussions sur la promotion de la santé *Promotion de la santé* (fall): 2–8.

MACDONALD, P. L., J. P. HORNICK, G. P. ROBERTSON, and J. E. WALLACE. 1991. *Elder Abuse and Neglect in Canada.* Toronto: Butterworths Canada Ltd.

MCKENZIE, P., L. TOD, and P. YELLEN. 1995. Community-based intervention strategies for cases of abuse and neglect of seniors: A comparison of models, philosophies and practice issues. In *Abuse and Neglect of Older Canadians: Strategies for Change,* ed. M. MACLEAN. Toronto: Thompson Educational Publishing Inc. pp. 55–62.

MAHEU, P., and GUBERMAN, N. 1992. Familles, personnes adultes dépendantes et aide naturelle, entre le mythe et la réalité. *La revue internationale d'action communautaire* 28(68): 40–51.

MAISON JEANNE SIMARD. 1994. *Projet pilote parrainé par la Maison Jeanne Simard.* Ottawa: Family Violence Prevention Division, Health Canada.

MINISTRY OF COMMUNITY AND SOCIAL SERVICES. 1985. *Report of a Survey of Elder Abuse in the Community.* Toronto (ON): Government of Ontario. Standing Committee on Social Development.

MOON, A. and O. WILLIAMS. 1993. Perceptions of elder abuse and help-seeking patterns among African American, Caucasian American and Korean American elderly women. *The Gerontologist* 33(3): 387–393.

MULLENDER, A., and D. WARD. 1991. *Self-Directed Group Work: Users Take Action for Empowerment.* London: Whiting and Birch Ltd.

MYERS, J.E. 1993. Personal empowerment. *Aging International* 20 (March): 3–8.

MYERS, J.E., and B. SHELTON. 1987. Abuse and older persons: Issues and implications for counsellors. *Journal of Counselling and Development* 65(7) (March): 376–380.

NAHMIASH, D. 1994a. *A Comparison of Social Welfare Services in the Community in Japan with Quebec.* Report to the Heiwa Nakajima Foundation. Tokyo, Japan.

_____. 1994b. Empowerment as a research concept: Its use and abuse. Paper for doctoral seminar. Quebec City: Laval University School of Social Work.

NAHMIASH, D., and M. REIS. 1995. Intervention: Most successful strategies. Project Care, Montreal. Unpublished.

NATIONAL ADVISORY COUNCIL ON AGING. 1990. *The NACA Position on Informal Caregiving.* Ottawa: Ministry of Supply and Services Canada.

NEYSMITH, S.M. 1995. Power in relationships of trust: A feminist analysis of elder abuse. In *Abuse and Neglect of Older Canadians: Strategies for Change,* ed. M. MACLEAN. Toronto: Thompson Education Publishing Inc. pp. 43–54.

NORTH SHORE COMMUNITY SERVICES. 1995. *Developing Community Response Networks: Report.* Ottawa: Family Violence Prevention Division, Health Canada.

_____. 1995b. *Elder Abuse Community Development Project: Program Impact Assessment.* Ottawa: Seniors Independence Program, Health Canada.

O'MALLEY, T. A. 1987. Abuse and neglect of the elderly: The wrong issue? *Journal of Long Term Health Care* 5: 25–28.

ONE VOICE. 1994. *Getting Together against Elder Abuse: Seniors Speak Out.* Ottawa: Health Canada, National Clearing House on Violence (September).

PAVEZA, G.J., D. COHEN, C. EISDORFER, S. FREELS, T. SEMLA, W.J. ASHFORD, P. GORELICK, R. HIRSCHMAN, D. LUCHINS, and P. LEVY. 1992. Severe family violence and Alzheimer's disease: Prevalence and risk factors. *The Gerontologist* 32(4): 493–497.

PEDRICK-CORNELL, C., and R. J. GELLES. 1982. Elder abuse: The status of current knowledge. *Journal of Legal Medicine* 3: 413–441.

PEPIN, J. I. 1992. Family caring and caring in nursing. *The Gerontologist* 24(2): 127–131.

PHILLIPS, L. R. 1983. Abuse and neglect of the frail elderly at home: An exploration of theoretical relationships. *Journal of Advanced Nursing* 8: 379–392.

PILLEMER, K. A. 1984. Social isolation and elder abuse. *Response* 8(4): 2–4.

_____. 1985. The dangers of dependency: New findings on domestic violence of the elderly. *Social Problems* 33: 146–158.

_____. 1986. Risk factors in elder abuse: Results from a case-control study. In *Elder Abuse: Conflict in the Family,* eds. K. A. PILLEMER and R. S. WOLF, Dover (MA): Auburn House Publishing Co. pp. 239–263.

PILLEMER, K. A., and D. FINKELHOR. 1985. Domestic violence against the elderly: A discussion paper. Paper presented at the Surgeon General's Workshop on Violence and Public Health, Leesburg (VA).

_____. 1988. The prevalence of elder abuse: A random sample survey. *The Gerontologist* 28(1): 51–57.

PILLEMER, K. A., and J. SUITOR. 1992. Violence and violent feelings: What causes them among family caregivers? *Journal of Gerontology* 47(4): S165–S172.

PILLEMER, K. A., and R. S. WOLF. 1986. Major findings from three model projects on elderly abuse. In *Elder Abuse: Conflict in the Family,* eds. K. A. PILLEMER, and R. S. WOLF. Dover (MA): Auburn House. pp. 212–238.

PITTAWAY, E., E. GALLAGHER, M. STONES, D. NAHMIASH, J. I. KOSBERG, E. PODNIEKS, L. STRAIN, and J. BOND. 1995. *Services for Abused Older Canadians.* Ottawa: Family Violence Prevention Division, Health Canada.

PODNIEKS, E., K. A. PILLEMER, J. NICHOLSON, J. SHILLINGTON, and A. FRIZZELL. 1990. *National Survey on Abuse of the Elderly in Canada.* Toronto: Office of Research and Innovation, Ryerson Polytechnical Institute.

QUINN, M. J., and S. K. TOMITA. 1986. *Elder Abuse and Neglect: Causes, Diagnosis and Intervention Strategies.* New York: Springer Publising Co.

RAPPAPORT, J. 1990. Research methods and the empowerment social agenda. In *Researching Community Psychology*, eds. P. TOLAN, C. KEYS, F. CHERTOK, and L. JASON. Washington, (DC): American Psychological Association.

REIS, M., and D. NAHMIASH. 1995a. *Final Report on Project Care.* Ottawa: Family Violence Prevention Division, Health Canada.

_____. 1995b. *When Seniors are Abused.* Toronto, Captus Press.

RENAUD, M. 1994. The future: Hygeia versus Panakeia. *Daedalus* 123(4): 317–344.

RISSEL, C. 1994. Empowerment: The holy grail of health promotion? *Health Promotion International* 9(1): 39–47.

ROBERTSON, G. B. 1995. Legal approaches to elder abuse and neglect in Canada. In *Abuse and Neglect of Older Canadians: Strategies for Change*, ed. M. MACLEAN. Toronto: Thompson Educational Publishing Inc. pp. 63–78.

ROSENBLATT, D. E. 1990. Documentation. In *Abuse, Neglect and Exploitation of Older Persons: Strategies for Assessment and Intervention*, eds. L. A. BAUMHOVER and S. C. BEAL. Baltimore: Health Professions Press. pp. 150–162.

ROSENTHAL, C. J. 1987. Aging and intergenerational relations in Canada. In *Aging in Canada: Social Perspectives*, ed. MARSHALL, 2nd ed. Markham (ON): Fitzhenry and Whiteside.

SADLER, P. M., and S. E. KURRLE. 1993. Australian service providers responses to elder abuse. *Journal of Elder Abuse and Neglect* 5(1): 55–75.

SAUNDERS, D. 1988. Wife abuse, husband abuse or mutual combat? In *Feminist Perspective on Wife Abuse*, eds. K. YLLO and M. BOGRAD. Newbury Park (CA): Sage Publishing. pp. 90–113.

SELECT COMMITTEE ON AGING. 1981. *Elder Abuse: An Examination of a Hidden Problem.* Committee Publication. Washington (DC): U.S. Government Printing Office. pp. 99–502.

SENGSTOCK, M. C., and M. HWALEK. 1987. A review and analysis of measures for the identification of elder abuse. *Journal of Gerontological Social Work* 10: 21–36.

SHELL, D. J. 1982. *Protection of the Elderly: A Study of Elder Abuse.* Winnipeg (MN): Manitoba Council on Aging, Association on Gerontology.

SOLOMON, B. B. 1976. *Black Empowerment: Social Work in Oppressed Communities.* New York: Columbia University Press.

STEINMETZ, S. K., and D. J. AMSDEN. 1983. Dependent elders, family and abuse. In *Family Relationships in Later Life*, ed. T. H. BRUBAKER. Beverly Hills (CA): Sage Publications Inc. pp. 178–192.

STEINMETZ, S. K. 1988. *Duty bound: Elder abuse and family care.* Newbury Park (CA): Sage Publications Inc.

STEVENSON, C. 1985. *Family Abuse of the Elderly in Canada.* Report for the Senior Citizens Bureau. Alberta Social Services and Community Health.

STONES, M. 1991. A lexicon for elder mistreatment. Paper prepared by the Provincial Working Committee on Elder Mistreatment. St. John (NF).

STONES, M. J. 1995. Scope and definition of elder abuse and neglect in Canada. In *Abuse and Neglect of Older Canadians: Strategies for Change*, ed. M. MACLEAN. Toronto: Thompson Educational Publishing Inc. pp. 150–164.

STRYCKMANN, J., and D. NAHMIASH. 1994. Payment for care: The case of Canada. In *Payment for Care: A Comparative Overview*, eds. A. EVERS, M. PJIL, and C. UNGERSON. European Center, Vienna: Avebury. pp. 307–320.

SONKIN, D. J., D. MARTIN, and E. A. WALKER. 1985. *The Male Batterer.* New York: Springer.

SYME, L. S. 1994. The social environment and health. *Daedalus: Journal of the American Academy of Arts and Sciences Health and Wealth* 123 (4): 79–86.

TATARA, T. 1993. Understanding the nature and scope of domestic elder abuse with the use of State aggregate data: Summaries of the key findings of a National Survey of State APS and aging agencies. *Journal of Elder Abuse and Neglect* 5(4): 35–59.

THÉRIAULT, C. 1994. Inventaire des perceptions des personnes âgées de 70 ans et plus, fréquentant un centre de jour, sur la violence exercée envers les personnes âgées (territoire du CLSC du Centre de la Mauricie). Mémoire présenté pour l'obtention du grade de maître en service social. Québec: Université Laval. École de service social.

VÉZINA, A., and J. ROY. In press. State-family relations in Quebec from the perspective of intensive home care services for the elderly. *Journal of Gerontological Social Work.*

WALLERSTEIN, N. 1992. Powerlessness, empowerment and health: Implications for health promotion. *American Journal of Health Promotion* 6(3): 197–205.

WATSON, E., C. PATTERSON, S. MACIBORIC-SOHOR, A. GREK, and L. GREENSLADE. 1995. Policies regarding abuse and neglect of older Canadians in health care settings. In *Abuse and Neglect of Older Canadians: Strategies for Change,* ed. M. MACLEAN. Toronto: Thompson Educational Publishing Inc. pp. 73–78.

WEILER, K., and K. C. BUCKWALTER. 1992. Abuse among rural mentally ill *Journal of Psychosocial Nursing and Mental Health Services* 30(9): 32–36.

WILKINSON, R. G. 1994. The epidemiological transition: From material scarcity to social disadvantage? *Daedalus* 123(4): 42–77.

WOLF, R. S., C. P. STRUGNELL, and M. A. GODKIN. 1982. *Preliminary Findings from Three Model Projects on Elderly Abuse.* Worcester (MA): University Centre on Aging, University of Massachusetts Medical Centre.

WOLF, R. S., and K. A. PILLEMER. 1989. *Helping Elderly Victims: The Reality of Elder Abuse.* New York: Columbia University Press.

_____. 1994. What's new in elder abuse programming? Four bright ideas. *The Gerontologist* 34(1): 126–129.

ZARIT, S. H., K. E. REEVER, and J. BACH-PETERSON. 1990. Relatives of impaired elderly: Correlates of feelings of burden. *The Gerontologist* 20: 649–655.

Series
Canada Health Action: Building on the Legacy
Papers Commissioned by the National Forum on Health

Volume 1
Determinants of Health
Children and Youth

Jane Bertrand
Enriching the Preschool Experiences of Children

Paul D. Steinhauer
Developing Resiliency in Children from Disadvantaged Populations

David A. Wolfe
Prevention of Child Abuse and Neglect

Christopher Bagley and Wilfreda E. Thurston
Decreasing Child Sexual Abuse

Barbara A. Morrongiello
Preventing Unintentional Injuries among Children

Benjamin H. Gottlieb
Strategies to Promote the Optimal Development of Canada's Youth

Paul Anisef
Making the Transition from School to Employment

Pamela C. Fralick and Brian Hyndman
Youth, Substance Abuse and the Determinants of Health

Gaston Godin and Francine Michaud
STD and AIDS Prevention among Young People

Tullio Caputo and Katharine Kelly
Improving the Health of Street/Homeless Youth

Series
Canada Health Action: Building on the Legacy
Papers Commissioned by the National Forum on Health

Volume 2

Determinants of Health

Adults and Seniors

Series
Canada Health Action: Building on the Legacy
Papers Commissioned by the National Forum on Health

Volume 3
Determinants of Health
Settings and Issues

Volume 4

Striking a Balance

Health Care Systems in Canada and Elsewhere

Series
Canada Health Action: Building on the Legacy
Papers Commissioned by the National Forum on Health

Volume 5

Making Decisions

Evidence and Information

Joan E. Tranmer, S. Squires, K. Brazil, J. Gerlach, J. Johnson, D. Muisner, B. Swan, Dr. R. Wilson
Using Evidence-Based Decision Making: What Works, What Doesn't

Paul Fisher, Marcus J. Hollander, Thomas MacKenzie, Peter Kleinstiver, Irina Sladecek, Gail Peterson
Decision Support Tools in Health Care

Charlyn Black
Building a National Health Information Network

Robert Butcher
Foundations for Evidence-Based Decision Making

Carol Kushner and Michael Rachlis
Consumer Involvement in Health Policy Development

Frank L. Graves and Patrick Beauchamp (EKOS Research Associates Inc.), and David Herle (Earnscliffe Research and Communications)
Research on Canadian Values in Relation to Health and the Health Care System

Thérèse Leroux, Sonia Le Bris, Bartha Maria Knoppers, with the collaboration of Louis-Nicolas Fortin and Julie Montreuil
The Feasibility of a National Canadian Advisory Committee on Ethics: Points to Consider

AGMV
MARQUIS
Québec, Canada
1998